Presented as a service
to the medical profession
by Sandoz Pharmaceuticals

makers of

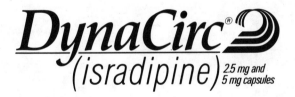

DynaCirc®
(isradipine) 2.5 mg and
5 mg capsules

Nephrology for the House Officer

Edited by

C. Craig Tisher, M.D.

Professor of Medicine and Pathology
Chief, Division of Nephrology, Hypertension and Transplantation
University of Florida College of Medicine
Gainesville, Florida

Christopher S. Wilcox, M.D. Ph.D.

Professor of Medicine and Pharmacology and Therapeutics
Director, Hypertension Service for the Health Science Center
University of Florida College of Medicine
Chief, Renal Section
Gainesville Veterans Administration Medical Center
Gainesville, Florida

WILLIAMS & WILKINS
BALTIMORE · HONG KONG · LONDON · MUNICH
PHILADELPHIA · SYDNEY · TOKYO

Editor: Michael G. Fisher
Associate Editor: Marjorie Kidd Keating
Copy Editor: Susan S. Vaupel
Design: Dan Pfisterer
Illustration Planning: Wayne Hubbel
Production: Raymond E. Reter

Copyright © 1989
Williams & Wilkins
428 East Preston Street
Baltimore, MD 21202, USA

Accurate indications, adverse reactions, and dosage schedules for drugs are provided in this book, but it is possible that they may change. The reader is urged to review the package information data of the manufacturers of the medications mentioned.

Printed in the United States of America

Library of Congress Cataloging in Publication Data

Nephrology for the house officer/edited by C. Craig Tisher, Christopher S. Wilcox.
   p. cm.
Includes bibliographies and index.
ISBN 0-683-08275-2
1. Nephrology. I. Tisher, C. Craig, 1936–   . II. Wilcox, Christopher, S.
[DNLM: 1. Kidney Diseases—handbooks. WJ 39 N439]
RC903.N45   1989
616.6'1—dc20
DNLM/DLC
for Library of Congress   89-9105
                                               CIP

91 92 93

4 5 6 7 8 9 10

To Audrae Tisher and Linda Wilcox

About the Editors

C. Craig Tisher, M.D., is Professor of Medicine and Pathology and Chief of the Division of Nephrology, Hypertension and Transplantation at the University of Florida College of Medicine. He received his M.D. degree from Washington University of St. Louis in 1961. Dr. Tisher is recognized both nationally and internationally for his writings in the fields of kidney pathology, anatomy, and physiology. He is the author of more than 80 peer-reviewed publications in both clinical and basic science research. Dr. Tisher has authored 30 chapters and served as the editor of 3 books in the fields of kidney pathology, anatomy, and clinical nephrology. He remains active in teaching, research, and patient care.

Christopher S. Wilcox, M.D., Ph.D., Professor of Medicine and Pharmacology and Therapeutics at the University of Florida College of Medicine, is Chief of the Renal Section, Gainesville Veterans Administration Medical Center, and Director of the Hypertensive Service for the Health Science Center. Dr. Wilcox qualified in medicine at Oxford University and obtained his Ph.D. degree in physiology from London University. He is a member of the Royal College of Physicians of London. He is the author of more than 40 peer-reviewed publications in both clinical and basic science journals in the fields of renal physiology, clinical pharmacology, and hypertension. In addition, he has authored 15 chapters and reviews. He has active research programs in kidney disease and hypertension.

Preface

Nephrology is a subspecialty of internal medicine that embraces both basic and clinical science. It encompasses a wide variety of disciplines including renal physiology and pathophysiology, renal anatomy and pathology, immunology, pharmacology, and molecular biology and biochemistry. This manual of clinical nephrology has been written to aid both the house officer and the medical student in the care of patients with disorders in which the kidney plays a central or dominant role. It will also be a valuable aide to physicians beginning a specialist career in nephrology and those whose primary area of responsibility is in another medical subspecialty.

Chapter 1, *Evaluation of Kidney Function*, provides a review of the current techniques that are available to examine the functional status of the kidney. Chapter 2, *Hematuria*, and Chapter 3, *Proteinuria and the Nephrotic Syndrome*, discuss the etiology, evaluation, pathophysiology, and management of two common signs of abnormal kidney function. Chapter 4, *Glomerulonephritis*, and Chapter 5, *Diabetic Nephropathy*, describe the diagnosis and management of two of the most common illnesses that lead to end-stage renal disease.

Chapters 5 through 10 provide succinct yet thorough discussions of the diagnosis and management of the major fluid and electrolyte disturbances and acid-base disorders. Chapter 11, *Renal Stone Disease*, Chapter 12, *Urinary Tract Obstruction*, and Chapter 13, *Urinary Tract Infection*, describe disease processes that can affect the upper or the lower urinary tract or both and often present difficult diagnostic problems. Chapter 14, *Tubulointerstitial Nephritis*, discusses a disease process with a variety of etiologies that can cause either acute or chronic renal failure. *Renal Cystic Disease*, Chapter 15, reviews the diagnosis and management of three entities, autosomal dominant polycystic kidney disease, medullary sponge kidney, and acquired polycystic kidney disease, that are seen principally in adult patients. Chapter 16, *AIDS and Kidney Disease*, outlines the appropriate guidelines for the management of acute and chronic renal failure in patients afflicted with HIV infections.

Chapters 17 through 20 provide a concise and well-organized outline for the diagnosis and treatment of patients with primary and secondary forms of hypertension. Hypertensive emergencies receive special attention in Chapter 20. Chapter 21, *Acute Renal Failure*, and Chapter 22, *Chronic Renal Failure*, outline the etiology, diagnosis, and proper treatment of renal failure. The techniques of hemo-dialysis, CAVH and peritoneal dialysis, and their use in the management of both acute and chronic renal failure are presented in Chapters 22 through 24. Chapter 25, *The Renal Transplant Patient*, outlines the proper approach to the management of the transplant recipient, especially in the clinical setting of an acute rise in the creatinine level. Chapter 26, *Nutrition in Renal Failure*, discusses a frequently neglected aspect of the care of patients with kidney disease. The use of drugs in renal failure is presented in Chapter 27 followed by a detailed discussion of the proper use of diuretics in hypertension, renal failure, and related disorders. The final chapter, *Anatomy of the Kidney*, provides an overview of important structural-functional relationships in the kidney.

All chapters in this manual were written by and reviewed extensively by the faculty, fellows, and staff of the Division of Nephrology, Hypertension and Transplantation at the University of Florida. Each chapter incorporates the knowledge and personal experience of the authors and their colleagues. The contents of this manual are intended to serve as a practical and useful guide in the recognition and treatment of kidney disease and related disorders.

Contributors

Nancy G. Ahlstrom, M.D.
  Clinical Fellow in Nephrology
C. Michael Bucci
  Physician's Assistant
Kevin A. Curran, M.D.
  Clinical Fellow in Nephrology
Patti Dean
  Renal Dietician
Edward D. Frederickson, M.D.
  Assistant Professor of Medicine
Nicolas J. Guzman, M.D.
  Senior Research Fellow in Nephrology
Paul B. Lim, M.D.
  Research Fellow in Nephrology
Kirsten M. Madsen, M.D., Ph.D.
  Associate Professor of Medicine and Anatomy and Cell Biology
John C. Peterson, M.D.
  Associate Professor of Medicine
Daniel R. Salomon, M.D.
  Associate Professor of Medicine
Gerald B. Stephanz, Jr., M.D.
  Research Fellow in Nephrology
C. Craig Tisher, M.D.
  Professor of Medicine and Pathology
Joel T. Van Sickler, M.D.
  Research Fellow in Nephrology
Christopher S. Wilcox, M.D., Ph.D.
  Professor of Medicine and Pharmacology and Therapeutics
Charles S. Wingo, M.D.
  Associate Professor of Medicine
Nicolie A. Thorn
  Editorial Assistant

Contents

Chapter 1

Evaluation of Kidney Function

Paul B. Lim

GENERAL CONSIDERATIONS

The clinical manifestations of kidney disease are frequently nonspecific and include a change in urine volume, dysuria, gross hematuria, hypertension, edema, lethargy, bleeding tendency, peripheral neuropathy, weight loss, fatigue, and anorexia. Therefore, the evaluation of a patient with suspected kidney disease is heavily dependent on laboratory assessment to develop an accurate database for both diagnosis and prognosis. This database must provide a quantitative measurement of kidney function and often includes evaluation of the anatomic structure of the urinary tract in order to answer the following questions:

- Is the functional integrity of the glomerular filtration barrier intact; i.e., is there evidence for proteinuria or hematuria?

- Is there any urogenital tract inflammation or pyuria?

- What is the overall rate of glomerular filtration; i.e., is there evidence for acute or chronic renal insufficiency?

- Are there abnormalities of tubular function; i.e., is there impairment of the ability to concentrate, dilute, or acidify urine, or the ability to conserve or excrete specific solutes?

- Are there gross abnormalities seen by direct or indirect imaging of the urinary tract; i.e., are there indications of abnormal kidney size or contour, obstructive lesions, mass lesions, or calcifications?

- Are there microscopic abnormalities seen in the urine sediment or on histologic tissue examination?

This chapter provides a review of some general screening studies commonly performed to evaluate kidney function.

URINALYSIS

COLLECTION AND HANDLING

A freshly voided midstream urine sample is obtained by a clean catch technique. A 10 ml aliquot is decanted into a centrifuge tube and is spun at 3000 RPM for 3-5 minutes. The supernatant is observed for color, the specific gravity is measured, and a dipstick is used to check the pH, glucose, hemoglobin, and protein. Thereafter, the urine supernatant is discarded. The sediment is resuspended in the residual drop of urine by gentle tapping of the centrifuge tube, is transferred by Pasteur pipette to a glass slide, and a cover slip is placed over the drop. Microscopic examination is performed to determine the presence of cells, casts, fat, bacteria, and crystals. Erythrocytes and casts degenerate quickly, especially in alkaline or dilute urine. Moreover, urine pH may change and bacteria may grow with prolonged standing. If examination of a freshly obtained and properly handled urine specimen reveals evidence of pyuria or bacteriuria, the specimen should be sent for bacteriologic culture. If the specimen has been contaminated inadvertently during handling, a new clean catch specimen must be sent.

EXAMINATION OF THE SUPERNATANT

Color

Normal urine is clear yellow, but when concentrated, it may be a deep yellow-brown. Other colors are seen in a variety of conditions as listed below.

Agents Affecting Urine Color

Appearance	Cause
Dark brown, yellow; foam on shaking	Bilirubin
Brown-black	Homogentisic acid (ochronosis)
	Melanin (melanoma)
Red	Porphyria
	Hemoglobinuria
	Myoglobinuria
	Rifampin
	Phenazopyridine (Pyridium)
	Beets
Green	Methylene blue
Turbid white	Pyuria
	Crystalluria

Specific Gravity

Specific gravity is defined as the weight of a unit volume of urine relative to an equal volume of distilled water. In contrast to osmolality, which depends on the number of osmotically active particles in solution, the specific gravity is determined by both the number and the mass of solute particles. Therefore, urea yields a specific gravity that is less than that anticipated for a given measured osmolality. In contrast, glucose, intravenous radiographic contrast agents, and protein yield a specific gravity that is greater than that expected for a measured osmolality. Within these limitations the specific gravity provides a rough approximation of urine osmolality. A urine that is isosmotic with plasma has an osmolality of 285 mOsm/kg H_2O and a urine specific gravity of 1.010. The urine specific gravity may be read directly from a refractometer by using 1 drop of urine, or it may be measured with a urinometer which requires 10 ml of urine. For screening purposes, a semiquantitative dipstick method to measure specific gravity is also available.

pH

Normally, the urine pH is below 7, but this varies with diet, respiration, and systemic acid-base balance. A urine pH >7.0 suggests a bicarbonate diuresis or the presence of urease-producing bacteria (*Proteus mirabilis*). Acidic urine is associated with uric acid stones, and alkaline urine, with struvite stones. In specific tests of renal acidification, a pH meter should be used. In most clinical settings, however, pH is read by dipstick.

Glucose

With use of a dipstick, glucose is detected through conversion to gluconic acid by glucose oxidase, which releases peroxide and oxidizes orthotoluidine to a blue color. In the absence of hyperglycemia, glucosuria may indicate proximal tubule dysfunction.

Hemoglobin

When a dipstick is used, the presence of heme is detected by its catalytic oxidation of orthotoluidine to a blue color. High urine levels of ascorbic acid can inhibit the oxidation reaction and result in a false negative dipstick test. A "trace" to "1+" reaction corresponds to a urinary erythrocyte concentration of 5,000-10,000 cells/ml. The absence of erythrocytes in the urinary sediment despite a positive dipstick test indicates hemoglobinuria or myoglobinuria.

Leukocytes

The detection of leukocyte esterase by dipstick indicates at least 4 leukocytes/high-power field.

Bacteriuria

Many types of bacteria can reduce nitrates to nitrites, resulting in a red color change in the presence of Griess' reagent. However, only 50% of bacteriuric specimens yield a positive nitrite test, so a negative dipstick result does not exclude bacteriuria.

Protein

Most normal adults excrete 40-80 mg of protein each day in the urine, while the upper limit of normal is 150 mg/24 hr. Of this amount, albumin comprises 40%; Tamm-Horsfall mucoprotein, 40%; immunoglobulins, 15%; and other plasma proteins, 5%. Detection of protein (predominantly albumin) by dipstick is based on a color change by tetrabromophenol from yellow to green to blue with increasing amounts of albumin in the urine sample. As a corollary, even large amounts of nonalbumin proteinuria, such as Bence Jones proteins, can be missed by dipstick methods. Alternatively, 2.5 ml of urine supernatant can be mixed with 7.5 ml of 3% sulfosalicylic acid which precipitates all proteins including globulins.

Factors Causing False Positive Tests

Dipstick Test	Sulfasalicylic Acid Test
Gross hematuria	Gross hematuria
Urine pH > 8.0	Radiographic contrast agents
Phenazopyridine	ß-Lactam antibiotics
Contamination with	Tolbutamide
antiseptic	Tolmetin
	Sulfonamide

Both methods can detect as little as 10-15 mg/dl of protein. However, interpretation must take into account the urine specific gravity; a 1+ result in a concentrated specimen with a specific gravity of 1.030 may have no significance, while a 1+ finding in a urine with a specific gravity of 1.002 may require further investigation.

A more accurate assessment of proteinuria is achieved by comparing the ratio of urine protein concentration to urine creatinine concentration on a randomly obtained urine specimen. The normal ratio should be < 0.15, while a ratio of 1.0 correlates with a daily protein excretion of 1 g/24 hr/1.73 m^2.

The most accurate quantitation of proteinuria is a 24-hour urine collection for total protein. The finding of more than 3.5 g/24 hr/1.73 m^2 of protein defines nephrotic range proteinuria. Any significant degree of proteinuria > 150 mg/24 hr requires further evaluation (see Chapter 3).

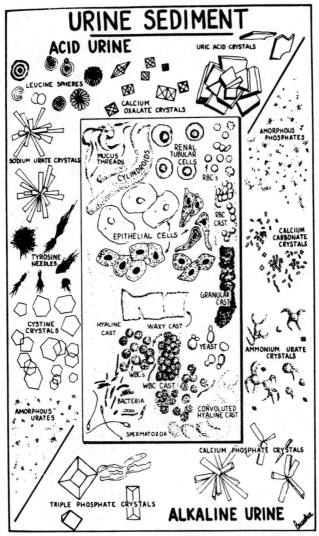

Figure 1-1. Microscopic examination of urine sediment. (Reproduced with permission from Johns Hopkins Hospital: The Harriet Lane Handbook, 11th ed., edited by Peter C. Rowe, M.D. Copyright © 1987 by Year Book Medical Publishers, Inc., Chicago.)

Erythrocytes

The normal range is 0-2 erythrocytes/high-power field. By phase-contrast microscopy, dysmorphic erythrocytes (varying shapes) are associated with glomerular bleeding, while a uniform red cell morphology suggests an extraglomerular source.

Casts

Casts are cylindrical molds of the renal tubular lumen. Most are composed of a protein matrix and trapped cellular elements. Factors favoring cast formation include urinary stasis, an acid pH, and high urine electrolyte concentrations.

Significance of Specific Types of Casts

Type of Cast	Interpretation
• Hyaline	Seen in concentrated urine, following fever, exercise, or diuretic use; does not contain cellular elements; not indicative of renal disease.
• Erythrocyte	Diagnostic of glomerular bleeding (glomerulonephritis).
• Leukocyte	Usually indicative of pyelo-nephritis but may also be seen in glomerulonephritis or interstitial nephritis.
• RTE	Seen in acute tubular necrosis, other tubulointerstitial diseases, and glomerulonephritis.
• Coarsely granular, or waxy	Represents progressive degeneration of cellular elements or aggregated proteins within a cast.
• Broad	Suggests stasis in collecting tubule draining diseased nephrons; may contain cellular elements; indicative of chronic renal failure.

Leukocytes

The normal range is 0-2 leukocytes/high-power field. Significant pyuria usually denotes a urinary tract infection. Persistent pyuria in the face of negative routine bacterial cultures should prompt consideration of chronic urethritis, prostatitis, interstitial nephritis, renal tuberculosis, calculi, papillary necrosis, or polycystic kidney disease. Eosinophiluria can be identified by Wright's or Hansel's stain, and its presence suggests an interstitial nephritis.

Renal Tubular Epithelial (RTE) Cells

RTE cells are 1.5-3 times the size of a leukocyte and have a large round nucleus. They are seen in association with acute tubular necrosis, glomerulonephritis, and pyelonephritis. In nephrotic proteinuria, degenerating tubular epithelial cells may be seen as "oval fat bodies" and have a "Maltese cross" appearance under polarized light.

Crystals

Factors determining crystal formation include the degree of supersaturation, the presence or absence of inhibitors, and the urine pH.

Clinical Significance of Crystals

Type of Crystal	Interpretation
• Cystine	Diagnostic of cystinuria.
• Calcium oxalate	In renal failure may indicate excessive absorption of dietary oxalate, primary hyperoxaluria, exposure to methoxyfluorane, high-dose vitamin C, or ingestion of ethylene glycol.
• Uric acid	May be seen with acute renal failure following massive tumor lysis.

ASSESSMENT OF GLOMERULAR FILTRATION

The glomerular filtration rate (GFR) provides a broad reflection of the functioning nephron mass. Decrements in GFR are used to identify renal failure and monitor its course. Parameters that are used to measure the GFR include the blood urea nitrogen concentration (BUN), the serum creatinine concentration (S_{Cr}), and the endogenous creatinine clearance (C_{Cr}).

BLOOD UREA NITROGEN (BUN)

Hepatic catabolism of amino acids generates ammonia which, after conversion to urea, is measured as the BUN. BUN is filtered, and normally approximately 50% of the filtered load is reabsorbed by the tubule. However, the percent reabsorbed varies inversely with urine flow rates, and in volume-depleted states the BUN is elevated out of proportion to the fall in GFR (prerenal azotemia)(see Chapter 17). Thus, the BUN is affected by many factors and is not a reliable index of the GFR.

$$BUN = \frac{urea\ production\ rate\ +\ tubular\ reabsorption\ rate}{GFR}$$

The accepted normal range for BUN is:

Conventional units
7-18 mg/dl

International units
2.5-6.4 mmol/L

Conditions That Affect the BUN Independent of GFR

Increased BUN	*Decreased BUN*
• High protein diet	• Malnutrition
• Gastrointestinal bleeding	• Liver disease
• Tissue trauma	• Sickle cell anemia
• Glucocorticoids	
• Tetracycline	
• Reduction of effective circulating blood volume	

SERUM CREATININE

Creatinine is formed nonenzymatically by the dehydration of muscle creatine, which proceeds at a relatively constant rate. It is reflective of the total muscle mass and is influenced additionally by dietary ingestion of creatinine contained in cooked meat (up to 3 mg/g). On a constant diet, S_{Cr} is a relatively reliable guide to GFR.

$$S_{Cr} = \frac{\text{constant creatinine production rate}}{\text{GFR}}$$

The accepted normal range for S_{Cr} is:

	Conventional units	International units
Males	0.6-1.2 mg/dl	53-106 μmol/L
Females	0.5-1.1 mg/dl	44-97 μmol/L

Conditions That Affect S_{Cr} Independent of GFR

Condition	Mechanism
Spurious or true elevation	
• Ketoacidosis	Noncreatinine chromogen
• Cefoxitin, cephalothin	Noncreatinine chromogen
• Ingested cooked meat	Gastrointestinal absorption of creatinine
• Drugs (aspirin, cimetidine, trimethoprim, triamterene, spironolactone, amiloride)	Inhibition of tubular creatinine secretion
Decrease	
• Increasing age	Physiologic decrease in muscle mass
• Cachexia	Pathologic decrease in muscle mass

ESTIMATION OF GFR

The Cockcroft-Gault formula can be used to estimate GFR based on a steady state S_{Cr}, weight, age, and sex:

$$\text{Males} \quad \text{GFR} = \frac{(140 - \text{age in yr}) \times (\text{kg lean body weight})}{(S_{Cr} \text{ in mg/dl}) \times 72}$$

Females   Value for males x 0.85

Since the S_{Cr} varies inversely with GFR, serial measurements of $1/S_{Cr}$ depict the rate of decline of GFR as a result of chronic renal disease.

CREATININE CLEARANCE

Under normal conditions, endogenous creatinine is generally handled like inulin by the kidney (i.e., freely filtered, not secreted, not reabsorbed, not metabolized). The creatinine clearance (C_{Cr}), therefore, is a close approximation of GFR determined by inulin clearance in the normal kidney.

$$C_{Cr} = GFR = \frac{(urine\ creatinine\ concentration)\ x\ (urine\ flow\ rate)}{S_{Cr}}$$

The normal range for C_{Cr} is:

	Conventional units	International units
Males	97-137 ml/min/1.73 m²	0.93-1.32 ml/sec/m²
Females	88-128 ml/min/1.73 m²	0.85-1.23 ml/sec/m²

The C_{Cr} declines with age by 1 ml/min/yr over age 40. In progressive renal failure, as the GFR approaches 20 ml/min/1.73 m², the proportion of creatinine excreted by tubular secretion increases. Thus, the C_{Cr} may overestimate the true GFR by as much as 40-50%. Another major source of error is a poorly timed or incomplete urine collection. The traditional urine collection is performed over 24 hours. The accepted normal range for a 24-hour urine creatinine is:

	Conventional units	International units
Males	14-26 mg/kg body wt/24 hr	124-230 μmol/kg/24 hr
Females	11-20 mg/kg body wt/24 hr	97-177 μmol/kg/24 hr

Therefore, a 24-hour urine volume with a total creatinine content of at least 15 mg/kg body weight in a female, or 20 mg/kg body weight in a male will ensure an adequate collection.

ASSESSMENT OF TUBULAR FUNCTION

Confronted with a filtered daily volume of 180 liters, a major task of the renal tubules is to reclaim fluid, sodium, chloride, and bicarbonate, while excreting the daily accumulation of nonvolatile acids.

RENAL HANDLING OF WATER

Normal urine tonicity can be in the range of 40-1200 mOsm/kg H_2O. The obligatory volume necessary to excrete a solute load of 600 mOsm varies from 0.5 to 15 liters, depending on the urine concentration. Impairment of urine concentrating ability can be caused by deficient antidiuretic hormone (ADH) release, inadequate tubular response to ADH, or loss of medullary hypertonicity. The formal test of concentrating capacity relies on demonstrating an appropriate renal response to a sufficient physiologic stimulus for endogenous ADH release (the water deprivation test; see Chapter 6).

For demonstration of impaired renal diluting capacity or inability to excrete a solute-free water load, it is sufficient to demonstrate that the urine is less than maximally dilute in the presence of a sustained reduction in plasma osmolality. Often seen in states of ADH excess, this can also occur in the setting of chronic renal insufficiency (decreased delivery of fluid and solute to the tubular diluting segments) and following use of loop diuretics (blockade of active transport systems in the thick ascending limb of Henle) (see Chapter 6).

RENAL HANDLING OF SALT

Renal "salt wasting" is typically seen in mild to moderate chronic renal insufficiency resulting from a variety of disease states. It should be suspected when there is clinical evidence of inappropriate polyuria in the context of prerenal azotemia. The hallmark is an inability to achieve sodium balance without a severe fall in total body sodium, reduction of effective circulating volume, and reduction of GFR. These patients should not be placed routinely on dietary salt restriction.

TESTS OF URINARY ACIDIFICATION

Proximal renal tubular acidosis is suspected when hyperchloremic metabolic acidosis is associated with glucosuria, amino aciduria, phosphaturia, or uricosuria. It can be excluded by finding a fractional urine bicarbonate excretion of <5%.

A variety of methods are available for formal assessment of the capacity for distal tubular acidification (see Chapter 9).

RADIONUCLIDE STUDIES

The renogram is a valuable noninvasive technique for measuring renal function. Several radiopharmaceutical preparations are available. Technetium diethylenetriamine pentaacetic acid ([99mTc]-DTPA) is freely filtered by the glomerulus and is not reabsorbed. It is used to estimate GFR. Technetium dimercaptosuccinate ([99mTc]-DMSA) is bound to the tubules and provides information on the location, size, and contour of functional renal tissue. Radioiodinated orthoiodohippurate ($[^{131}I]$-OIH) is secreted into the tubules with a renal extraction efficiency of 80-90% and is used to assess renal plasma flow. Competition for tubular secretion by penicillin, probenecid, and certain intravenous radiographic contrast media can interfere with a hippurate scan. The relative function of each kidney can be measured, and a kidney that contributes < 8% to overall renal function can be regarded as being at end stage.

Indications for a Nuclear Renogram

- To quantify total renal function through measurement of overall GFR and renal plasma flow
- To quantify the percentage contribution of each kidney to overall renal function
- To detect obstruction
- To demonstrate presence or absence of normal renal parenchyma in evaluation of suspected mass lesions
- To evaluate renovascular disease

PATIENT PREPARATION AND COMPLICATIONS

Before the test the patient should be hydrated orally with 500 ml of water. The bladder is emptied immediately before, immediately after, and 1 hour after the test. Urine flow rates should be in the range of 1.5-4.0 ml/min. Adverse reactions to the intravenous injection of radiopharmaceutical agents are rare. The gonadal radiation dose is 30-140 mrad, and the whole-body dose is in the range of 8-100 mrad, depending on the particular scan performed. (A single view chest radiograph typically delivers a gonadal dose of 0.01 mrad.)

ULTRASONOGRAPHY

Ultrasound is a powerful tool for noninvasive imaging of the kidney. Image resolution is 1-2 cm, depending on the acoustic property of the tissue examined. Renal structures usually identified include cortex, medulla, renal pyramids, and a distended collecting system or distended ureter. Interposed bone or gas can cast acoustic shadows that hamper adequate imaging of renal anatomy. A kidney length < 9 cm is abnormal and indicates significant renal disease. A difference in size between the two kidneys of more than 1½ cm indicates a unilateral or asymmetric renal disease.

Simple cysts contain no internal echoes, have a sharply defined smooth internal wall, and have increased "through transmission" of sound energy posteriorly. Other hypoechoic renal mass lesions to consider include lymphoma, melanoma, infarct, hematoma, and xanthogranulomatous pyelonephritis. Complex cysts or solid lesions require further investigation. Ultrasound has become the procedure of choice in the early diagnosis of adult polycystic kidney disease.

Hydronephrosis is easily seen as a multiloculated fluid collection within the renal sinus. However, ultrasound does not assess renal function, and false positive images can occur with anatomic variants such as an extrarenal pelvis, in vesicoureteric reflux, and in pregnancy.

Indications for Renal Ultrasound

- To measure renal size
- To screen for hydronephrosis
- To characterize renal mass lesions
- To evaluate the perirenal space for abscess or hematoma
- To screen for adult polycystic kidney disease
- To localize the kidney for invasive procedures
- To assess residual bladder volume in excess of 100 ml

PATIENT PREPARATION AND COMPLICATIONS

The bladder is usually emptied prior to scanning. There is no radiation exposure or contrast agent required, and there are no known adverse effects of ultrasound.

INTRAVENOUS UROGRAPHY

The intravenous pyelogram (IVP) has been the traditional imaging procedure for the urinary tract. It provides an overview of the kidneys, ureters, and bladder. The nephrogram is formed by opacification of the renal parenchyma, and its density depends on the GFR, the dose of radiographic contrast agent, and the rate of intravenous injection. Although it is not able to provide absolute quantitative functional data, the IVP can demonstrate differential function between the right and left kidneys by the rate of appearance of the nephrogram phase. Filling of the pelvicaliceal system produces the pyelogram.

The normal renal size as measured by urography is > 11 cm, as a result of radiographic magnification of 30%. The left kidney is generally longer than the right kidney by up to 1½ cm. As an estimate, a normal kidney seen on plain film should occupy 3.5 lumbar vertebral bodies in height. Information of interest includes renal size, position, number, the presence of calcifications, distorting intrinsic or extrinsic mass lesions, adequacy of parenchymal thickness, abnormalities of cortical contour or papillary appearance, dilatation or blunting of calices, abnormal position or course of the ureters, reflux, and congenital variants.

Indications for an IVP

- To obtain a detailed definition of the pelvicaliceal system
- To assess renal size and contour
- To detect and locate calculi
- To provide qualitative assessment of function of each kidney

---

PATIENT PREPARATION AND COMPLICATIONS

Patients are generally given nothing by mouth for several hours prior to the study. Laxatives are often given for 2 days before the study.

The gonadal radiation dose may be as high as 800 mrad. Minor adverse reactions (flushing, nausea) are common. More serious reactions (vomiting, urticaria, angioneurotic edema, bronchospasm, hypotension) occur in about 5% of patients. Life-threatening events (cardiac arrest, convulsion, coma, pulmonary edema) occur in 0.01% of patients. Circumstances that predispose to postcontrast acute renal failure include advanced age (>60 years), chronic renal insufficiency, dehydration, diabetes mellitus, multiple myeloma, hyperuricemia, and large doses of or repeated exposure to hypertonic contrast agents. This complication could frequently be averted by correction of dehydration and use of intravenous mannitol, 12.5-25 g, given prior to the injection of contrast.

The traditional radiographic contrast agents such as metrizoate, iothalamate, and diatrizoate have osmolalities of 1400-1700 mOsm/kg H_2O. Newer nonionic agents such as metrizamide, iopamidol, and iohexol have become available and have an average osmolality of 600 mOsm/kg H_2O. Their use may result in fewer cases of acute renal failure, but they are also more expensive.

A history of a previous mild allergic reaction to radiographic contrast agents should prompt steroid prophylaxis with prednisone (50 mg orally every 6 hours x 3 doses), with the third dose given 1 hour before the study. A severe prior reaction may preclude any further exposure to these agents.

COMPUTED TOMOGRAPHY

Computed tomography (CT) is usually requested as an adjunctive study for further investigation of abnormalities discovered on ultrasound or IVP. CT is performed without contrast when the object is to demonstrate hemorrhage or calcification. The routine study is otherwise performed following radiographic contrast administration which is given intravenously by drip infusion or by rapid injection.

The radiographic contrast media are filtered by the glomeruli and concentrated in the tubules, thus allowing parenchymal enhancement and visualization of neoplasms or cysts. In addition, renal vessels and the position of the ureters can be identified. CT is useful in the evaluation of mass lesions or fluid collections in the kidney or retroperitoneal space, particularly when ultrasound examination is hindered by intra-abdominal gas or by obesity.

Generally Accepted Indications for CT

- To evaluate a renal mass and differentiate a solid neoplasm from a cyst, abscess, or hematoma when this cannot be defined by ultrasonography
- To more accurately display calcification patterns within a solid lesion
- To stage a renal neoplasm in preparation for surgery, chemotherapy, or radiation therapy
- To provide followup for tumor recurrence after primary therapy
- To evaluate a nonfunctioning kidney when the cause cannot be established by other means
- To confirm the presence of an angiomyolipoma
- To search for suspected calculi not revealed by other methods
- To study upper tract obstruction resulting from retroperitoneal fibrosis or tumor
- To delineate the extent of renal trauma
- To guide percutaneous needle aspiration or biopsy

PATIENT PREPARATION AND COMPLICATIONS

Patients should be able to cooperate to minimize artifact secondary to respiratory motion. No bowel preparation is needed. When possible, oral radiographic contrast agents are given to identify bowel loops. The radiation exposure is comparable to that of a routine IVP.

MAGNETIC RESONANCE IMAGING

The rapidly evolving new modality of magnetic resonance imaging (MRI) can be performed in the coronal, sagittal, or transaxial planes. Radiographic contrast agents are not yet used routinely but are under development.

Renal cortex can be readily distinguished from medulla. The loss of the corticomedullary demarcation on MRI is a nonspecific feature associated with glomerulonephritis, hydronephrosis, renal vascular occlusion, renal failure, and renal allograft rejection. Renal cysts are seen easily and yield data comparable to that obtained via CT. However, a major drawback is that foci of calcification cannot be detected by MRI. In the staging of known solid renal lesions, MRI may be superior to CT in the ability to detect tumor thrombus in major vessels and in distinguishing renal hilar collateral vessels from hilar lymph nodes. However, some renal neoplasms that may appear "isointense" or homogeneous with surrounding normal renal parenchyma may be missed with currently available noncontrasted MRI. MRI can be of help in differentiating adrenal mass lesions and in the evaluation of patients with pheochromocytoma.

Suggested Indications for MRI

- As an alternative or addition to CT in staging known renal cell carcinoma or in the detection of angiomyolipoma
- As a replacement for CT in evaluation of suspected renal mass lesions in patients who are intolerant of intravenous radiographic contrast agents
- In the evaluation of a hypertensive patient with an adrenal mass

COMPLICATIONS

MRI does not require the use of ionizing radiation, and there are no known harmful effects of exposure to either static magnetic fields or radio waves at the intensities used clinically. Potential hazards that exclude some patients as candidates for MRI include the presence of <u>pacemaker devices</u>, which can malfunction, or critically located ferromagnetic <u>surgical clips</u>, which may be subjected to torque forces. In addition, magnetizable objects left unsecured in the proximity of an intense magnetic field may become dangerous flying missiles. Conductive materials such as <u>metallic necklaces</u> may heat and cause skin burns. However, low resistance metallic devices such as skull plates or joint prostheses do not cause excessive tissue heating.

ARTERIOGRAPHY AND VENOGRAPHY

Contrast imaging of the arterial and venous vasculature is useful to assess primary disease of renal blood vessels, to diagnose renal infarction, or to seek distortions induced in the vascular tree by parenchymal renal pathology. This is most commonly performed by percutaneous cannulation of femoral or brachial vessels or, in selected cases, by digital subtraction angiography.

MODALITIES

<u>Arteriography</u> is useful in the evaluation of atherosclerotic or fibrodysplastic stenotic lesions of the renal arteries, aneurysms, arteriovenous fistulae, vasculitis, and mass renal lesions. <u>Venography</u> is performed to diagnose renal vein thrombosis. <u>Angiography</u> is often combined with interventional diagnostic procedures such as determination of selective renal vein renin

activity or with therapeutic procedures such as percutaneous transluminal balloon angioplasty or renal embolization.

COMPLICATIONS

Complications of this procedure include puncture site hemorrhage, retroperitoneal hemorrhage, arterial obstruction, rupture of an arterial aneurysm, arterial dissection, inadvertent distal arterial embolization of cholesterol plaques resulting in tissue ischemia, arteriovenous fistulae, and radiographic contrast-related adverse reactions. Significant complications may occur in 1.8% of patients, and there is a mortality rate of 0.03%.

RENAL BIOPSY

In consultation with a nephrologist, the percutaneous needle biopsy can be helpful for establishing a diagnosis, assessing prognosis, monitoring disease progression, and selecting a rational therapy.

INDICATIONS

Acute Renal Failure

In a patient in whom the underlying cause of acute renal failure is not evident at presentation or who fails to recover normal renal function following 3-4 weeks of supportive therapy, biopsy may be necessary to distinguish acute tubular necrosis from a host of renal diseases that may require alternative management (see Chapter 21).

Nephrotic Syndrome

In the adult patient without evidence of systemic disease, many nephrologists would recommend biopsy to look for primary glomerular diseases. The most frequently encountered entities include membranous glomerulonephritis, focal segmental glomerulosclerosis, membrano-proliferative glomerulonephritis, IgA nephropathy, amyloidosis, and minimal change disease (see Chapters 3 and 4).

Proteinuria

In the setting of persistent nonnephrotic proteinuria of 2 g/24 hr/1.73 m^2 or more, or in the presence of an abnormal urine sediment, or if there is documented functional deterioration, biopsy may detect early underlying renal disease. Orthostatic proteinuria does not require biopsy.

Hematuria

Biopsy may be helpful in patients with microscopic hematuria persisting for longer than 6 months, with a history of episodic gross hematuria, or with a family history of hematuria, particularly when there is associated abnormal urine sediment or proteinuria. Secondary causes of hematuria must be excluded. Common findings include Alport's syndrome and IgA nephropathy. Biopsy is usually not helpful in isolated microscopic hematuria (see Chapter 2).

Systemic Disease

A variety of systemic disorders may be associated with kidney involvement. These include diabetes mellitus, systemic lupus erythematosus, Schönlein-Henoch purpura, polyarteritis nodosa, Goodpasture's syndrome, Wegener's granulomatosis, and dysproteinemias. Biopsy is often performed to confirm the diagnosis, to establish the extent of renal involvement, and to guide management.

Transplant Allograft

Biopsy is helpful in differentiating rejection from acute tubular necrosis, drug-induced interstitial nephritis, hemorrhagic infarction, and de novo or recurrent glomerulonephritis (see Chapter 25).

CONTRAINDICATIONS

Commonly accepted contraindications to percutaneous needle biopsy include a solitary or ectopic kidney (except for transplant allografts), horseshoe kidney, the presence of an uncorrected bleeding disorder, severe uncontrolled hypertension, renal infection, renal neoplasm, or an uncooperative patient. Relative contraindications may include pregnancy, severe obesity, hydronephrosis, end-stage kidneys, and congenital anomalies.

PATIENT PREPARATION AND COMPLICATIONS

Percutaneous renal biopsy is an _inpatient_ procedure. Routine admission laboratory tests should include a prothrombin time, partial thromboplastin time, complete blood count, platelet count, blood type and antibody screen for possible crossmatch should the need for transfusion arise, and a urinalysis to rule out urinary tract infection. If coagulation parameters are abnormal, a bleeding time should be performed. Intravenous access must be secured, and the line kept patent with an appropriate intravenous fluid. The biopsy is commonly performed under ultrasound or fluoroscopic guidance. Postbiopsy, the patient must remain at strict bedrest for 24 hours. Frequent vital signs are recorded to monitor evidence of hypovolemia resulting from hemorrhage. Serial hematocrits are obtained 4-6 hours after the biopsy and again the following morning. Aliquots of each voided urine are saved to observe for gross hematuria.

The most frequent complication is bleeding that is usually self-limited. Significant bleeding requiring transfusion, percutaneous arterial embolization of a bleeding vessel, or nephrectomy is uncommon, with an occurrence rate of 2.1%. The mortality rate of 0.07% is comparable to that of percutaneous liver biopsy or coronary angiography.

When percutaneous needle biopsy is technically not feasible and a histologic diagnosis is imperative, an open biopsy performed by a urologic surgeon in the operating room under general anesthesia should be considered.

SUGGESTED READING

Cockcroft DW, Gault MH. Prediction of creatinine clearance from serum creatinine. Nephron 1976;16:31-41.

Davidson AJ, Hartman DS. Imaging strategies for tumors of the kidney, adrenal gland, and retroperitoneum. Cancer J Clin 1987;37:151-164.

Hricak H, Crooks L, Sheldon P, Kaufman L. Nuclear magnetic resonance imaging of the kidney. Radiology 1983;146:425-432.

Levey AS, Perrone RD, Madias NE. Serum creatinine and renal function. Ann Rev Med 1988;39:465-490.

Mitch WE, Walser M, Buffington GA, Lemann J. A simple method of estimating progression of chronic renal failure. Lancet 1976;2:1326-1328.

Schoolwerth AC. Hematuria and proteinuria: their causes and consequences. Hosp Prac 1987;22:45-62.

Tisher CC, Croker BP. Indications for and interpretation of renal biopsy: evaluation by light, electron, and immunofluorescence microscopy. In: Schrier RW, Gottschalk CW, eds. Diseases of the Kidney. 4th ed. Boston: Little, Brown and Co, 1988:527-556.

Tisher, CC. Clinical indications for kidney biopsy. In: Tisher CC, Brenner BM, eds. Renal Pathology with Clinical and Functional Correlations. 1st ed. Philadelphia: JB Lippincott Co, 1989:2-10.

Chapter 2

Hematuria

Nicolas J. Guzman
Charles S. Wingo

DEFINITION

Hematuria is defined as the presence of abnormal quantities of erythrocytes in the urine. Careful examination of the sediment from a freshly voided urine may show up to 3 erythrocytes per 10 to 20 high-power fields. Although this value is commonly accepted as the upper limit of normal, approximately 10% of normal subjects will excrete up to 10 erythrocytes per high-power field. However, in an otherwise normal subject, the persistent excretion of more than 3 erythrocytes per high-power field is an indication for evaluation of the genitourinary tract.

DETECTION OF HEMATURIA

Gross hematuria is easily detected by visual inspection. Microscopic hematuria can be detected by direct microscopic inspection of the urinary sediment or by the use of orthotoluidine-impregnated paper strips ("dipstix") which gives positive results with urine containing as little as 3 to 5 erythrocytes per high-power field. This method, however, also detects hemoglobinuria and myoglobinuria. Occasionally, calcium oxalate crystals, yeast, and air bubbles can be mistakenly identified as erythrocytes on microscopic examination. The paper strip method will be negative in all of these cases. Normally large numbers of erythrocytes will be found in urine samples obtained by urethral catheterization and in voided specimens from menstruating females.

LOCALIZATION OF HEMATURIA

Relationship Between Clinical Findings and Origin of Hematuria

	Renal Parenchyma	*Urinary Tract*
• Pain	Usually dull flank pain	Commonly suprapubic pain with dysuria, or colicky flank pain
• Blood clots	Absent in glomerular diseases; may occur with trauma, tumors, and vascular anomalies	Commonly present
• Cellular casts	Commonly present in glomerular diseases	Absent
• Proteinuria >150 mg/dl	Commonly present	Absent
• RBC shape	Usually distorted	Normal

ETIOLOGY

The following display outlines the more common causes of hematuria.

Common Causes of Hematuria

RENAL PARENCHYMA

Glomerular Diseases
- Primary glomerulonephritis
- Glomerulopathies associated with systemic disease including:
  systemic lupus erythematosus, vasculitis, Wegener's granulomatosis, Goodpasture's syndrome, Schönlein-Henoch purpura, thrombotic microangiopathies, diabetes mellitus
- Infection including:
  postinfectious glomerulonephritis, infective endocarditis, "shunt" nephritis
- Hereditary
  Alport's syndrome

Vascular Disease
- Malignant hypertension
- Renal thromboembolic disease
- Loin-pain hematuria syndrome
- Vascular anomalies

Tubulointerstitial Disease
- Hereditary diseases including:
  polycystic kidney disease, medullary sponge kidney
- Hypersensitivity interstitial nephritis
- Papillary necrosis due to:
  analgesic nephropathy, sickle cell disease or trait,
  diabetes mellitus, obstructive uropathy
- Acute bacterial pyelonephritis

Tumors
- Renal cell carcinoma, Wilms' tumor

TRAUMA

URINARY TRACT DISEASE

Renal Pelvis
- Transitional cell carcinoma
- Calculi
- Trauma
- Vascular anomalies

Ureter
- Calculi
- Transitional cell carcinoma
- Retroperitoneal fibrosis
- Vascular anomalies

Bladder
- Carcinoma
- Cystitis including:
  infectious, drug-induced, radiation-induced,
  hypersensitivity
- Postobstructive decompression
- Vascular anomalies
- Trauma
- Schistosomiasis
- Marathon runner's hematuria

Prostate
- Benign prostatic hypertrophy
- Carcinoma of the prostate
- Acute and chronic prostatitis

Urethra
- Acute and chronic urethritis
- Trauma and foreign bodies
- Polyps
- Carcinoma of the urethra or penis
- Vascular anomalies

SYSTEMIC COAGULATION DISORDERS

EVALUATION OF HEMATURIA

Initial routine laboratory studies should include coagulation tests and urine cultures. If pyuria is present, a Gram stain of the urine should be performed and further studies withheld until results of the cultures become available. Sterile pyuria coupled with hematuria suggests renal tuberculosis.

Once **infectious** etiologies have been excluded, a plain abdominal X-ray film should be obtained and carefully reviewed for the presence of renal or pelvic calcifications and masses. If this study is negative, a cystoscopy with biopsy of all suspicious lesions should be performed. All biopsy material should be sent for culture as well as for pathological examination. If the bladder appears normal, the origin of both ureters should be inspected for hematuria and selective ureteric urine samples should be obtained and sent for culture and cytology. If cystoscopy is nondiagnostic, or if the abdominal plain film reveals a renal mass or calcifications, a renal ultrasound should be considered. This study is helpful in the evaluation of renal masses for solid or cystic features or to identify renal calculi. Further identification and characterization of structural and vascular lesions usually requires an intravenous pyelogram (IVP), retrograde pyelography, a computed tomography (CT) scan, an angiogram, or a combination of these studies. Indications for these studies are reviewed in Chapter 1.

Glomerular causes of hematuria (see Chapter 4) should be considered in all patients in whom complete evaluation fails to provide a definitive diagnosis. If the creatinine clearance is greater than 30 ml/min, a renal biopsy should be performed. In addition, renal biopsy should be strongly considered in those patients presenting with hematuria associated with proteinuria or red blood cell (RBC) casts, rather than going through the extensive evaluation outlined above.

Despite extensive investigations, the cause of the hematuria will remain unknown in 10 to 15% of all patients.

DIFFERENTIAL DIAGNOSIS OF HEMATURIA OF RENAL PARENCHYMAL ORIGIN

Glomerular Causes

Renal involvement in systemic diseases, such as systemic lupus erythematosus, Schönlein-Henoch purpura, and various types of vasculitis, is commonly associated with hematuria. The presence of fever, arthralgias, a skin rash, or purpura suggests the presence of a systemic disorder. Positive serologic tests for **collagen-vascular disease**, or hypocomplementemia and cryoglobulinemia usually point to the cause of the hematuria. **Wegener's granulomatosis** and **Goodpasture's syndrome** present commonly with pulmonary involvement and hemoptysis. Antiglomerular basement membrane antibodies are characteristic of Goodpasture's syndrome.

Postinfectious glomerulonephritis is characterized by a history of recent skin or throat infection and elevated titers of antistreptolysin O, antihyaluronidase, or anti-DNase. Fever associated with the appearance of a heart murmur should suggest the diagnosis of infective endocarditis, particularly in patients with prosthetic heart valves and a history of recent dental procedures, as well as in intravenous drug abusers. Blood cultures will usually demonstrate the causative organism. Echocardiography may disclose the presence of vegetations.

Hereditary nephritis or Alport's syndrome very commonly presents with hematuria. The diagnosis is suggested by a family history of kidney disease, kidney failure, deafness, and ocular abnormalities. Audiometry is abnormal in half of these patients.

Vascular Causes

Renal vein thrombosis can sometimes present as hematuria. These patients will commonly have a history of nephrotic syndrome and their laboratory evaluation may show a hyperchloremic metabolic acidosis, proteinuria, and glycosuria. The diagnosis is made by selective renal venography.

Sudden back pain and hematuria, particularly in a patient with atrial fibrillation or a recent myocardial infarction, suggest renal arterial embolism. Renal angiography is the procedure of choice to identify this condition.

Tubulointerstitial Disease

Patients with polycystic kidney disease usually give a family history of kidney failure. Physical examination may disclose an abdominal mass. The diagnosis can be made with an IVP or renal ultrasound.

Hypersensitivity interstitial nephritis is suspected when a patient with recent drug exposure presents with hematuria and sterile pyuria. Urticaria may or may not be present. Peripheral eosinophilia is common, and eosinophiluria, when present, is a helpful clue.

Papillary necrosis is usually an acute and more dramatic condition. It should be considered whenever hematuria occurs in a patient with analgesic nephropathy, sickle cell disease or trait, and diabetes mellitus complicated by acute pyelonephritis with obstruction.

Acute bacterial pyelonephritis usually presents with fever, back pain, and pyuria with bacteriuria.

Treatment

Hematuria rarely produces enough blood loss to require volume replacement. The passing of blood clots can, however, cause severe pain and urinary obstruction, which may require urethral catheterization and saline irrigation. In cases of severe hematuria caused by structural lesions of the urinary tract, a surgical therapeutic approach may be indicated. Correction of a coagulopathy, if present, is essential. In most cases, the treatment of hematuria is directed toward the primary cause.

SUGGESTED READING

Abitol CL. The evaluation of a patient with hematuria. Medical Times 1983;111:63-69.

Benson G, Brewer E. Hematuria: algorithms for diagnosis II. JAMA 1981;246:993-995.

Brewer E, Benson G. Hematuria: algorithms for diagnosis I. JAMA 1981;246:877-880.

Brown SH, MacDougall ML, Wiegmann TB. Microscopic hematuria. Kansas Medicine 1986;87:99-101.

Glassock RJ. Hematuria and pigmenturia. In: Massry SG, Glassock RJ, eds. Textbook of Nephrology. 2nd ed. Baltimore: Williams & Wilkins, 1989:491-500.

Chapter 3

Proteinuria and the Nephrotic Syndrome

Daniel R. Salomon

DEFINITION

Proteinuria refers to the presence of protein in the urine. Normal adults may excrete up to 150 mg of protein each day. Greater values usually imply a disease state. The nephrotic syndrome refers to a combination of abnormal findings that includes:

- Urine protein excretion of $\geq$ 3.5 g 24 hr/1.73 m^2.
- Hypoalbuminemia (serum albumin less than 3.0 g/dl).
- Peripheral edema (occasionally anasarca with ascites).
- Hypercholesterolemia (fasting level greater than 200 mg/dl).

INCIDENCE

Proteinuria greater than 150 mg/24 hr is common in patients with even mild renal insufficiency, congestive heart failure, diabetes mellitus, severe obesity, severe or malignant hypertension, the elderly, and pregnant women. In contrast, the nephrotic syndrome, which implies glomerular disease or glomerulonephritis, is uncommon in a general hospital population (i.e., less than 1% of patients).

ETIOLOGY

The differential diagnosis of proteinuria includes etiologies in which the primary pathology involves the kidney directly (e.g., Renal Parenchymal Origin) and etiologies in which another primary systemic disorder is associated with increased urine protein excretion (e.g. Other Causes) (see display on p. 27). Making this distinction is important in deciding how to design a diagnostic plan. The differential diagnosis of nephrotic syndrome includes many of the same etiologies listed for proteinuria under Renal Parenchymal Origin. However, the nephrotic syndrome is caused only by renal disease which results in significant damage to the glomeruli and their basement membranes. Thus, proteinuria may represent an early stage in the progression of a renal disease toward the nephrotic syndrome.

Differential Diagnosis of Proteinuria and Nephrotic Syndrome

Proteinuria	Nephrotic Syndrome
• Renal Parenchymal Origin	
Chronic renal disease	Glomerulonephritis
Diabetes mellitus	Primary forms
Obstructive/reflux nephropathy	Secondary forms
Interstitial nephritis	Diabetes mellitus
Glomerulonephritis	Connective tissue disease
Primary forms	Systemic infections
Secondary forms	Viral
Connective tissue disease	Bacterial
Renal transplantation	Neoplasia
Amyloidosis	Drug toxicity
Drug toxicity	NSAIDS
Sickle cell disease	Gold
Acute pyelonephritis	Penicillamine
Orthostatic proteinuria	Phenytoin
	Serum sickness
• Other Causes	Congestive heart failure
Essential hypertension	Constrictive pericarditis
Congestive heart failure	Sarcoidosis
Acute febrile illness	Massive obesity
Serum sickness	Ulcerative colitis
Normal pregnancy	Hereditary diseases
Severe obesity	Hypothyroidism
Neoplasia	Amyloidosis

NORMAL PHYSIOLOGY

GLOMERULAR BASEMENT MEMBRANE

The anatomical barrier to protein loss in the kidney is the glomerular basement membrane (GBM). The GBM possesses fixed negatively charged sites that restrict the filtration of negatively charged macromolecules such as albumin.

SIZE BARRIER TO PROTEIN LOSS

The GBM excludes plasma proteins on the basis of molecular size and shape. In general, a protein with a molecular weight greater than 70,000 will be poorly filtered. For example, less than 1% of the plasma albumin (M.W. 67,000) crosses the GBM during the passage of plasma through the glomerulus.

CHARGE BARRIER TO PROTEIN LOSS

The GBM has a net negative charge which repulses most plasma proteins including albumin and the immunoglobulins which are negatively charged.

TUBULAR REABSORPTION OF PROTEIN

A small amount of albumin and several other plasma proteins do escape across the GBM (approximately 500-1500 mg/24 hr). The proximal tubule reabsorbs the majority of this filtered protein that is catabolized subsequently. Thus, a normal individual will excrete only 25-150 mg of protein each day in the urine.

PATHOPHYSIOLOGY
STRUCTURAL DAMAGE TO THE GLOMERULAR BASEMENT MEMBRANE

Renal disease often results in structural damage to the GBM, which impairs its barrier function. For example, in certain forms of glomerulonephritis the deposition of antibodies or immune complexes in the GBM in concert with complement activation and local inflammation results in membrane disruption. A reduction or even neutralization of the negative charge barrier has also been documented in glomerulonephritis. In diabetes mellitus the local deposition of abnormal glycosylated material may result in the disruption of the integrity of the GBM. In renal diseases associated with various vascular lesions, the GBM may be damaged by the destruction of capillary endothelium or as the consequence of tissue ischemia.

DAMAGE TO THE TUBULAR REABSORPTION PROCESS

Proteinuria may also result from damage to the proximal tubule resulting in inadequate reabsorption of the filtered protein load, but this does not exceed 1500 mg/24 hr. Interstitial nephritis, acute tubular necrosis, reflux nephropathy, and amyloidosis are the most common renal diseases associated with this mechanism. Renal vein thrombosis may also result in tubular damage.

HEMODYNAMIC CAUSES OF INCREASED PROTEIN LOSS

The pathophysiology of proteinuria in congestive heart failure, hypertension, and perhaps pregnancy relates to an increase in the transglomerular capillary pressure which increases glomerular protein filtration.

OTHER CAUSES OF PROTEINURIA

In certain neoplastic conditions proteinuria may be the result of filtration of low molecular weight proteins produced by the malignant cells (e.g., lysozyme in acute monomyelocytic leukemia or the Bence Jones proteinuria of multiple myeloma).

CONSEQUENCES OF DECREASED PLASMA ONCOTIC PRESSURE

Several important physiological changes occur when urinary protein excretion exceeds several grams each day. A reduction in plasma albumin concentration decreases the plasma oncotic pressure which opposes the loss of plasma fluid into the interstitial space, resulting in peripheral edema, ascites, and anasarca. The reduction of plasma oncotic pressure also increases sodium reabsorption and this, in turn, enhances the development of ascites and peripheral edema.

ROLE OF THE RENIN-ANGIOTENSIN SYSTEM

The loss of plasma fluid into the interstitial space causes contraction of the intravascular volume which activates the renin-angiotensin system and increases plasma aldosterone levels. Aldosterone increases total body salt and water and exacerbates peripheral edema and ascites.

LOSS OF OTHER PLASMA PROTEINS

Albumin is only one of several important plasma proteins which are lost in the urine. The loss of several vitamin D-binding proteins results in the depletion of activated vitamin D metabolites and contributes to the development of osteomalacia. The loss of lipid carrier proteins results in hyperlipidemia. Several studies of patients with the nephrotic syndrome have confirmed an increased risk of atherosclerosis and ischemic cardiac disease. The loss of thyroid-binding globulins and thyroid hormones may alter standard thyroid function test results; however, levels of free thyroid hormone remain normal and there is no alteration in thyroid hormone-dependent metabolism.

A HYPERCOAGULABLE STATE AND RENAL VEIN THROMBOSIS

The loss of antithrombin III and other proteins involved in the clotting and fibrinolytic cascades can lead to a relative hypercoagulable state. There is an increased incidence of peripheral venous thrombosis and, most importantly, renal vein thrombosis. Renal vein thrombosis may increase urinary protein excretion further and be complicated by pulmonary embolization.

CLINICAL PRESENTATION

SIGNS

Peripheral edema is the hallmark of significant proteinuria or the nephrotic syndrome. This will not occur until plasma albumin concentrations fall below 3 g/dl. The development of **ascites** and the progression of the peripheral edema to **anasarca** are a matter of time and the severity of the hypoalbuminemia. Some patients will present with a reduced blood pressure or **orthostatic hypotension** as a result of a contracted intravascular volume. **Hypertension** in association with an abnormal urinalysis or decreased renal function suggests glomerulonephritis, diabetes mellitus, or connective tissue disease. Retinal vascular changes consistent with long-standing hypertension would indicate that the hypertension is not a primary event associated with the renal dysfunction or proteinuria. The development of **acute tachypnea, tachycardia,** and **hypotension** strongly suggests a pulmonary embolus, although an acute myocardial infarction must also be excluded. Chronic or exertional tachypnea suggests pulmonary edema associated with severe hypoalbuminemia, large pleural effusions, or increased respiratory effort due to a restriction of diaphragmatic motion by ascites. Vertebral compression fractures or poorly healing stress fractures may be signs of the osteomalacic bone disease. Renal vein thrombosis may cause microscopic or gross hematuria.

SYMPTOMS

Many patients complain of feeling bloated or tight as a result of peripheral edema. Patients with ascites will note abdominal fullness and a reduced tolerance to food intake. Dyspnea may be associated with pulmonary edema, pulmonary emboli, or reduced diaphragmatic motion. The osteomalacic bone disease is usually asymptomatic unless associated with a vertebral compression fracture. Renal vein thrombosis may cause flank pain but it is most often asymptomatic.

INVESTIGATIONS

ROUTINE TESTS

Dipstick Protein Analysis

A positive protein by dipstick performed as a routine screening procedure is a common means of identifying patients with proteinuria. It is critical to determine the specific gravity of the urine since the dipstick detection of protein in a highly concentrated urine (i.e., specific gravity of 1.025 or greater) has uncertain diagnostic significance. It is important to note that Bence Jones proteins are not detected by dipstick.

24-Hour Urine Collection

The 24-hr urine collection is the only reliable way to quantify proteinuria. The patient should be instructed carefully as compliance is critical. Upon rising on the first morning the patient should void and discard the urine. Subsequently, all urine is saved until the next morning at which time the patient's first void is saved and the collection is complete. The creatinine clearance should also be determined as a key assessment of the patient's renal function. It is also a measure of patient compliance because the amount of creatinine produced and excreted every day is a function of the size and sex of the patient. A 24-hr urine with a total creatinine content of at least 15 mg/kg body weight in a female, or 20 mg/kg body weight in a male, will ensure an adequate collection (see Chapter 1). More than one complete 24-hr urine collection should be performed to provide an accurate baseline for determining the course of the proteinuria, response to therapy, etc.

Orthostatic Proteinuria

Orthostatic proteinuria is a benign condition that does not require further diagnostic evaluation and usually remits spontaneously. The most practical test for this entity is to split the 24-hr urine into two 12-hr collections. The first 12-hr specimen is collected during the day when the patient is active and upright. The second 12-hr collection is obtained overnight while the patient is at rest or sleeping. A positive result is significant proteinuria in the first 12 hr (patient active) and a protein excretion of less than 75 mg in the second 12 hr (patient inactive).

Microscopic Analysis

The microscopic analysis of a centrifuged urine specimen for the presence of cellular elements and urinary casts is a critical test. Hematuria, pyuria, and cellular casts suggest the diagnosis of glomerulonephritis. The presence of oval fat bodies is common in the nephrotic syndrome. They are seen best under polarized light where they appear to contain a miniature maltese cross. The microscopic analysis in patients with glomerulonephritis will be described in greater detail in Chapter 4.

Blood Chemistries

A decreased serum albumin (<3 g/dl) and total serum protein (<6 g/dl) are typical in patients with nephrotic-range proteinuria but may also be seen in patients with lesser amounts of proteinuria if associated with poor protein intake, increased protein catabolism (stress, surgery, steroids, systemic illness), or liver disease. Elevations of cholesterol (>200 mg/dl) and triglyceride levels (>300 mg/dl) are part of the nephrotic syndrome. An elevated serum creatinine and blood urea nitrogen (BUN) are important indicators of renal insufficiency.

Hematology

Anemia is common in renal disease but may be associated with many of the other diseases that cause proteinuria. Leukocytosis or leukopenia may be associated with various infections or neoplasias. For example, the presence of anemia and the rouleaux phenomenon ("stacking" of red blood cells) suggests multiple myeloma, while the presence of anemia, thrombocytopenia, and many mature or atypical lymphocytes suggests a viral infection with glomerulonephritis.

Special Tests

Erythrocyte sedimentation rate (ESR). The ESR rate is virtually always elevated in patients with the nephrotic syndrome because of the loss of plasma proteins and, thus, is of little diagnostic value.

Complement levels (C3, C4, and CH50). These are decreased in postinfectious glomerulonephritis, membranoproliferative glomerulonephritis, and systemic lupus erythematosus.

Serum and urine protein electrophoresis. These tests are employed either to detect a monoclonal protein characteristic of multiple myeloma or amyloidosis including the presence of light chains in the urine (e.g., Bence Jones proteins) or to assess the selectivity of proteinuria. If albumin is the predominant protein excreted, the patient has "selective" proteinuria. This is associated with minimal change disease and early or mild forms of focal segmental and membranous glomerulonephritis. In contrast, more extensive GBM injury results in "nonselective" proteinuria with the excretion of both albumin and the larger globulin fractions of plasma (including IgG as a major protein). This is associated with advanced focal segmental and membranous glomerulonephritis, with various forms of proliferative glomerulonephritis, diabetes mellitus, and amyloidosis.

Immunoelectrophoresis. This test is used to identify the monoclonal antibody in multiple myeloma or to demonstrate a polyclonal gammopathy which is often seen with acute or chronic infection.

Determinations of antinuclear antibody (ANA) and rheumatoid factor (RF) status. These tests may establish the diagnosis of systemic lupus erythematosus or other connective tissue diseases. RF may be present in subacute endocarditis.

Viral titers, IgM, and IgG. These titers include cytomegalovirus and Ebstein-Barr virus. An elevated IgM titer is diagnostic of acute infection, while a rise in IgG titer in comparison with a previous sample may be strongly suggestive of a viral infection.

Viral cultures of urine and blood. These cultures are particularly useful for the diagnosis of cytomegalovirus infection.

Cryoglobulins and immune complexes. These serum components are associated with vasculitis and various forms of acute glomerulonephritis.

Hepatitis serology. Viral hepatitis, particularly the "serum type" with a positive test for hepatitis B surface antigen, may be associated with a glomerulonephritis presumably due to immune complex deposition in the glomeruli.

Endocrine function tests. These include a glucose tolerance test and thyroid function tests.

Renal Ultrasound

The renal ultrasound has replaced the intravenous pyelogram (IVP) for the noninvasive determination of renal size and the detection of urinary tract abnormalities. Renal size may be increased with renal vein thrombosis, with acute pyelonephritis or glomerulonephritis, in amyloidosis, or in diabetic nephropathy. It is usually decreased in chronic renal disease. Obstructive or reflux uropathy may be suggested by the presence of a dilated ureter or renal pelvis, a kidney stone, or a significant postvoid residual in the bladder. Any finding suggestive of obstruction must be pursued with other urologic tests including an IVP, diuretic renogram, and cystoscopy (see Chapter 12).

Fluorescein Angiography of the Retina

It is important to establish the presence of microvascular disease in the retina of patients with diabetes mellitus (specifically microaneurysms and capillary proliferation) since this is highly suggestive that diabetes is the cause of the proteinuria. An abnormal fundus, which can sometimes only be shown by fluorescein angiography, is sufficient evidence to conclude that diabetes mellitus is a major factor in renal injury and proteinuria (see Chapter 5).

Renal Biopsy

The renal biopsy remains the gold standard for establishing the diagnosis of renal disease and proteinuria. If a diagnosis can be definitively established by the studies described above, the biopsy may be deferred. In some patients the biopsy may still be indicated to establish the extent of renal involvement as a guide to therapy or prognosis (e.g., lupus nephritis). If the kidney is small or scarred and there is significant renal insufficiency, the risk of the biopsy may outweigh the benefit. This decision should be deferred to a nephrologist (see Chapter 1).

MANAGEMENT

This section will be restricted to a discussion of the management of problems common to all patients with proteinuria or the nephrotic syndrome as listed below:

- Protein loss
- Peripheral edema and ascites
- Bone disease
- The hypercoagulable state and renal vein thrombosis
- Hyperlipidemia

PROTEIN LOSS

The development of hypoalbuminemia is a primary cause of peripheral edema, pleural effusions, and ascites. A protein restricted diet (0.5-0.6 g/kg/day) or an angiotensin-converting enzyme inhibitor, such as captopril, lisinopril, or enalapril, will often decrease glomerular filtration rate (GFR) and reduce protein loss. These approaches can be used in combination.

Urine protein excretion may become sufficient to cause negative nitrogen balance and protein malnutrition. When the protein loss exceeds 10 g/24 hr, we suggest addition of protein to the diet in amounts equivalent to the daily losses.

PERIPHERAL EDEMA AND ASCITES

A key to success in managing edema is dietary salt restriction. A reduction in the use of processed and canned foods which are typically high in salt, and replacement of cooking with table salt with spices or salt substitutes which contain potassium, is a good first step. However, most patients eventually require a diuretic. A thiazide is helpful to control mild edema in patients with preserved renal function, but a loop diuretic is required for refractory edema associated with pleural effusions or ascites. The principles of diuretic administration are described in Chapter 28.

Activation of the renin-angiotensin system by intravascular volume loss in the hypoalbuminemic patient leads to secondary hyperaldosteronism which exacerbates the edema by increasing sodium reabsorption in the distal nephron. Thus, the use of an aldosterone antagonist such as spironolactone or a potassium-sparing diuretic such as amiloride or triamterene is rational and also reduces the hypokalemia which is a common side effect of the other diuretics. The addition of a diuretic such as metolazone or hydrochlorothiazide that acts distal to the loop of Henle may greatly potentiate the diuretic activity of a loop diuretic. However, this strategy must be used cautiously. Many patients with the nephrotic syndrome already have a contracted intravascular volume due to the loss of plasma fluid into the interstitial space. Overzealous use of diuretics can contract the intravascular volume further, lower the GFR, and promote salt retention and diuretic resistance. Diuretic therapy provides largely symptomatic treatment for the nephrotic syndrome. Therefore, the goal should be the control of peripheral edema, but not its elimination.

BONE DISEASE

Chronic urinary loss of vitamin D metabolites can cause osteomalacic bone disease. Although this is usually asymptomatic unless associated with a vertebral compression fracture, it can be documented by biopsy in many patients. It is very important to preserve bone integrity in patients with progressive renal disease in whom many other metabolic abnormalities will eventually impact on the bone (see Chapter 22). Replacement therapy should be initiated with vitamin D_2 unless significantly reduced renal or hepatic function suggests the need for the $1,25(OH)_2$ form of vitamin D. An initial dose of 50,000 units each day should be followed carefully by weekly serum calcium determinations for at least 3 weeks before adjusting the dosage. The goal should be to maintain the serum ionized calcium level in the normal range.

THE HYPERCOAGULABLE STATE AND RENAL VEIN THROMBOSIS

Renal vein thrombosis should be treated by immediate hospitalization and heparin therapy. After 1 week of heparin the patient should be converted to warfarin (Coumadin[R]) and treated for at least 6 months. Many patients require prolonged Coumadin[R] for therapy because of recurrent thrombosis.

HYPERLIPIDEMIA

All patients with hypercholesterolemia and hypertriglyceridemia should be maintained on a low fat diet, a weight control plan, and regular exercise. In patients who remain hyperlipidemic, an endocrinologist should be consulted concerning pharmacologic intervention because of the documented increase in cardiovascular events in nephrotic hyperlipidemic patients.

FOLLOW-UP

Renal function and protein excretion must be followed closely, especially during the initiation of diuretic therapy. A sudden change suggests a renal vein thrombosis requiring immediate diagnosis and therapy. Office visits twice each month are reasonable. Once the patient is stable the visits can be reduced to every 2 months.

OUTCOME

The outcome of proteinuria and the nephrotic syndrome is largely dependent on the etiology. Patients with **proteinuria** and renal insufficiency will often continue to lose renal function and eventually may require dialysis therapy. Patients with the **nephrotic syndrome** have some form of glomerular lesion by definition and, thus, many will eventually develop renal insufficiency.

SUGGESTED READING

Appel GB, Blum CB, Chien S, Kunis CL, Appel AS. The hyperlipidemia of nephrotic syndrome. N Engl J Med 1985;312:1544-1548.

Fine LG. Preventing the progression of human renal disease. Have rational therapeutic principles emerged? Kidney Int 1988;33:116-128.

Skorecki KL, Nadler SP, Badr KF, Brenner BM. Renal and systemic manifestations of glomerular disease. In: Brenner BM, Rector FC Jr, eds. The kidney. Philadelphia: WB Saunders Company, 1986:891-921.

Chapter 4

Glomerulonephritis

Daniel R. Salomon

DEFINITION

Glomerulonephritis is an inflammatory process involving the glomerulus, although other components of the renal parenchyma may be affected. Glomerular inflammation, usually the direct result of an immune response, leads to injury of any of three major elements of the glomerulus: the basement membrane, the mesangium, or the capillary endothelium. In fact, different forms of glomerulonephritis are characterized by the predominant pattern of inflammation that occurs in the glomerulus (see Pathophysiology). Glomerulonephritis may be a primary kidney disease such as acute postinfectious proliferative glomerulonephritis or the consequence of a systemic disease such as systemic lupus erythematosus.

Primary and Secondary Forms of Glomerulonephritis*

Primary	*Secondary*
• Membranous	• Systemic lupus erythematosus
• Focal glomerular sclerosis	• Infections
• Primary IgA (Berger's)	• Systemic vasculitis
• Idiopathic crescentic	• Schönlein-Henoch purpura
• Membranoproliferative	• Goodpasture's syndrome
• Focal proliferative	• Heredofamilial diseases
• Minimal change disease	• Liver disease
• Acute postinfectious	• Neoplasia

*Order of approximate clinical incidence in adults.

INCIDENCE

Patients with glomerulonephritis constitute about 5% of the average nephrologist's office practice. However, in a patient population requiring chronic hemodialysis or transplantation, a history of glomerulonephritis will be the stated cause of end-stage renal disease in approximately 40%.

PATHOGENESIS

The definition of glomerulonephritis depends on identification of specific histopathologic patterns of glomerular injury. This requires a knowledge of the normal structure of the glomerulus. Figure 29-3 depicts the mesangium surrounded by four capillary loops and a layer of epithelium marking the beginning of the urinary space. Important structures include the two mesangial cells (M) which are surrounded by mesangial matrix, the endothelial cell (En) which lines the glomerular capillary, the dark band of glomerular basement membrane (GBM), and the epithelial cell (Ep) with its many foot processes attached to the urinary side of the GBM.

MESANGIAL CELLS

The kidney is constantly exposed to foreign antigens. Mesangial cells can take up and process antigen and antigen-antibody immune complexes. When mesangial cells are overwhelmed by this task, antigens and immune complexes accumulate and distort the normal glomerular architecture leading to mesangial expansion often with immune deposits. Some immune complexes activate complement in the mesangium, which causes inflammation and tissue injury and may also stimulate proliferation of mesangial cells.

ENDOTHELIAL CELLS

Endothelial cells separate the intravascular space from the mesangium and the GBM. This endothelial cell lining is interrupted by many small "windows" called fenestrae which permit the passage of large antigens and even immune complexes into the mesangial area. These antigens and immune complexes are also deposited in the subendothelial space adjacent to the GBM where they represent subendothelial immune deposits. Mesangial cells stimulated by these immune deposits extend processes out along the GBM beneath the endothelial cell in an attempt to engulf these subendothelial deposits--a process called **mesangial interposition**. Finally, if the endothelium is injured by the activation of complement or acute inflammation, endothelial cell proliferation, thrombosis, or even necrosis of the capillary system may occur.

GLOMERULAR BASEMENT MEMBRANE

Although an integral component of the glomerular capillary wall, the GBM is not present between the mesangial space and the endothelial cells. The GBM is composed of three layers which form a complex network of transmembrane passages through which protein movement is restricted by both size and charge (see Chapter 3 for discussion). Therefore, both antigens and immune complexes may be trapped **within** the GBM. Injury caused by inflammation in this location results in proteinuria. The GBM shares some antigenic sites with the pulmonary capillary basement membrane, which explains the linear deposition of anti-GBM antibody in the glomerulus associated with hemorrhagic pulmonary disease in Goodpasture's syndrome.

EPITHELIAL CELLS

Epithelial cells extend foot processes over the outer surface of the GBM. In an animal model of glomerulonephritis investigators have identified a protein antigen expressed on the surface of the epithelial cells which is the target of circulating IgG antibodies that are filtered to form immune complexes in the subepithelial space. This is called in situ immune complex formation and may be the mechanism responsible for membranous glomerulonephritis. Complement activation and acute inflammation are less likely in the subepithelial site, thus limiting glomerular injury. However, in other forms of acute glomerulonephritis the GBM may leak activated lymphocytes, macrophages, soluble inflammatory mediators, and red blood cells into the urinary space. The result is epithelial cell proliferation, fibrin activation, fibroblast transformation, and crescent formation.

With virtually all forms of glomerular injury there is a healing phase characterized by scarring or fibrosis of the glomeruli, so-called **glomerulosclerosis** which may be global or segmental in character.

CLINICAL PRESENTATION

The display on the next page lists some common symptoms and signs of glomerulonephritis. However, many patients may not have any symptoms or overt signs at presentation. The first suspicion of glomerular disease often comes from a routine urinalysis revealing proteinuria or too many cells, from the development of unexplained hypertension or anemia, or from an elevation in the serum creatinine concentration. At the other extreme are patients with a systemic disease that is often complicated by a glomerulonephritis in which a careful physician will screen closely and frequently for renal involvement. A classic example is systemic lupus erythematosus.

Symptoms and Signs of Glomerulonephritis

Symptoms	Signs
• Nausea	• Proteinuria
• Headache	• Hematuria
• Flank pain	• Pyuria
• Dysuria	• Cellular casts
• Malaise	• Renal failure
• Anorexia	• Hypertension
• Weakness	• Anemia
• Visual changes	• Edema
	• Hemoptysis

The concept of nephritic and nephrotic presentations is useful in subdividing patients with glomerulonephritis.

NEPHRITIC

This presentation can include an active urinary sediment with red blood cells (RBCs), white blood cells (WBCs), and cellular casts, proteinuria, anemia, decreased complement, microangiopathic changes, and rapidly decreasing renal function. It is often associated with acute hypertension, flank pain, arthralgias, edema, and fever.

NEPHROTIC

This presentation includes a benign urinary sediment or microscopic hematuria, proteinuria, and relatively stable renal function, with edema.

Types of Glomerulonephritis Commonly Associated with Nephritic or Nephrotic Presentations

Nephritic Presentation	*Nephrotic Presentation*
• Systemic lupus erythematosus • Primary IgA (Berger's) nephropathy • Focal proliferative • Idiopathic crescentic • Acute postinfectious • Membranoproliferative • Systemic vasculitis • Schönlein-Henoch purpura • Goodpasture's syndrome	• Membranous • Focal glomerular sclerosis • Primary IgA (Berger's) nephropathy • Minimal change disease • Membranoproliferative • Heredofamilial disease • Neoplasia • Liver Disease • Infections • Systemic lupus erythematosus

INVESTIGATIONS

Investigations Performed to Evaluate a Patient with Suspected Glomerulonephritis

Initial Evaluation	*Advanced Evaluation*
• Urinalysis • 24-hr urine protein excretion • Creatinine clearance • Urine protein electrophoresis • Serum protein electrophoresis • Renal and electrolyte profile • CBC • Erythrocyte sedimentation rate	• Complement levels • ANA • ASO titer • Anti-GBM antibody • Cryoglobulins • C3 Nephritic factor • Renal ultrasound • Renal biopsy

URINALYSIS

The urine may reveal gross hematuria. The dipstick examination will often be positive for both hemoglobin and protein. Microscopically there may be numerous RBCs and WBCs. Nephritic patients will have RBC and WBC casts (cellular casts), while nephrotic patients will usually have only granular and hyaline casts and oval fat bodies.

24-HR URINE PROTEIN

Abnormal protein excretion (defined as greater than 150 mg/24 hr) is present with either a nephritic or nephrotic presentation. Three 24-hr collections should be performed to determine the average protein excretion to provide an important baseline for assessing disease course and the effect of any therapy. However, the total amount of protein excretion is of little diagnostic value. Moreover, while abnormal protein excretion indicates glomerular injury, it does not diagnose glomerulonephritis (see Chapter 3).

CREATININE CLEARANCE

Creatinine clearance should be determined along with the 24-hr protein collections. A decrease in renal function may also decrease protein excretion. Therefore, urine protein excretion can be expressed as mg protein/ml creatinine clearance.

URINE AND PLASMA PROTEIN ELECTROPHORESIS

Urine and plasma samples from older patients with significant proteinuria should be tested to exclude a monoclonal or Bence Jones protein indicative of multiple myeloma or some other neoplasia.

RENAL AND ELECTROLYTE PROFILE

Determination of baseline renal function is critical in both diagnosis and management. Although any form of glomerulonephritis may result in renal failure, typically, the acute and proliferative forms (i.e., idiopathic crescentic, Schönlein-Henoch purpura, vasculitis, acute postinfectious) will present with renal dysfunction.

COMPLETE BLOOD COUNT (CBC) AND PLATELET COUNT

Anemia, particularly if acute and associated with microangiopathic changes demonstrated on the blood smear, suggests an acute or proliferative glomerulonephritis (nephritic presentation). Thrombocytopenia may be associated with microangiopathy or vasculitis, and it is also suggestive of systemic lupus erythematosus or an acute viral infection.

ERYTHROCYTE SEDIMENTATION RATE (ESR)

This is a nonspecific measure of inflammatory states resulting in hepatic release of acute phase proteins (i.e., infection), the production of abnormal immunoglobulins including cryoglobulins (i.e., systemic lupus erythematosus) or diseases resulting in the consumption of fibrinogen (i.e., vasculitis). However, an hematocrit below 30% elevates the ESR directly by decreasing blood viscosity.

COMPLEMENT LEVELS

A decrease in the C3 component of complement reflects activation of the classic pathway and is seen most commonly in systemic lupus erythematosus, idiopathic crescentic, membranoproliferative, and acute postinfectious glomerulonephritis. A reduction in the C4 component reflects the activation of the alternate pathway in membranoproliferative glomerulonephritis.

ANTINUCLEAR ANTIBODIES (ANA)

This is the most useful test for systemic lupus erythematosus. If the ANA is positive, most laboratories will now perform an entire panel of tests including assays for anti-single stranded DNA.

ANTISTREPTOLYSIN-O TITER (ASO)

This antibody reflects immunity to Group A streptococci, and its presence indicates a recent infection particularly if serial determinations confirm at least a two-fold rise in titer. About 90% of patients with acute streptococcal infection will demonstrate a rise in titer within 3 to 5 weeks and then a slow decline over several months. Many laboratories will routinely offer an ASO panel which also includes antibody titers for antistreptokinase (ASKase), anti-hyaluronidase (AHase), and anti-nicotyladenine dinucleotidase (ANADase). A false-positive test for the ASO titer can occur in patients with high cholesterol levels which commonly accompany the nephrotic syndrome. Throat cultures are positive in only 25% of patients with acute poststreptococcal glomerulonephritis.

ANTI-GLOMERULAR BASEMENT MEMBRANE ANTIBODY (ANTI-GBM)

This antibody is specific for anti-GBM nephritis including Goodpasture's syndrome and is present in 95% of such patients.

CRYOGLOBULINS

These are abnormal immunoglobulins or immune complexes that precipitate in the cold. The best known cryoglobulin is rheumatoid factor, which is a circulating IgM anti-IgG immune complex. Cryoglobulins are associated with the following conditions:

- Multiple myeloma
- Waldenstrom's macroglobulinemia
- Sjögren's syndrome
- Lymphoma
- Systemic lupus erythematosus
- Bacterial endocarditis
- Chronic infections
- Systemic vasculitis
- Neoplasia

There is also an entity of essential cryoglobulinemia that may present with a vasculitis-like clinical picture and acute glomerulonephritis.

C3 NEPHRITIC FACTOR (C3Nef)

This is present in 60% of patients with membranoproliferative glomerulonephritis (type II) although it may also be present in other forms of acute proliferative glomerulonephritis. It is an IgG auto-antibody that binds to an enzyme activated by the alternative pathway of complement. This enzyme, called C3 convertase, causes the degradation of C3. The C3Nef prevents the inhibition of the enzyme and, thus, results in continued degradation of native C3.

RENAL ULTRASOUND

This is the simplest way to determine kidney size and exclude urinary tract obstruction, stones, tumors, cysts, or other anatomical abnormalities. In the differential diagnosis of significant proteinuria, the presence of small or scarred kidneys would suggest chronic renal disease, while kidneys of normal size and appearance are more likely to be seen in acute glomerulonephritis.

RENAL BIOPSY

The renal biopsy remains the gold standard for the definitive diagnosis of any form of glomerulonephritis. It provides the only reliable way of establishing the extent of renal injury and, thus, a means of determining the prognosis and potential response to therapy. A renal biopsy should be considered in any patient with suspected glomerulonephritis in whom the specific diagnosis is unknown (see Chapter 1 for a discussion of indications for renal biopsy).

DIFFERENTIAL DIAGNOSIS AND MANAGEMENT

MINIMAL CHANGE DISEASE

This disease presents with the nephrotic syndrome, normal renal function, and highly selective proteinuria. There is no diagnostic clinical or laboratory finding. Thus, the diagnosis requires a kidney biopsy. Children are very responsive to corticosteroid therapy. Though the disease may remit spontaneously or with corticosteroids in adults, it may also progress slowly to end-stage renal disease.

IDIOPATHIC MEMBRANOUS GLOMERULONEPHRITIS

Patients present with proteinuria or the nephrotic syndrome, and hematuria. Impaired renal function and hypertension may be present also. The biopsy specimen reveals subepithelial immune deposits which are positive by immunofluorescence microscopy for IgG immunoglobulin and C3 and thickened basement membranes. These patients will often maintain renal function for many years. Initial management should focus on the nephrotic syndrome (see Chapter 3). Oral corticosteroid administration may result in a remission of proteinuria, but not a cure. It is unclear whether corticosteroids alter or delay the long-term development of renal failure in adults.

FOCAL GLOMERULAR SCLEROSIS

Classically patients present with nephrotic-range proteinuria or the nephrotic syndrome. Renal function may be modestly impaired with some RBCs in the urine. Hypertension is common especially in the presence of diminished renal function. Histologically there is focal segmental or global sclerosis of glomerular capillary tufts and the immunofluorescence microscopy is positive for IgM immunoglobulin and C3 in the areas of glomerulosclerosis. Though a primary form of glomerulonephritis in many patients, focal glomerulosclerosis is also associated with heroin abuse, analgesic abuse, reflux nephropathy, massive obesity, and AIDS. Most of these patients will go on to end-stage renal disease within 5 to 10 years. Some reports advocate oral corticosteroid administration with or without azathioprine (Imuran), although most patients will not respond and long-term benefit is doubtful.

IGA (BERGER'S) NEPHROPATHY

This disease often presents with episodic gross hematuria, frequently in association with stressful exercise or an apparent viral upper respiratory infection. Microscopic hematuria and abnormal protein excretion are very common. There is a male predominance in the Western world, while the disease is much more common in both sexes in the Far East. Uncommonly, patients will present with rapidly progressive renal failure (3 months to 3 years). More typical is a slow progression of renal insufficiency over many years. The key biopsy finding is mesangial expansion and the deposition of IgA immunoglobulin as demonstrated by immunofluorescence microscopy. There is no established role for corticosteroid or other immunosuppressive therapy. Currently it is thought that this form of glomerulonephritis represents an immunological response to an ingested antigen.

SCHÖNLEIN-HENOCH PURPURA

This disease classically presents with palpable purpura caused by a leukocytoclastic vasculitis, arthralgias, and abdominal symptoms including colic, nausea, and melena. Renal insufficiency is common with a nephritic presentation. Males are affected in greatest numbers and the disease is more common in the pediatric population. The renal biopsy findings are essentially the same as those of IgA nephropathy, though the clinical presentations of these two entities are clearly distinct. Most patients will recover their renal function completely and seldom go on to end-stage renal disease.

IDIOPATHIC CRESCENTIC AND GOODPASTURE'S SYNDROME

Both entities present with a nephritic clinical picture. Goodpasture's syndrome includes an interstitial pulmonary infiltrate and hemoptysis and is associated with an anti-GBM antibody in the circulation. The renal biopsy demonstrates crescentic glomerulonephritis with extensive glomerular injury. The Goodpasture's form also includes the linear deposition of the antibody on the GBM. High dose or pulse corticosteroid therapy has been advocated, particularly when the biopsy reveals extensive and active inflammation. Patients with Goodpasture's syndrome should also be plasmapheresed to remove the circulating antibody, and cytotoxic drugs are usually added as an adjunctive therapy. Goodpasture's syndrome will often respond to this therapy and the prognosis is good in selected patients. In contrast, idiopathic crescentic glomerulonephritis will often progress to end-stage renal disease, though the early use of corticosteroids may delay this evolution.

MEMBRANOPROLIFERATIVE GLOMERULONEPHRITIS

This entity presents either insidiously or with a nephritic picture. There is no characteristic clinical feature, but laboratory evidence of a persistent decreased complement level, an elevated ESR, and positive tests for C3Nef or ASO titers are very useful. The biopsy reveals a hypercellular glomerulus with thickened basement membranes and mesangial expansion and interposition. Pathologists refer to a type I pattern with subendothelial immune deposits and a type II pattern with electron dense deposits within the GBM. The use of antiplatelet drugs including dipyridamole (Persantine[R]) and acetylsalicylic acid has been advocated. Immunosuppressive therapy has little value. Though some patients may experience a spontaneous remission, the majority will progress to end-stage renal disease.

PROLIFERATIVE GLOMERULONEPHRITIS

Patients usually present with a nephritic clinical picture. It is often associated with acute infections (bacterial or viral) and certain drugs, but it may also be idiopathic. Laboratory evidence of cryoglobulins, decreased complement, and an elevated ESR are helpful diagnostically; however, a kidney biopsy is still required for diagnosis. The biopsy reveals proliferation of mesangial and glomerular epithelial cells, acute inflammation including the deposition of complement and immunoglobulins, and the presence of polymorphonuclear leukocytes. Diagnosis and effective therapy of the primary disease will often result in resolution of the glomerulonephritis.

SYSTEMIC LUPUS ERYTHEMATOSUS (SLE)

Patients may present with either a nephrotic or a nephritic clinical picture. Though many patients will already have the classic clinical and laboratory evidence of SLE at the time of renal presentation, it is not uncommon to employ the renal biopsy to establish the diagnosis. Laboratory evidence of disease activity includes decreased complement levels, the presence of cryoglobulins, elevated ESR, anemia, leukopenia, and a positive ANA. Five types of renal biopsy patterns have been classified by the World Health Organization in SLE: I) normal; II) mesangial proliferative; III) focal and segmental proliferative; IV) diffuse proliferative; and V) membranous. It is important to note that each type of glomerular disease has a different prognosis and that a patient may progress from one type to another. It is interesting that patients who progress to end-stage renal disease will often have no further clinical manifestations of SLE even if they are transplanted successfully.

SYSTEMIC VASCULITIS

Patients with renal involvement in systemic vasculitis present with a nephritic clinical picture. Systemic vasculitis is a general term referring to acute, immune-mediated inflammation of the blood vessels, typically involving arteries and arterioles, though also involving capillaries and veins. The spectrum includes polyarteritis nodosa (PAN), Wegener's granulomatosis, and hypersensitivity angiitis. Laboratory evidence of an elevated ESR is typical, but complement levels are not decreased. There is a characteristic angiographic picture in PAN. Wegener's granulomatosis is often associated with nodular pulmonary infiltrates and sometimes with sinusitis. A kidney biopsy is often required for diagnosis, though in some patients a tissue diagnosis can be obtained from biopsy of lung, skin, or other organs. High dose corticosteroids and cyclophosphamide are indicated in most of these patients. The prognosis is variable, though long remissions and even cures are not rare.

SUGGESTED READING

Adler S, Couser W. Review: immunologic mechanisms of renal disease. Am J Med Sciences 1985;289:55-60.

Eddy AA, Michael AF. Immunopathogenetic mechanisms of glomerular injury. In: Tisher CC, Brenner BM, eds. Renal pathology with clinical and functional correlations. 1st ed. Philadelphia: JB Lippincott, 1989;6:111-155.

Fine LG. Preventing the progression of human renal disease. Have rational therapeutic principles emerged? Kidney Int 1988;33:116-128.

Glasscock R, Cohen A, Adler S, Ward H. Secondary glomerular diseases. In: Brenner BM, Rector FC Jr, eds. The kidney. 3rd ed. Philadelphia: WB Saunders Co, 1986;23:1014-1084.

Chapter 5

Diabetic Nephropathy

C. Craig Tisher

DEFINITION

Nephropathy is a complication of diabetes mellitus that leads to end-stage renal disease in approximately 10% of diabetic patients. The likelihood of developing nephropathy and renal failure in type I or insulin-dependent diabetes mellitus (IDDM) is 30-50%, whereas in type II or non-insulin-dependent diabetes mellitus (NIDDM) it is strikingly different, being only 20%.

INCIDENCE

Some 2 to 4% of the United States population or 5-10 million individuals have diabetes mellitus. The yearly incidence is approximately 700,000 individuals, and the yearly incidence rate is about 0.3%. In 1981, diabetes mellitus ranked sixth in causes of death by disease in the United States of which approximately 3500 deaths could be attributed to renal failure. At present approximately 25% of all patients hospitalized for the treatment of end-stage renal disease have diabetes as the underlying cause. The prevalence of diabetic nephropathy increases with the duration of the disease. Poor glycemic control, smoking, and hypertension also appear to be associated with a greater prevalence of renal disease.

OUTCOME

In those patients who develop renal disease, the time of progression to end stage is highly variable (see subsequent section on Clinical Presentation and Pathophysiology). Both dialysis and transplantation are regularly offered to patients with renal failure resulting from diabetic nephropathy. In those individuals the combined 3-year survival rate is approximately 50%.

CLINICAL PRESENTATION AND PATHOPHYSIOLOGY

IDDM

The progression of renal disease in IDDM can be divided into 5 stages as described by Mogensen.

Stage I (Hyperfiltration-Hypertrophy Stage)

The characteristic clinical features relative to the kidney at **initial** presentation include:

- Hyperfiltration [increase in glomerular filtration rate (GFR) that is 20-50% above age-matched control subjects]
- Hypertrophy of the kidneys (visible by X-ray)
- Glucosuria with polyuria
- Microalbuminuria (>20 but <200 μg/min)

With insulin treatment of several weeks duration the hyperfiltration and hypertrophy correct in the majority of patients, and the microalbuminuria (determined by a radioimmunoassay technique) falls below 20 μg/min.

Stage II (Silent Stage)

- Normal or near normal microalbuminuria (<20 μg/min)
- Normalization of elevated GFR in majority of patients
- Development of structural damage in the kidney (see explanation below)

Those patients destined to develop diabetic nephropathy often manifest a persistently elevated GFR (>150 ml/min) and poor metabolic control. From 30 to 50% of diabetic patients will proceed into Stage III and beyond and develop structural damage in the kidney.

Stage III (Incipient Nephropathy Stage)

- Persistent hyperfiltration early, but GFR starts to decrease later
- Microalbuminuria (20 μg/min to 200 μg/min which correlates with an excretion rate of 30 to 300 mg/24 hr).
- Early hypertension

This stage can last for several years and the level of protein excretion can be decreased and the decline in GFR can be slowed with improved control of hypertension and hyperglycemia.

Stage IV (Overt Nephropathy Stage)

- Fixed and reproducible proteinuria (>0.5 g/24 hr detectable with dipstick).
- Hypertension
- Declining GFR

Stage V (End-Stage Renal Failure)

In those patients with IDDM who progress to end-stage renal failure, the duration of time required to develop overt diabetic nephropathy (Stage IV) is highly variable but averages 15-17 years. However, subsequent progression to end stage (Stage V) is relatively predictable and averages 5-7 years. There is increasing clinical evidence that aggressive control of hypertension can retard the progression of diabetic nephropathy in IDDM (see later section on Management).

NIDDM

Far less is known regarding the development of diabetic nephropathy in type II diabetes mellitus. At diagnosis, microalbuminuria is frequently present and is often reversible with proper metabolic control. In contrast to type I disease, hyperfiltration is present only rarely and there is no evidence of glomerular hypertrophy. It is clear, however, that in comparison with an age-matched population, the presence of microalbuminuria in NIDDM carries a worse prognosis.

Other manifestations of renal disease in any diabetic patient include:

- Bacteriuria
- Cystitis
- Acute pyelonephritis
- Papillary necrosis
- Perinephric abscess
- Atonic bladder with hydronephrosis

PATHOLOGY

The histopathologic alterations observed in diabetic nephropathy typically affect the glomeruli, the vasculature, and the tubulo-interstitial compartment.

Summary of Histopathology of Diabetic Nephropathy

Glomerular Lesions

- Diffuse intercapillary glomerulosclerosis
- Nodular intercapillary glomerulosclerosis
- Capsular drop lesion
- Fibrin-cap lesion
- Glomerular basement membrane thickening

Vascular Lesions

- Subintimal hyalin arteriolosclerosis
- Benign arteriosclerosis

Tubular and Interstitial Lesions

- Hyaline droplets in proximal tubules (representing reabsorbed protein in lysosomes)
- Glycogen deposits in the pars recta of the proximal tubule (so-called Armanni-Ebstein change)
- Tubular atrophy
- Interstitial fibrosis

Nodular intercapillary glomerulosclerosis, while not pathognomonic of diabetic nephropathy, is the most characteristic of the renal lesions observed in this disease. However, a very similar lesion can be observed in light chain deposition disease. Therefore, caution must be exercised when this lesion is found in patients with proteinuria in the absence of hyperglycemia.

PATHOGENESIS

The pathogenesis of diabetic nephropathy is undoubtedly multifactorial and remains to be clearly elucidated. However, one important factor is the presence of glomerular hyperfiltration early in the disease which, if persistent, is more likely to be associated with renal failure later. An abnormal metabolic milieu must also be present for the development of the characteristic renal lesions. These hemodynamic and metabolic abnormalities are associated with a complex set of events that eventually result in renal destruction and include abnormal glycosylation of proteins that form the glomerular basement membrane and mesangial matrix; hyperperfusion of the glomerular capillaries with an associated increase in the transcapillary pressure gradient; and growth of the glomerular capillaries. The combination of these events, if left unchecked, leads to progressive glomerulosclerosis and hypertrophy of residual nephrons which, in turn, undergo eventual destruction as the kidney reaches end-stage. Improved control of hyperglycemia and reduction in intraglomerular and systemic hypertension can delay the progression of these functional and histologic changes.

INVESTIGATIONS

The presence of proteinuria, with or without hypertension and renal insufficiency, in a patient with diabetes mellitus of several years duration is diabetic nephropathy until proven otherwise. The presence of diabetic retinopathy, which is observed in over 90% of those patients with diabetic nephropathy, strengthens the diagnosis. Thus, in the absence of diabetic retinopathy, causes other than diabetic nephropathy should be entertained to explain the presence of proteinuria. However, only one-fourth to one-third of those patients with diabetic retinopathy have clinically detectable renal disease.

There are other situations in which renal disease other than diabetic nephropathy should be considered in the diabetic patient. For instance, the sudden onset of the nephrotic syndrome, especially early in the course of diabetes mellitus, or renal insufficiency in association with an active urinary sediment (red blood cells, white blood cells, red cell casts, granular casts) may indicate the presence of a primary glomerular disease (e.g., mimimal change disease, membranous glomerulonephritis or focal glomerular sclerosis, etc.). In these situations a percutaneous renal biopsy is often indicated to establish the diagnosis, determine the prognosis, and aid in management.

Occasionally, a patient may present with proteinuria and on kidney biopsy be found to have pronounced subintimal hyalin arteriolosclerosis in the absence of other renal lesions. Diabetes mellitus should be considered and excluded in this situation.

MANAGEMENT

IDDM

The management of the renal disease associated with IDDM depends on which point in the disease course you encounter the patient.

Hypertension

Today most physicians would agree that the single most important factor in the management of diabetic renal disease is the control of hypertension. Intraglomerular hypertension is thought by many to cause progressive glomerular destruction. Although lowering systemic blood pressure can lower intraglomerular pressures, angiotensin-converting enzyme inhibitors such as captopril or enalopril lower intraglomerular hypertension more predictably by reducing post-glomerular vascular resistance. Lowering the blood pressure in the hypertensive diabetic patient can slow the rate of decline in GFR by 5 to 6 ml/min/year.

Cardioselective β-blockers are preferable to nonselective agents such as propranolol to avoid masking symptoms of hypoglycemia. Vasodilator agents such as prazosin and calcium channel blockers are also useful in the control of hypertension in the diabetic patient.

Hyperglycemia

At the onset of diabetes mellitus, before insulin therapy is initiated (hyperfiltration-hypertrophy stage), the GFR is elevated and the kidneys are enlarged. With institution of insulin therapy and proper diet, both the GFR and the size of the kidney usually decrease. Since studies in animals and long-term clinical observations provide evidence that failure to correct the elevated GFR increases the likelihood of the development of progressive renal disease later, proper control of blood glucose levels early in the disease is important. Experimental studies have also demonstrated that normalization of blood glucose levels will reduce microalbuminuria especially in patients in the so-called incipient nephropathy stage (Stage III). It is unclear at present whether the ability to retard or reverse the progressive renal histologic changes with tight control of blood glucose levels in hyperglycemic animals will also be possible in patients with diabetic renal disease. Nevertheless, proper control of blood glucose levels in any diabetic patient would appear to be a reasonable treatment goal.

Urinary Tract Infection

In general asymptomatic bacteriuria(> 100,000 organisms per ml) should be treated in the diabetic patient. The development of acute pyelonephritis, especially if associated with obstruction, can result in papillary necrosis which can be life threatening (see Chapter 13 for management of urinary tract infections).

Renal Insufficiency

Once it has been established that renal insufficiency in a diabetic patient is due to the underlying disease and not to a superimposed or secondary problem which may be reversible, management is essentially the same as in any patient with renal insufficiency (see Chapter 20). Blood pressure control is essential. Earlier studies suggest that dietary protein restriction can retard the progression of renal failure. This will require testing in large prospective clinical trials.

Transplantation and Dialysis

Hemodialysis and continuous ambulatory peritoneal dialysis offer a 3-year survival rate of approximately 50%. In the younger diabetic patient, and especially in the absence of severe peripheral vascular disease, renal transplantation offers the best chance for survival. The 3-year patient survival with a living related donor allograft is close to 85%. Unfortunately, the disease does recur in the transplanted kidney and can cause destruction of the graft in 5 to 10 years or less. Often the successful rehabilitation of the transplant patient depends largely on the rate of progression of the disease in other organs.

SUGGESTED READING

Kimmelstiel P, Wilson C. Intercapillary lesions in glomeruli of kidney. Am J Path 1936;12:83-97.

Mogensen CE. Microalbuminuria as a predictor of clinical diabetic nephropathy. Kidney Int 1987;31:673-689.

Mogensen CE, Christensen CK. Predicting diabetic nephropathy in insulin-dependent patients. N Engl J Med 1984;311:89-93.

Parving H, Smidt UM, Andersen AR, Svendsen PA. Early aggressive hypertensive treatment reduces rate of decline in kidney function in diabetic nephropathy. Lancet 1983;1:1175-1179.

Tisher CC, Hostetter TH. Diabetic nephropathy. In: Tisher CC, Brenner BM, eds. Renal pathology with clinical and functional correlations. 1st ed. Philadelphia: JB Lippincott, Vol 2 1989:1309-1334.

Chapter 6

Disorders of Water Metabolism

Joel T. Van Sickler
Charles S. Wingo

INTRODUCTION

Regulation of water homeostasis is dependent on: 1) intact thirst mechanism; 2) appropriate renal handling of water and solute; and 3) intact antidiuretic hormone (ADH) release and response. Serum tonicity is maintained within a limited range (285 to 295 mOsm/ kg H_2O) due primarily to regulation of water balance. Derangements are largely reflected by changes in the serum sodium concentration (S_{Na}).

HYPONATREMIA

DEFINITION

Hyponatremia is a S_{Na} below 135 mEq/l (135 mmol/l).

INCIDENCE

This is the most frequent electrolyte abnormality in hospital-ized patients and has an incidence of 1%.

GENERAL PHYSIOLOGIC PRINCIPLES

Total body Na content depends on the balance between Na intake and renal excretion. Dietary Na restriction can reduce Na excretion to < 5 mEq/day, while a large Na intake normally provokes a natri-uresis. Total body Na will vary by no more than 2 to 5% and S_{Na} remains quite constant.

Total body water (TBW) constitutes 60% of the body weight. Some 40% of TBW is intracellular and 20% is extracellular. Of the latter, 5% is plasma water and 15% is interstitial water. Approximately 95% of Na and attendant anions (chloride and bicarbonate) are localized in the extracellular fluid (ECF).

Sodium and its anions are the main determinants of plasma osmo-lality; thus, 2 times S_{Na} will approximate the serum osmolality (S_{osm}). The incorporation of blood urea nitrogen (BUN) and glucose is important when these concentrations are increased. Thus, S_{osm} is defined by the equation:

$$S_{osm} \text{ (mOsm/kg } H_2O) = 2 \text{ [Na(mEq/l)]} + \frac{BUN \text{ (mg/dl)}}{2.8} + \frac{glucose \text{ (mg/dl)}}{18}$$

The estimated and measured values of S_{osm} should agree within 10-15 mOsm/kg H_2O. A greater difference implies either an error in measurement or the presence of another osmotically active agent (e.g., mannitol, ethanol, ethylene glycol, etc). Because the intracellular (IC) and extracellular (EC) osmolality are equal, reduction in EC osmolality simultaneously reduces IC osmolality. This can result in cellular edema (e.g., cerebral edema and neurologic abnormalities).

The principal determinant of S_{Na} is TBW rather than total body Na. Changes in total body Na alter EC volume (ECV), whereas changes in S_{Na} reflect altered regulation of water excretion. Normally, changes of only 2% in S_{osm} are detected by osmoreceptors in the hypothalamus which regulate ADH release from the neurohypophysis. The maximal ADH action reduces urine output to 500 ml/day and increases urine osmolality to 800-1400 mOsm/kg H_2O. Complete absence of ADH causes a large diuresis (15-20 liters/day) with a urine osmolality of 40 to 80 mOsm/kg H_2O. ECV changes of 10% or greater also regulate ADH secretion. In fact, volume-mediated stimulation of ADH secretion can override osmotic stimuli and cause water retention irrespective of S_{osm}.

PATHOPHYSIOLOGY

Hyponatremia is caused by 1) excess water intake (water intoxication) with normal renal function or 2) a continued solute-free water intake with a decreased renal capacity for solute-free water excretion. Water excretion can be divided into two components:

- The osmolar clearance (C_{osm}) is the urine volume (isotonic to plasma) that is needed to excrete the solute load.
- The solute-free water clearance (C_{H_2O}) is the urine volume from which solute has been removed during the elaboration of a hypotonic urine.

Therefore, urine volume = $C_{osm} + C_{H_2O}$

Elimination of water requires:

- Adequate glomerular filtration without excessive proximal reabsorption in order to deliver tubular fluid to the diluting sites of the nephron (ascending limb of Henle and early distal convoluted tubule).
- Normal function of the diluting segments of the nephron.
- Suppression of ADH to prevent solute-free water from being reabsorbed by the collecting ducts.

CLASSIFICATION OF HYPONATREMIC DISORDERS

Follow the diagnostic tree shown in Figure 6-1. The initial evaluations require measurement of S_{osm} and assessment of the ECV status (see display on page 54).

Evaluation of ECV Status

	Physical Findings	Laboratory Findings
• Hypovolemic	Poor skin turgor Dry mucous membranes Absent/decreased sweat	Hematocrit and $S_{protein}$ increased Elevated BUN/creatinine
	Postural hypotension	U_{Na} <20 mEq/l
• Euvolemic	Normal examination	Normal
• Hypervolemic	Distended neck veins Peripheral or sacral edema	Decreased hematocrit and $S_{protein}$ Decreased BUN/creatinine
	Normal or increased BP	U_{Na} less helpful

ISO-OSMOLAR HYPONATREMIA

Pseudohyponatremia occurs with hyperlipidemia (usually triglyceridemia exceeding 1500 mg/dl) and hyperproteinemias (e.g., Waldenström's macroglobulinemia and multiple myeloma) when the water content of plasma is decreased by the increased solid.

HYPEROSMOLAR HYPONATREMIA

Hypertonic infusions of glucose, mannitol, or glycine can cause osmotic shifts of ICF to the EC space. The following formulas are useful:

- Glucose - for every 100 mg/dl of glucose over 100 mg/dl, the serum Na will fall by 1.6 mEq/l

- Glycine - for every 100 mg/dl rise in blood glycine, the serum Na will fall by 3.8 mEq/l

HYPOOSMOLAR HYPONATREMIA

HYPOVOLEMIC HYPONATREMIA

This condition implies renal or nonrenal loss of Na.

Renal Sodium Losses (see Figure 6-1)

Diuretic administration. This is the most frequent cause and can be the result of two mechanisms: 1) Inhibition of NaCl reabsorption in the distal nephron by thiazides inhibits urinary dilution, but, unlike loop diuretics, thiazides do not inhibit urine concentration. Therefore, hyponatremia is more common and more severe during thiazide therapy. 2) Proximal tubular NaCl reabsorption is increased (due to volume contraction and decreased GFR), which diminishes fluid delivery to the diluting segment.

Figure 6-1 **Hyponatremia**

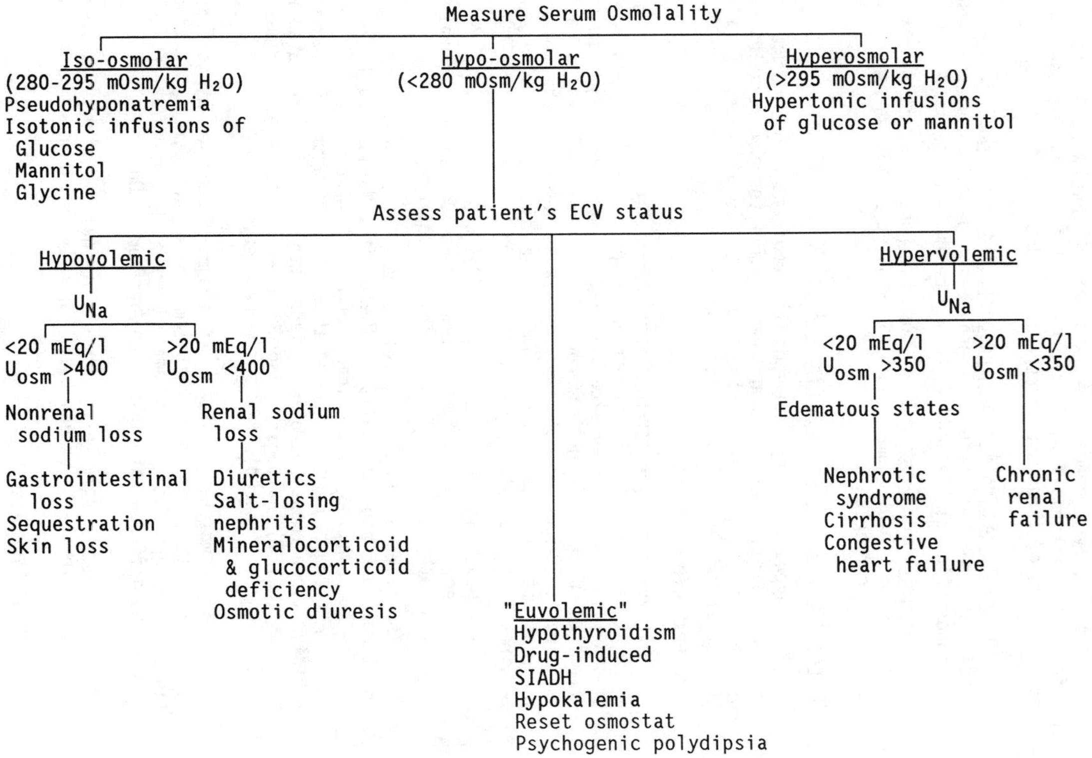

Measure Serum Osmolality

Iso-osmolar
(280-295 mOsm/kg H_2O)
Pseudohyponatremia
Isotonic infusions of
Glucose
Mannitol
Glycine

Hypo-osmolar
(<280 mOsm/kg H_2O)

Hyperosmolar
(>295 mOsm/kg H_2O)
Hypertonic infusions
of glucose or mannitol

Assess patient's ECV status

Hypovolemic
U_{Na}

<20 mEq/l
U_{osm} >400

>20 mEq/l
U_{osm} <400

Nonrenal
sodium loss

Renal sodium
loss

Gastrointestinal
loss
Sequestration
Skin loss

Diuretics
Salt-losing
nephritis
Mineralocorticoid
& glucocorticoid
deficiency
Osmotic diuresis

"Euvolemic"
Hypothyroidism
Drug-induced
SIADH
Hypokalemia
Reset osmostat
Psychogenic polydipsia

Hypervolemic
U_{Na}

<20 mEq/l
U_{osm} >350

>20 mEq/l
U_{osm} <350

Edematous states

Nephrotic
syndrome
Cirrhosis
Congestive
heart failure

Chronic
renal
failure

Salt-losing nephritis. This can be seen in patients with chronic renal failure given a salt-deficient intake or in patients with relatively preserved renal function, but with a disease which affects the interstitium (e.g., polycystic kidney disease, medullary cystic disease, chronic pyelonephritis, etc.).

Mineralocorticoid and glucocorticoid deficiencies. A combination of volume depletion with enhanced proximal tubular reabsorption and nonosmotic stimulation of ADH may be implicated.

Osmotic diuresis. This causes hyponatremia primarily by abstraction of fluid from cells. Subsequently, Na excretion increases and S_{Na} is corrected.

Nonrenal Sodium Losses (see Figure 6-1)

In hypovolemic hyponatremia the contracted ECV reduces the GFR and enhances proximal tubular reabsorption thereby reducing delivery of fluid to the distal diluting segments. In addition, there is nonosmotic stimulation of ADH secretion.

EUVOLEMIC HYPONATREMIA

"Euvolemic" hyponatremia occurs in patients without hypovolemia or edema, although TBW is increased by approximately 3-5 liters. This disorder is due to 1) an excessive secretion of ADH; 2) a potentiated effect of ADH; or 3) an inappropriate action of ADH. The causes are detailed in Figure 6-1. An important cause is the syndrome of inappropriate ADH secretion. This is a diagnosis of exclusion and requires that the following be **absent:**

- Hypovolemia
- Edema
- Hypothyroidism
- Renal failure
- Drug ingestion causing hyponatremia
- Addison's disease

The urine is inappropriately concentrated for the degree of hyponatremia and hypo-osmolality. The urinary Na is usually >20 mEq/l. Failure to excrete a water load can establish the diagnosis of SIADH but may produce dangerous hyponatremia. Syndrome of inappropriate antidiuretic hormone secretion (SIADH) generally is associated with 1) malignancies; 2) pulmonary disorders; and 3) central nervous system (CNS) disorders (see display on the next page).

Reset osmostat. This is an uncommon cause of hyponatremia due to down regulation of the hypothalamic-pituitary axis. S_{Na} concentrations, although decreased, remain stable during a water load thus helping to differentiate this disorder from SIADH.

Psychogenic polydipsia. Some emotionally disturbed patients can drink sufficiently to exceed their capacity to excrete free water.

Drugs (see display).

Causes of SIADH

- Pulmonary Disorders

  Pneumonia   Asthma
  Abscess   Acute respiratory failure
  Tuberculosis   Aspergillosis

- Tumors

  Oat cell carcinoma of the lung
  Hodgkin's and non-Hodgkin's lymphoma
  Other carcinomas (e.g., duodenum, pancreas)
  Thymoma

- Central Nervous System Disorders

  Meningitis   Seizures
  Encephalitis   Acute psychosis
  Brain abscess   Delirium tremens
  Head trauma   Multiple sclerosis
  Tumors   Hydrocephalus
  Subarachnoid hemorrhage   Shy-Drager syndrome
  Subdural hemorrhage   Guillain-Barré syndrome
  Acute intermittent porphyria   Stroke

Drug-Induced Hyponatremia

- Drugs that potentiate ADH action

  Tolbutamide
  Acetaminophen
  Nonsteroidal anti-inflammatory drugs (NSAIDS)
  ADH analogues

- Drugs that cause ADH release

  Clofibrate
  Vincristine
  Carbamazepine
  Narcotics
  Barbiturates

- Drugs that potentiate ADH action and stimulate release

  Chlorpropamide
  Cyclophosphamide
  Thiazide diuretics

HYPERVOLEMIC HYPONATREMIA

Patients with edema (e.g., congestive heart failure, nephrotic syndrome, and cirrhosis with ascites) can have an increase in TBW that is greater than total body Na. A reduced "effective" circulatory plasma volume not only decreases GFR and enhances proximal tubular reabsorption thereby decreasing delivery of filtrate to the diluting segment but also stimulates ADH release. The urine Na concentration is <15 mEq/l and the urine osmolality is >350 mOsm/kg H_2O. In addition, chronic renal failure can cause hyponatremia because the reduced GFR diminishes solute delivery to the diluting segment.

CLINICAL PRESENTATION

Severe, acute hyponatremia (S_{Na} < 120 mEq/l) has a mortality of approximately 50%. Chronic hyponatremia has a lower mortality (< 10%) which is due to compensatory electrolyte loss from cells which decreases cellular water content.

Most patients with hyponatremia are asymptomatic. The severity of the symptoms depends on the rate of decline in the S_{Na} concentration. Although early symptoms are related to the gastrointestinal tract, neurological manifestations are more frequent and serious (see display that follows). Severe symptoms which can cause death such as seizures or coma are usually seen at a S_{Na} < 120 mEq/l.

Symptoms and Signs of Hyponatremia

• Lethargy	• Seizures
• Nausea	• Coma
• Vomiting	• Abnormal reflexes
• Agitation	• Hypothermia
• Hallucinations	• Cheyne-Stokes respiration
• Weakness	• Pseudobulbar palsy
• Headache	

TREATMENT

Severe symptomatic hyponatremia (e.g., seizures, coma) is a medical emergency. The aim is to raise the S_{Na} to >120 mEq/l by using hypertonic NaCl solutions. During correction of hyponatremia, an occasional patient may develop a very severe complication termed central pontine myelinolysis (CPM; destruction of the medullary sheaths in the center of the base of the pons). Clinical manifestations vary from minimal dysfunction to flaccid quadriplegia and death. This rare complication is probably caused by overzealous correction of hyponatremia leading to hypernatremia. A recent prospective study defined four risk factors for CPM:

- Raising the S_{Na} to normal or hypernatremic levels within 48 hr.

- Increasing the S_{Na} > 25 mEq/l in the first 48 hr.

- Presence of hypoxic-anoxic episodes.

- Elevation of the S_{Na} to hypernatremic levels in patients with liver disease.

Generally the S_{Na} should not be corrected faster than 1.5-2.0 mEq/l/hr. The following is a useful protocol for correction of severe life-threatening hyponatremia.

- Admit patients to an intensive care unit for monitoring of electrolytes, blood pressure (BP), neurologic status, and renal function.

- Initiate a salt and water diuresis with loop diuretics (e.g., furosemide, 1 mg/kg body weight).

- Measure urinary Na and K losses hourly and replace with 3% NaCl (513 mEq Na/l) and KCl until S_{Na} is > 120-125 mEq/l.

- Maintain a urinary output of approximately 1 l/hr.

If symptoms are less severe, an infusion of 0.9% NaCl solution and a loop diuretic can be used.

HYPOVOLEMIC HYPONATREMIA

Initial therapy should include discontinuation of diuretics, correction of gastrointestinal fluid losses, and expansion of ECV with 0.9% NaCl. When Na depletion is predominant (more salt loss than water), the Na deficit can be calculated as illustrated in this example:

A 70-kg person who now weighs 65 kg has a S_{Na} of 130 mEq/l

The normal TBW is 60% of 70 kg = 42 liters

A 5-kg weight loss (which is water) decreases TBW to 37 liters

Normal total body Na = 42 l with 140 mEq/l = 5880 mEq

Current total body Na = 37 l with 130 mEq/l = 4810 mEq

Therefore Na deficit = 5880 - 4810 = 1070 mEq.

One-third of the Na deficit can be given as 0.9% NaCl over 6 hr and the remainder over 24 to 48 hr. Potassium deficits will need to be corrected if vomiting, diarrhea, or diuretics caused the volume contraction.

EUVOLEMIC HYPONATREMIA

The hyponatremia can usually be treated by restriction of water intake to 1 l/day. The volume of water excess needed to be removed to correct the hyponatremia should be calculated:

A 75-kg person has a S_{Na} of 115 mEq/l.

The current TBW is 60% of 75 kg = 45 liters.

A normal S_{Na} = 140 mEq/l

$$\frac{\text{Actual } S_{Na} \text{ mEq/l}}{\text{Normal } S_{Na} \text{ mEq/l}} \times \text{current TBW} = \text{normal TBW}; \quad \text{therefore,}$$

$$\frac{115 \text{ mEq/l}}{140 \text{ mEq/l}} \times 45 \text{ liters} = 36.9 \text{ liters}$$

Current TBW - normal TBW = excess water; therefore,

45 liters - 36.9 liters = 8.1 liters excess water

Symptomatic patients are managed as described above. When the cause of SIADH is not reversible, drugs can be used to create a state of nephrogenic diabetes insipidus. The drugs include:

- Demeclocycline-(600 to 1200 mg/day). The side effects include sensitivity and a reversible decline in GFR. It is contraindicated in patients with liver disease.

- Lithium carbonate-(300 mg 3 times a day). Toxicity (e.g., diarrhea, vomiting, ataxia, tremor, etc.) can occur; therefore, drug levels must be monitored. This is contraindicated in patients with renal or cardiovascular disease.

HYPERVOLEMIC HYPONATREMIA

Initial treatment should include salt and fluid restriction if the hyponatremia is due to the primary disease; or if secondary to diuretics, then liberalize salt intake and reduce diuretic dosage.

HYPERNATREMIA

DEFINITION

A serum Na concentration > 145 mEq/l.

INCIDENCE

Hypernatremia is less frequent than hyponatremia but occurs in about 1% of elderly hospitalized patients.

PATHOPHYSIOLOGY

Hypernatremia implies a relative deficiency of TBW compared to total body Na. Normally, a small increase in S_{osm} stimulates secretion of ADH and, thereby, increases renal water retention. Since the hypertonicity also stimulates thirst, even patients with a complete absence of ADH secretion (central diabetes insipidus) can maintain their S_{osm}. Severe hypernatremia results when water intake is prevented.

ETIOLOGY

Hypernatremia can be readily classified according to the total body Na content and the state of hydration.

Decreased Total Body Sodium

Loss of hypotonic body fluid results in EC volume depletion and hypernatremia. The usual signs of hypovolemia are present: poor skin turgor, postural hypotension, tachycardia, dry mucous membranes, and flat neck veins. Hypotonic fluid losses can occur from:

Extrarenal sources. Skin or gastrointestinal losses are common; the renal response leads to a high urine osmolality (>800 mOsm/kg H_2O) and a low urinary Na (<10 mEq/l).

Renal sources. Polyuria and hypotonic fluid loss can occur during osmotic diuresis with glucose and mannitol. An osmotic diuresis due to urea can occur in severely catabolic patients fed protein-rich meals or given large concentrations of amino acids with hyperalimentation. Usually, however, osmotic agents shift fluid to the EC compartment resulting in hyponatremia. The urine may be either hypotonic or isotonic and the urinary Na is usually > 20 mEq/l.

Normal Total Body Sodium

Losses of water without Na can result in hypernatremia. Evidence of volume contraction usually does not occur unless the water losses are extreme. The usual causes include:

Extrarenal water loss. Both cutaneous and pulmonary losses of water can result in hypernatremia. A common clinical problem is the tachypneic, febrile patient whose insensible fluid losses are inappropriately replaced with physiologic saline. The urinary osmolality (U_{osm}) is high and urinary Na is a function of Na intake.

Renal water losses. This is a more frequent cause of water loss and is due to central diabetes insipidus, nephrogenic diabetes insipidus, and an uncommon disorder termed "essential" hypernatremia. Central diabetes insipidus (CDI) is characterized by a failure to synthesize or secrete ADH resulting in an inability to concentrate urine maximally. Patients with complete CDI have profound polyuria resulting in polydipsia. Approximately half of the patients have idiopathic CDI (usually diagnosed in childhood). The rest are due to a variety of causes listed below:

Causes of Central Diabetes Insipidus

• Head trauma	• Granulomatous disease
• Posthypophysectomy	• Histiocytosis
• Suprasellar and intrasellar neoplasms	• Vascular insults
	• Infections

The diagnosis is often delayed because the only symptom the patient has is thirst. CDI can be differentiated from other causes of polyuria by performing a **fluid deprivation test** followed by exogenous ADH administration.

Fluid Deprivation Test

- During the test strict urinary output, weight, and vital signs must be obtained to prevent severe volume contraction.

- Patients with mild polyuria (<10 l/day) should have fluids withheld the night preceding the test (e.g., 6 p.m.); patients with severe polyuria (> 10 l/day) should be fluid deprived only during the day (e.g., 6 a.m.) to allow close observation. The time to achieve a maximal U_{osm} varies from 4 to 18 hr.

- S_{osm} should approach 295 mOsm/kg H_2O after fluid deprivation and before ADH administration.

- Urine osmolality is measured at baseline and then hourly, until two urine osmolalities vary by <30 mOsm/kg H_2O or 3% to 5% of the body weight is lost.

- Five units of vasopressin is administered subcutaneously and 1 hr later a final urine osmolality is obtained.

Table 6-1 provides approximate values of urinary osmolality which are helpful in establishing the diagnosis.

Table 6-1 Response to Fluid Deprivation and ADH Administration

Condition	U_{osm} after Fluid Deprivation	U_{osm} after ADH Administration	Percent Change
Normal	1000-1120	unchanged	0
Complete CDI	150-180	400-500	>50
Partial CDI	420-480	510-580	>10
Nephrogenic DI	150-200	unchanged	0
Compulsive water drinking	700-780	700-820	<5

Treatment for CDI is hormonal replacement.

Preparation	Dose	Duration of Action
Aqueous vasopressin	5-10 units subcutaneously	3-6 hr
Vasopressin tannate in oil	5 units intramuscularly	24-72 hr
DDAVP	400-1600 units intranasally	per 24 hr

Nephrogenic diabetes insipidus (NDI) is characterized by impaired urinary concentrating ability despite maximal synthesis and release of ADH. NDI can be caused by 1) a failure to generate a maximal hypertonic medullary and papillary interstitium and/or 2) a failure of ADH to increase the water permeability of the collecting ducts. While both congenital and acquired forms of this disorder occur, the acquired form is most common (see display below). The hallmark of diagnosis is the failure to concentrate urine in response to exogenous ADH.

Therapy for acquired NDI should be directed at the primary disorder. Thiazide diuretics and a low salt intake produce volume depletion, reduce GFR, and enhance proximal tubular reabsorption resulting in less delivery of filtrate to the diluting segment and, thereby, decreased polyuria.

Acquired Causes of Nephrogenic Diabetes Insipidus

- Chronic renal disease
  Medullary cystic disease
  Polycystic kidney disease
  Obstructive uropathy
  Pyelonephritis
  Severe chronic renal failure

- Pharmacologic agents
  Demeclocycline
  Lithium
  Glyburide
  Tolazamide
  Propoxyphene
  Methoxyflurane
  Amphotericin B
  Vinblastine
  Colchicine

- Electrolyte disorders
  Hypercalcemia
  Hypokalemia

- Dietary abnormalities
  Poor protein intake
  Excessive water intake
  Poor salt intake

- Miscellaneous
  Amyloidosis
  Sarcoidosis
  Multiple myeloma
  Sjögren's syndrome
  Sickle cell disease

Modified from Schrier RW, Disorders of water metabolism. Renal and Electrolyte Disorders. Boston: Little, Brown, 1986: 33.

Increased Total Body Sodium

This is usually due to exogenous administration of hypertonic Na-containing solutions (e.g., $NaHCO_3$ administered to patients with a metabolic acidosis, or hypertonic NaCl solutions used in dialysate).

CLINICAL PRESENTATION

Signs and symptoms include restlessness, seizures, lethargy, coma, hyperreflexia, spasticity, muscle twitching, and death. Dehydration of brain cells leads to capillary and venous congestion, cerebral vessel tears, venous sinus thrombosis, and subcortical/subarachnoid hemorrhages.

The mortality in children is 7 to 29% in chronic and 43% in acute hypernatremia. Adults with acute hypernatremia have mortality rates as high as 60%.

TREATMENT

Decreased Total Body Sodium

Initially patients should receive isotonic NaCl until volume contraction has been corrected. Thereafter, hypotonic solutions using D_5W or 0.45% NaCl can be used.

Normal Total Body Sodium

Pure water loss should be replaced with D_5W. The water deficit can be calculated, assuming TBW is 60% of body weight. For example, in a 70-kg patient, 70 kg x .60 = 42 liters of TBW.

If the measured S_{Na} = 160 mEq/l, then calculate the water needed to lower S_{Na} to normal (i.e., 140 mEq/l).

$$\frac{\text{measured serum Na concentration}}{\text{required serum Na concentration}} \times TBW = \text{ideal body water}$$

$$\frac{160 \text{ mEq/l}}{140 \text{ mEq/l}} \times 42 \text{ l} = 47.9 \text{ l}$$

47.9 - 42 = 5.9 l, which represents the water deficit that must be corrected to improve the hypernatremia.

Normally the fluid deficit should be replaced over 48 hr. The S_{osm} should decrease by approximately 1-2 mOsm/kg H_2O/hr. Faster rates of correction can cause seizures. Frequent electrolyte monitoring is mandatory.

Increased total Body Sodium

These patients are total body Na and water overloaded, although they have a disproportionate increase in Na. The treatment is to remove excess salt and water using diuretic therapy.

SUGGESTED READING

Anderson RJ. Hospital-associated hyponatremia. Kidney Int 1986;29: 1237-1247.

Arieff AI, Guisado R. Effects on the central nervous system of hypernatremic and hyponatremic states. Kidney Int 1976;10:104-116.

Marsden PA, Halperin ML. Pathophysiological approach to patients presenting with hypernatremia. Am J Neph 1985;5:229-235.

Robertson GL, Berl T. Water metabolism. In: Brenner BM, Rector FC Jr, eds. The kidney. Philadelphia: WB Saunders Co, 1986:385-432.

Schrier RW. Pathogenesis of sodium and water retention in high-output and low-output cardiac failure, nephrotic syndrome, cirrhosis, and pregnancy. N Engl J Med 1988;319:1065-1072, 1127-1134.

Sterns RH. Severe symptomatic hyponatremia: treatment and outcome. Ann Intern Med 1987;107:655-664.

Chapter 7

Potassium Disorders
Gerald B. Stephanz, Jr.
Charles S. Wingo

Hypokalemia (serum K <3.5 mEq/l or mmol/l) and hyperkalemia (serum K >5.0 mEq/l or mmol/l) are common and potentially lethal.

PHYSIOLOGY

The daily potassium (K) load is 50-150 mEq. Approximately 90% of the K ingested is normally eliminated in the urine, with a small portion excreted in the stool and the sweat. However, when renal function is compromised, the gastrointestinal tract can eliminate up to 30% of the intake; enteric losses of K in diarrheal conditions can be substantial. K secretion by the colon and the sweat glands is stimulated by aldosterone.

The serum K concentration (S_K) is a general indicator of total body K. However, because only about 2% of total body K is in the extracellular fluid and 98% is in cells, small losses or gains by cells can cause large changes in the S_K.

ACID-BASE BALANCE

Metabolic acidosis promotes hyperkalemia, whereas alkalosis promotes hypokalemia. Strong mineral acids (HCl, NH_4Cl) raise S_K more than organic acids (lactic, beta-hydroxy-butyric).

INSULIN

Insulin deficiency impairs cellular K uptake and promotes hyperkalemia, probably through lack of stimulation of Na-K-ATPase. Increased S_K stimulates pancreatic insulin release, while hypokalemia has an inhibitory (diabetogenic) effect.

CATECHOLAMINES

Catecholamines, particularly the beta-2-agonists (e.g., terbutaline), stimulate the cellular Na-K pump and can result in moderate hypokalemia.

ALDOSTERONE

Aldosterone stimulates cellular K uptake and facilitates renal K excretion. It stimulates the Na-K pump, not only in the kidney (collecting duct) but in other organs as well; a deficiency frequently causes hyperkalemia (e.g., Addison's disease).

RENAL REGULATION OF POTASSIUM

Almost 90% of the K eliminated in the urine is due to secretion in the cortical collecting duct (see Chapter 29). However, several factors influence renal K secretion, primarily through the collecting duct. Adrenal insufficiency impairs K excretion and causes sodium wasting, while primary or secondary hyperaldosteronism causes sodium reabsorption and hypokalemia. High levels of glucocorticoids as seen in Cushing's syndrome, exogenous adrenocorticotrophic hormone (ACTH) administration, or ectopic ACTH-producing tumors are associated with renal K loss and hypokalemia.

K secretion by the collecting duct is stimulated by a high S_K, increased tubular fluid flow, and diuretics. Reduction of dietary K intake results in renal conservation of K both by decreasing K secretion in the cortical collecting duct and enhancing reabsorption in the medullary collecting duct. Maximal renal K conservation in man requires up to 3 weeks.

APPROACH TO THE HYPOKALEMIC PATIENT

The search for the etiology of hypokalemia should begin with a careful history and physical examination concentrating on the drug history and the state of hydration (vomiting and diarrhea).

Differential Diagnosis of Hypokalemia

- Artifactual [high white blood cell count (WBC), leukemia]
- Redistribution (cellular shift)
    - Insulin administration
    - Periodic paralysis (familial, thyrotoxic)
    - Refeeding (intravenous hyperalimentation)
    - Beta adrenergic agonists (epinephrine, terbutaline)
    - Alkalosis
    - Theophylline toxicity
- Inadequate dietary intake
    - Alcoholism
    - Starvation (anorexia nervosa)
- Gastrointestinal losses
    - Vomiting/nasogastric drainage
    - Diarrhea and chronic laxative abuse
    - Uterosigmoidostomy (urinary diversion)
    - Villous adenoma
- Renal losses
    - Drugs
        - Diuretics
        - Glucocorticoids
        - Antibiotic/antifungal/chemotherapeutic agents
            - Penicillins (carbenicillin)
            - Amphotericin B (renal tubular acidosis)
            - Aminoglycosides
            - Cis-platinum

Mineralocorticoid excess
Adenoma/hyperplasia
Malignant and renovascular hypertension
Glycyrrhizic acid intoxication
True licorice excess
Chewing tobacco abuse
Cushing's syndrome
Adrenal enzyme deficiency syndromes
- Bartter's syndrome
- Renal tubular acidosis
- Acute leukemia (lysozymuria)
- Hypomagnesemia
- Fanconi's syndrome
- Diuretic phase of acute tubular necrosis (ATN)
- Postobstructive diuresis

The clinical manifestations of hypokalemia are usually present at levels <2.5 mEq/l (see accompanying display) or with a rapid fall in serum K.

Clinical Manifestations of Hypokalemia

Cardiac
- Predisposition to digoxin toxicity
- Ventricular irritability
- Abnormal electrocardiogram (ECG)
    T wave flattening
    U waves
    ST segment depression
- Cardiac necrosis

Neuromuscular
- Skeletal
    Weakness, cramps, tetany
    Paralysis
    Rhabdomyolysis
- Gastrointestinal
    Constipation
    Ileus
- Encephalopathy (liver disease)

Renal
- Polyuria (nephrogenic diabetes insipidus)
- Polydipsia

Endocrine/metabolic
- Carbohydrate intolerance
- Decreased aldosterone levels

A diagnostic approach to hypokalemia is detailed in Figures 7-1 and 7-2. Measurements of blood pressure (BP), blood and urinary electrolytes, and determination of the acid-base status (by arterial blood gas) are of central importance.

It is first necessary to determine whether hypokalemia is artifactual, the result of redistribution of K, or a representation of true K depletion. Artifactual values may be seen in leukemic patients with a WBC of 100,000-250,000; the WBCs can extract K from the plasma if left at room temperature (if left in the cold, hyperkalemia). To avoid spurious values, plasma from leukemic patients should be separated quickly. The clinical setting and blood pH will determine whether hypokalemia is secondary to redistribution.

Laboratory Tests in Investigation of Hypokalemia

• Routine	• Additional
Serum electrolytes	Serum magnesium
Urinary electrolytes	Aldosterone
Blood pH	Renin
WBC	Cortisol

TREATMENT OF HYPOKALEMIA

Although S_K is not an exact indicator of the total body K deficit, a decrease (below 4 mEq/l) of 0.27 mEq/l is approximately equivalent to 100 mEq/l K deficit (up to a total deficit of 500 mEq/l). Serum K levels of <2.0 mEq/l may reflect deficits of more than 1000 mEq/l.

Four factors should be taken into account in the correction:

- **Acid-base status**--correction of coexisting metabolic acidosis without concomitant K replacement can cause the serum K to fall lower.

- **Intravenous glucose administration** can cause K levels to fall; in life-threatening hypokalemia, initial K replacement should be given in glucose-free solutions.

- **Overzealous administration of K** can result in hyperkalemia.

- **Coexisting hypomagnesemia** prevents correction of hypokalemia.

Intravenous K is reserved for patients unable to take K orally or in severe life-threatening situations, e.g., paralysis, digitalis intoxication (with arrhythmias), hypokalemic-induced hepatic coma, and those with ECG abnormalities.

Oral therapy is preferred because it rarely causes "overshoot" hyperkalemia (in the presence of normal renal function). Oral supplementation is generally given in doses of 20-120 mEq/day. Over the counter salt substitutes are an economical source of K and contain 3.5-7.5 mEq/g (5 g is approximately 1 teaspoon).

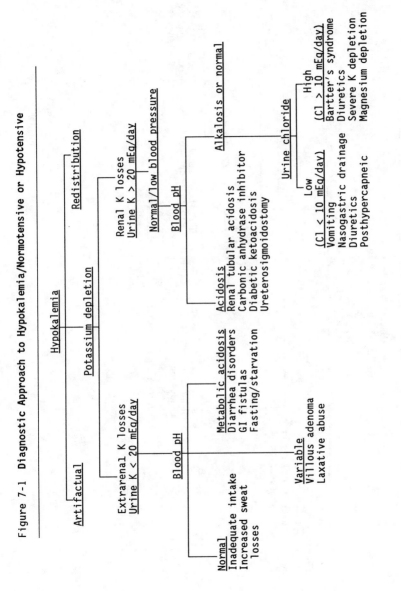

Figure 7-1 Diagnostic Approach to Hypokalemia/Normotensive or Hypotensive

Figure 7-2 Diagnostic Approach to Hypokalemia/Hypertensive Patient

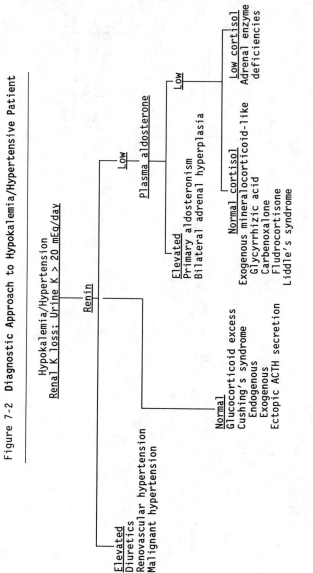

K is available as K chloride (KCl), K phosphate, and K bicarbonate, gluconate, acetate, or citrate. In general, KCl is appropriate to correct K depletion and is the only preparation effective when there is chloride depletion (metabolic alkalosis).

Oral K supplements come in a variety of liquids, powders, and tablets, containing 5-40 mEq K/dose. Liquid preparations are associated with gastrointestinal irritation; enteric coated preparations, in contrast to wax matrix KCl tablets, are associated with gastrointestinal (GI) ulcerations.

Intravenous K can be given safely at rates of 10 mEq/hr by peripheral vein without ECG monitoring and in concentrations of up to 30 mEq/l (to avoid pain/phlebitis). If the serum K is <2.5 mEq/l in association with ECG abnormalities and/or severe neuromuscular complications, doses of 40 mEq/hr can be given through a central venous catheter with continuous ECG monitoring-**doses of this magnitude are rarely necessary.** Frequent determinations of S_K are the best guide to replacement therapy (every 4-6 hr). Once indications for intravenous/emergent therapy have resolved, less aggressive therapy should be given.

Therapeutic measures in the treatment of chronic hypokalemia include the use of oral K supplements and the K-sparing diuretics spironolactone, triamterene, and amiloride. The use and potential complications of these agents are discussed in Chapter 27; combined use of K supplements and K-sparing diuretics is contraindicated.

APPROACH TO THE HYPERKALEMIC PATIENT

Hyperkalemia results from transcellular shifts or K retention (see Figure 7-3).

Key points in the history include diet, medications, past or family history of renal disease, and an assessment of urine volume. Careful questioning for symptoms of prostatism is appropriate in men. Helpful signs of neuromuscular irritability include weakness, paresthesias, and flaccid paralysis. ECG findings in hyperkalemia are detailed below.

ECG Findings in Hyperkalemia

- ECG abnormalities (in order of appearance and progression)
  Peaking/tenting T waves
  Flattening of P waves
  Prolongation of PR interval
  Widening of QRS complex (to sine wave)
  Ventricular fibrillation/cardiac arrest

LABORATORY/DIAGNOSTIC EVALUATION OF HYPERKALEMIA

The first step is to rule out artifactual hyperkalemia by drawing a fresh sample through a large bore needle without prolonged tourniquet time. The WBC and platelet count should also be evaluated.

Figure 7-3 Diagnostic Approach in Hyperkalemia

Hyperkalemia

Spurious
Hemolysis
Thrombocytosis
Leukocytosis
Mononucleosis
("leaky red
blood cells")

Redistribution
Acidosis
Diabetic ketoacidosis
Beta-adrenergic blockade
Arginine HCl
Succinylcholine
Periodic paralysis
Digitalis overdose

Increased intake or tissue release
Intravenous/oral administration
Hemolysis
Rhabdomyolysis
Tumor lysis
Stored blood administration

Potassium excess

GFR > 20 ml/min

Aldosterone
deficiency
Addison's disease
Hereditary
Adrenal enzyme defects
Hyporeninemic
hypoaldosteronism
Drugs
Heparin
Nonsteroidal anti-
inflammatory medications
Angiotensin-converting
enzyme inhibitors
Cyclosporine
Spironolactone

GFR < 20 ml/min
Acute renal failure
Chronic renal failure

Tubular hyperkalemia
without aldosterone deficiency
Acquired
Obstructive uropathy
Renal transplant
Systemic lupus erythematosus
(SLE)
Amyloidosis
Sickle cell nephropathy
Drugs
K-sparing diuretics

With platelet counts greater than 1,000,000, artifactual elevations in the measured K can be seen from K released during clotting. Spurious hyperkalemia can be seen with a WBC >500,000 from K release during coagulation. An ECG should be performed for any serum K value >6.0 mEq/l.

The accompanying display lists laboratory and diagnostic tests helpful in establishing the etiology of hyperkalemia. Bladder catheterization (to rule out bladder neck obstruction) and renal ultrasonography (to rule out hydronephrosis or small kidneys of end-stage renal disease) are often important in the acute evaluation.

Laboratory/Diagnostic Tests in Hyperkalemia

- Electrolytes
- Serum creatinine/blood urea nitrogen (BUN)
- Arterial blood gasses (pH)
- WBC
- Platelet count
- Hematocrit [if low, may indicate chronic renal failure (CRF)]
- Serum phosphate (if high, may indicate CRF/rhabdomyolysis)
- Creatinine clearance
- ECG
- Bladder catheterization
- Renal ultrasound

TREATMENT OF HYPERKALEMIA

Hyperkalemia is life threatening because of cardiac toxicity. Drugs used in the acute treatment of hyperkalemia, doses, and onset of action are listed below. Simultaneous use of all of these measures is indicated if ECG abnormalities exist. If hyperkalemia is of such severity to require all of these measures, emergent dialysis should be considered.

Drug Therapy of Hyperkalemia (See Text)

Drug	Dose	Onset of Action
Calcium gluconate	10-30 ml (10% solution)	1-2 min
Calcium chloride	10-30 ml (10% solution)	1-2 min
Sodium bicarbonate	50 mEq ampules	15-30 min
Glucose/insulin	25-50 g glucose IV/5 units regular insulin (repeat every 15 min)	15-30 min
Sodium polystyrene Sulfonate (Kayexalate)	Enema 50-100 g; oral 40 g (see text)	60-120 min

Calcium rapidly antagonizes the effects of K on cardiac conduction, but the effect lasts for only 15-20 minutes. The dose listed above can be repeated once, but further doses are generally ineffective unless hypocalcemia is present. Sodium bicarbonate ($NaHCO_3$) administration can be repeated every 15 minutes as needed if ECG changes persist. Alternatively, two ampules of $NaHCO_3$ can be mixed with 1 l of $D_{10}W$ (with 25-50 units of regular insulin per liter) and infused at a rate of 300-500 ml for the first half hour (rate titrated to serum K levels thereafter). $NaHCO_3$ administration has risks of circulatory overload and hypernatremia.

Sodium polystyrene sulfonate (Kayexalate) is a Na-K exchange resin that removes approximately 1 mEq K/g resin orally and 0.5 mEq K/g resin by enema. Oral doses are usually given in a hyperosmotic sorbitol solution (20%) to promote rapid gastrointestinal transit and should be repeated every 2-4 hr until the S_K is normal. If the patient is nauseated, retention enemas are preferred. Approximately 50-100 g of the resin in water are placed through a Foley catheter inserted rectally; the balloon is inflated to ensure retention for 30-60 min. Enemas should be repeated every 2-4 hr as needed. Both oral and enema administration can precipitate circulatory overload secondary to Na absorption.

Dialysis may be employed, especially in situations where hyperkalemia is compounded by volume overload, severe uremia, and acidosis (see Chapter 23). Hemodialysis can remove K at a rate of 25-30 mEq/hr while peritoneal dialysis can remove 10-15 mEq K/hr.

Treatment of chronic hyperkalemia (chronic renal failure, hyperalemic renal tubular acidosis) first entails dietary restriction of K to 40-60 mEq/day. Diuretic therapy (loop diuretics, metolazone) is beneficial, especially if patients have mild volume expansion but K-sparing diuretics are contraindicated. Oral bicarbonate therapy can also be employed, with initial doses of $NaHCO_3$ of 650 mg 3 times a day titrated upward to maintain a serum CO_2 of 20-22 mEq/l. Sodium polystyrene sulfonate can be used orally in doses of 15-60 g 4 times a day. Finally, fludrocortisone acetate (Florinef[R]) can be given in initial doses of 0.1-0.4 mg daily in patients without evidence of volume expansion, hypertension, or circulatory overload. Frequently, higher doses may be necessary. Hypertension and sodium retention complicate its use.

SUGGESTED READING

Gabow PA, Peterson LN. Disorders of potassium metabolism. In: Schrier RW, ed. Renal and electrolyte disorders. Boston: Little, Brown, and Company, 1986:207-249.

Magner PO, Robinson L, Halperin RM, Zettle R, Halperin ML. The plasma potassium concentration in metabolic acidosis: a re-evaluation. Am J Kid Dis 1988;11:220-224.

Narins RG, Jones ER, Stom MC, Rudnick MR, Bastl CP. Diagnostic strategies in disorders of fluid, electrolyte and acid-base homeostasis. Am J Med 1982;72:496-519.

Ponce SP, Jennings AE, Madias NE, Harrington JT. Drug-induced hyperkalemia. Medicine 1985;64:357-370.

Tannen RL. Potassium disorders. In: Kokko JP, Tannen RL, eds. Fluids and electrolytes. Philadelphia: WB Saunders Company, 1986:150-228.

Chapter 8

Acid-Base Disorders

Charles S. Wingo
Kevin A. Curran

DEFINITION

Acidosis is a manifestation of a disease process which, if left unopposed, results in acidemia (pH <7.35). Alkalosis is a manifestation of a disease process which, if left unopposed, results in alkalemia (pH >7.45). Acidosis can be subdivided into metabolic (a primary reduction in plasma bicarbonate concentration) and respiratory (a primary increase in pCO_2) types. Likewise, alkalosis can be divided into metabolic (a primary increase in plasma bicarbonate concentration) and respiratory (a primary decrease in pCO_2) types. Simple acid-base disorders are due to a **single** primary change in either pCO_2 or $[HCO_3]$. Except for chronic respiratory alkalosis, simple acid-base disorders result in an abnormal blood pH. Certain terms that are frequently confused are defined below:

- pH-a measure of acidity and approximately equal to $\log [H]^{-1}$.

- pCO_2-the partial pressure (in mm Hg, Torr) of CO_2 in a solution.

- Total CO_2-moles of CO_2 that can be released from a solution by adding a strong acid. The $[HCO_3]$ approximates the total CO_2 content.

INCIDENCE

In order of decreasing frequency the incidence of simple acid-base disorders is metabolic alkalosis > respiratory alkalosis > respiratory acidosis > metabolic acidosis.

ETIOLOGY

The simple acid-base disorders are listed in Table 8-1 with the primary causes and compensatory changes.

Table 8-1 Simple Acid-Base Disturbances and Predicted Compensations

Disorder	Mechanism	Primary Change	Compensatory Change	Expected Compensatory Response*
Metabolic acidosis	1) Excessive acid production or retention 2) Excessive base loss	↓ [HCO_3]	↓ pCO_2	$pCO_2 = 1.5 \times [HCO_3] + 8\ (\pm2)$ or pCO_2 = last two digits of pH
Metabolic alkalosis	1) Excessive base intake or retention 2) Excessive acid loss	↑ [HCO_3]	↑ pCO_2	$pCO_2 = 0.9 \times [HCO_3] + 16\ (\pm5)$ or pCO_2 = last two digits of pH
Respiratory acidosis				
Acute	1) Decreased CO_2 elimination	↑ pCO_2	↑ [HCO_3]	$[H] = 0.75\ pCO_2 + 9\ (\pm4)$ $\Delta[HCO_3] = 0.1\ \Delta pCO_2$
Chronic	1) Decreased CO_2 elimination			$[H] = 0.3\ pCO_2 + 28\ (\pm3)$ $\Delta[HCO_3] = 0.4\ \Delta pCO_2$
Respiratory alkalosis		↓ pCO_2	↓ [HCO_3]	
Acute	1) Increased CO_2 elimination			$[H] = 0.75\ pCO_2 + 9\ (\pm4)$ $[HCO_3] = \Delta0.2\ pCO_2$
Chronic	1) Increased CO_2 elimination			$[H] = 0.30\ pCO_2 + 28\ (\pm4)$ $\Delta[HCO_3] = \Delta0.5\ pCO_2$

*The following equations can be used to predict the expected steady-state relation between the primary and the compensatory change. For example, a reduction in [HCO_3] due to severe diarrhea (metabolic acidosis) to 15 mEq/l will produce a secondary change in pCO_2. With 95% confidence the pCO_2 will be: $pCO_2 = 1.5 \times 15 + 8\ (\pm2) = 30.5 \pm 2$ or 28.5 to 32.5 mm Hg. By coincidence the last two digits of the pH roughly approximate the predicted pCO_2.

PATHOPHYSIOLOGY

Acid-base homeostasis is maintained within a narrow range through a series of reversible chemical buffers and physiologic pulmonary and renal compensations. Intracellular and extracellular buffers which counteract changes in pH include CO_2/HCO_3, phosphate, protein (particularly hemoglobin), and bone. Although all body buffers participate in acid-base regulation, it is convenient to think in terms of the bicarbonate buffer system since all extracellular buffers are essentially in equilibrium. This relationship may be expressed in terms of the Henderson-Hasselbalch equation as follows:

$$pH = 3.5 + \log [HCO_3^-]/[H_2CO_3]$$

It is frequently more convenient to utilize the linear form of this equation (Henderson equation):

$$[H] = 24 \times \frac{pCO_2}{[HCO_3^-]}$$

The normal pH of 7.4 is equivalent to a [H] of 40 nM. This can be conveniently remembered as the last two digits of the normal pH (7.40). The following display gives the actual [H] for each 0.1 pH unit between 7.00 and 7.70. Note that between 7.20 and 7.50 each 0.1 increase in pH results in a decrease of [H] by approximately 10 nM.

Relationship Between pH and [H]

pH	7.00	7.10	7.20	7.30	7.40	7.50	7.60	7.70
[H]	100 nM	79 nM	63 nM	50 nM	40 nM	32 nM	25 nM	20 nM

COMPENSATION TO PRIMARY ACID-BASE DISORDERS

Physiologic compensation to changes in pH involves changes in both alveolar ventilation (pCO_2) and in renal acid excretion (Fig. 8-1). Complete respiratory compensation to metabolic acidosis requires 12-24 hr. The kidney reacts much more slowly to changes in systemic pH to affect net acid excretion. Net acid excretion is defined as the rate of ammonium plus titratable acid excretion minus the rate of bicarbonate excretion. Renal excretion of an alkali load requires 24-48 hr, whereas full renal compensation to an acid load requires 72 hr.

APPROACH TO ACID-BASE DISORDERS

Evaluating a patient with an acid-base disturbance requires consideration of both the clinical presentation and the laboratory data. A good history can greatly simplify a complex set of blood gas and electrolyte data.

The nomagram in Figure 8-2 provides the 95% confidence limits for steady-state simple acid-base disorders. The arterial blood gas is the cornerstone of diagnosis and management of most acid-base disturbances, but several caveats should be considered.

- An arterial pH within the confidence band for a simple disorder is compatible with a mixed acid-base disturbance.

- Patients with pure acid-base disturbances may lie outside the 95% confidence limits until full ventilatory or metabolic compensation has occurred.

- Systemic pH, pCO_2, bicarbonate, and electrolytes should be evaluated simultaneously and the calculated HCO_3 of the blood gas data should be compared to the total CO_2 content; differences >2 mEq/l suggest an error in pH or pCO_2 measurement.

- A blood gas value represents a specific point in time; identical values can be obtained for different acid-base disturbances moving in different directions.

- Nomograms such as Figure 8-2 may lead to the wrong diagnosis if the clinical presentation is ignored.

METABOLIC ACIDOSIS

Metabolic acidosis represents a primary decrease in plasma bicarbonate concentration and decreases blood pH. This can occur by one of three methods. **First**, a strong acid, which is buffered by bicarbonate, may be added to body fluids. **Second**, there can be direct loss of bicarbonate by the gastrointestinal (GI) tract or kidneys. **Third**, the extracellular fluid (ECF) can be rapidly diluted by a non-bicarbonate-containing solution.

The **compensatory response** to acidosis is an increase in ventilation which returns pH toward normal. When fully compensated after 12-24 hr, the pCO_2 closely approximates the last two digits of the serum pH. If this is not the case, a mixed acid-base disturbance should be considered.

CLINICAL PRESENTATION

Nausea, vomiting, and abdominal pain are frequent with metabolic acidosis, particularly diabetic ketoacidosis. Respiratory compensation produces rapid, deep (Kussmaul's) respirations. Severe acidosis can be associated with decreased myocardial contractility, hypotension, pulmonary edema, and tissue hypoxia.

The arterial blood gas reveals a low pH, a low plasma bicarbonate, and usually a low pCO_2. Electrolytes reveal a low total CO_2.

The first step in determining the etiology of a metabolic acidosis is calculation of the anion gap (AG). AG = [Na] - ([Cl] + [HCO_3]). A normal anion gap ranges between 8 and 16 nM providing the albumin and globulin concentrations are normal. Table 8-2 provides the differential diagnosis of an elevated AG acidosis, key clinical features, supporting laboratory data, and a brief outline of specific treatment options.

Table 8-2 Differential Diagnosis of Elevated Anion Gap Metabolic Acidosis

Etiology		Clinical Features	Laboratory	Treatment
K	Diabetic ketoacidosis	Fruity breath Possible history of diabetes mellitus	Increased Glu >300 mg/dl Serum and/or urine ketones	IV insulin IV saline (0.9% and 0.45%) depending on volume status
U	Uremia	Oliguria, uremic breath Pericarditis	Increased BUN and Cr Low urine output	Consider dialysis
S	Salicylate intoxication	Tinnitus History of acute or chronic salicylate ingestion Hyperventilation—especially in children and elderly	Positive urine ferric chloride test Increased salicylate (may be therapeutic level in chronic ingestion—may have accompanying respiratory alkalosis) Increased prothrombin time	Diuresis & alkalinization of urine NaHCO₃ therapy Hemodialysis
S	Starvation ketosis	None	Serum and/or urine ketones	
M	Methanol ingestion	History	Methanol levels evaluated osmole gap	Ethanol infusion Dialysis
A	Alcoholic lactic acidosis	Characteristic smell History ETOH abuse often with binge	Increased alcohol level Serum lactate increased	Phosphorus repletion
U	Unmeasured osmoles Ethylene glycol Aldehydes Paraldehydes	May have accompanying renal failure, hypotension, sepsis	Ethylene glycol level Evaluate osmole gap Calcium oxalate crystals in urine	Dialysis
L	Lactic acidosis	Sepsis and shock	Lactate level	Correction of underlying etiology

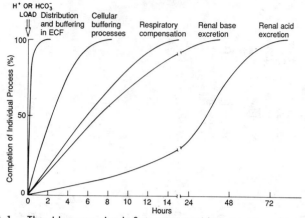

Figure 8-1 The time required for compensation to an acid or alkali load. Respiratory compensation is not complete for 10-12 hr and renal compensation to an acid load may require 72 hr. (From Cogan MG, Rector FC Jr, Seldin, DW. Acid-base disorders. 2nd ed. In: Brenner BM, Rector FC Jr, eds. The Kidney. Philadelphia: WB Saunders Co, 1981;17:899.)

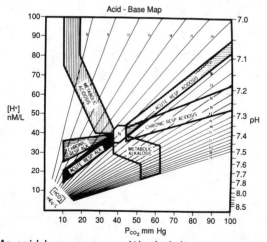

Figure 8-2 An acid-base nomagram with shaded areas representing the confidence limits after full compensation. (From Goldberg M, Green SB, Moss ML, et al. Computer-based instruction and diagnosis of acid-base disorders. J Am Med Assoc 1973;223:269-275.)

Normal AG metabolic acidosis with increased serum chloride concentrations is generally due to gastrointestinal or renal bicarbonate wasting. Specific causes are listed below.

Differential Diagnosis of Normal Anion Gap Metabolic Acidosis

• Gastrointestinal tract bicarbonate loss from diarrhea, pancreatic or biliary fistulas, or an immature ileostomy all yield fluid losses with a higher $[HCO_3]$ than serum and potassium depletion.

• Urinary diversion (i.e., ureterosigmoidostomy) with urine retention in the colon causes chloride and water reabsorption and bicarbonate secretion.

• Ingestion of chloride salts or chloride-containing anion exchange resins, i.e., $CaCl_2$, $MgCl_2$, or cholestyramine is associated with exchange of chloride for bicarbonate across the GI tract.

• Renal bicarbonate loss (RTA, see Chapter 9)

Chronic respiratory alkalosis may mimic the electrolyte pattern of a normal anion gap metabolic acidosis (i.e., low $[HCO_3]$ and increased plasma chloride). However, in uncomplicated metabolic acidosis the serum pH will be <7.35.

Therapy for these disorders involves treatment of the primary process. The choice between intravenous or oral bicarbonate depends on the specific etiology for the acidosis. Uremic acidosis, which typically has an elevated AG, should be treated with HCO_3 therapy. If a nonrenal mechanism of acidosis is present and renal function is normal, alkali therapy is not indicated generally for a serum pH >7.10 since overcorrection of acidemia, or metabolism of the organic anions, can lead to a metabolic alkalosis that can further complicate therapy. Most formulas overestimate the base requirement unless acid production is continuous as in lactic acidosis. Thus, we prefer to use the following more conservative estimate of bicarbonate deficit and reassess the patient's condition on a regular basis.

$[HCO_3](mEq) = 0.20 \times weight\ (kg) \times (desired\ [HCO_3] - observed\ [HCO_3])$

RESPIRATORY ACIDOSIS

Respiratory acidosis represents an increase in pCO_2 which decreases pH. The increased pCO_2 is generally due to failure of CO_2 excretion, usually alveolar hypoventilation, rather than increased CO_2 production. Causes of respiratory acidosis are listed in the display on page 82.

The increased CO_2 results in an increased carbonic acid concentration. In respiratory acidosis carbonic acid is buffered primarily by intracellular buffers such as hemoglobin or phosphate resulting in a small increase in plasma bicarbonate concentration. The kidneys compensate by increasing acid secretion which generates bicarbonate.

Chloride excretion is increased, which reduces plasma chloride concentration. The renal response takes longer than 24 hr to develop fully.

Causes of Respiratory Acidosis

Decreased alveolar ventilation and CO_2 removal from the lungs
- Obstruction
  Bronchospasm/stenosis
  Chronic bronchitis
  Emphysema (advanced)
  Aspiration

- Primary depression of respiratory center
  Drugs - all central nervous system (CNS) depressants, barbiturates, ethanol, etc.
  Trauma - epidural/subdural hematoma
  Neoplastic - primary or metastatic disease
  Infection - brain abscess, meningitis
  Vascular - cerebral infarction, subarachnoid hemorrhage

- Mechanical - structural defect
  Pneumothorax/hemothorax/ascites/obesity
  Flail chest
  Adult respiratory distress syndrome
  Severe pneumonia

- Mechanical - neuromuscular defect
  Primary muscular disease, periodic paralysis, severe hypokalemia, hypophosphatemia
  Neuromuscular
         Myasthenia gravis
         Motor-neuron disease
         Guillain-Barré syndrome
  Drugs
         Curare, succinyl choline, aminoglycosides
         Organophosphates
  Toxins
         Botulism, tetanus

- Decreased afferent stimulation of respiratory center
  Sleep apnea

Decreased tissue removal or pulmonary exchange of CO_2
- Cardiac arrest

- Circulatory shock

- Pneumonia

- Severe pulmonary edema

- Massive pulmonary embolus

CLINICAL FEATURES

Patients present with respiratory distress, dyspnea, or obtundation. If severe, patients may complain of headaches or show signs of increased intracranial pressure due to the vasodilatory properties of CO_2 which increase cerebral blood flow. The pCO_2 is elevated and the pH decreased (see Table 8-1).

The treatment of a respiratory acidosis is restoration of adequate ventilation.

RESPIRATORY ALKALOSIS

Respiratory alkalosis results from a decrease in pCO_2 caused by increased alveolar ventilation.

Causes of Respiratory Alkalosis

- Increased CNS drive for respiration
  Anxiety - hyperventilation
  CNS infection/infarction/trauma
  Drugs - salicylates/nicotine/aminophylline
  Fever/sepsis - especially Gram-negative sepsis
  Pregnancy/progesterone
  Liver disease

- Increased stimulation of chemoreceptors
  Anemia
  Carbon monoxide toxicity
  Pulmonary edema/pneumonia
  Pulmonary emboli
  Reduced inspired O_2 tension - high altitude

- Increased mechanical ventilation - iatrogenic

The initial response to alkalemia is buffering with intracellular protons. The renal compensation, which occurs over several days, decreases net acid excretion and plasma bicarbonate concentration, and restores pH toward normal.

CLINICAL PRESENTATION

Patients will often present with hyperventilation and signs of hypocapnia. These include perioral and extremity paresthesias, muscle cramps, hyperflexia, seizures, or cardiac arrhythmias.

The arterial blood gas measurement reveals a decreased pCO_2 and an increased pH. Plasma bicarbonate will be decreased. Serum CO_2 will be decreased and serum chloride may be increased. Some of these changes of chronic respiratory alkalosis may mimic non-anion gap acidosis, and the metabolic compensation often restores systemic pH to nearly normal.

The only effective therapy is to eliminate the cause of the hyperventilation.

METABOLIC ALKALOSIS

Metabolic alkalosis is due to a primary increase in plasma bicarbonate concentration and an increase in blood pH. This bicarbonate excess can result from ECF hydrogen ion loss, addition of bicarbonate or its precursors to the ECF, or loss of fluid with chloride content greater than that of bicarbonate. The major causes of metabolic alkalosis, listed below, can be divided into two large groups due to either Cl depletion or potassium (K) depletion. Uncomplicated K depletion in humans produces only a mild metabolic alkalosis. However, with excess aldosterone production, hypokalemia produces severe metabolic alkalosis.

Causes of Metabolic Alkalosis

- Chloride responsive metabolic alkalosis - frequently observed with volume contraction (urine [Cl] <10 mEq/l without diuretics)
     Vomiting/nasogastric suction
     Villous adenoma
     Diuretic therapy - e.g., loop & thiazide diuretics (urine Cl >10 mEq/l)
     Posthypercapnia state

- Chloride-resistant metabolic alkalosis - frequently observed with excessive mineralocorticoid effect and hypokalemia (urine [Cl] >20 mEq/l)
     Primary hyperaldosteronism
     Other causes of excessive mineralocorticoid effect
          Licorice
          Cushing's syndrome/disease
          Congenital adrenocorticoid excess or ectopic ACTH
     Diseases associated with high plasma renin activity
     Potassium depletion
     Bartter's syndrome
     • Milk-alkali syndrome
     • Acute alkali load

The administration of bicarbonate or bicarbonate precursors such as lactate, citrate, or acetate results in excess ECF bicarbonate. In the presence of normal GFR the majority of the bicarbonate load is excreted so only a mild alkalosis develops.

Certain gastrointestinal diseases and diuretics can induce the loss of fluid containing chloride in a greater concentration than bicarbonate leading to ECF volume contraction and a rise in bicarbonate concentration.

The bicarbonate generated is buffered with hydrogen ion derived from intracellular phosphate and protein buffers. Alveolar hypoventilation elevates pCO_2; this compensation is usually limited to a rise in pCO_2 to 55-60 mm Hg, since hypoxia stimulates ventilation. Moreover, even with normal renal function and adequate K and Cl intake, several factors may limit bicarbonate excretion. Development of metabolic alkalosis often leads to ECF volume contraction and intense Cl conservation. The attendant reduction in luminal chloride delivery to the collecting duct may limit $Cl-HCO_3$ exchange while excessive mineralocorticoid activity also stimulates renal generation of bicarbonate.

CLINICAL PRESENTATION

Patients may have muscle cramps or weakness and hyperreflexia. Alveolar hypoventilation can lead to signs of hypoxia and severe alkalemia can lead to cardiac arrhythmias.

Both plasma $[HCO_3]$ and pH are increased. Respiratory compensation increases pCO_2 and may also decrease pO_2. Hypochloremia and hypokalemia are almost invariably present. Volume contraction can increase blood urea nitrogen (BUN) and serum creatinine.

Treatment of chloride-responsive metabolic alkalosis requires administration of sodium chloride and potassium. In cases of sodium-chloride unresponsive alkalosis, the effect of mineralocorticoid excess must be corrected or potassium chloride must be provided. Amiloride or spironolactone can be used to treat hyperaldosteronism not amenable to surgical therapy.

MIXED ACID-BASE DISORDERS

Patients may present with two or even three acid-base disorders. The first step in diagnosis is to define the primary (predominant) disorder and the pulmonary or renal compensation (see Table 8-1). Identification of the primary disturbance can be made by the pH. A pH <7.35 indicates a primary acidosis, while a pH >7.45 indicates a primary alkalosis. "Overcompensation" does not occur for primary acid-base disturbances; however, mixed disorders can yield a "normal" pH. Since identical laboratory data can result from different combinations of acid-base disturbances, the history and physical examination must be used to narrow the differential diagnosis.

A low HCO_3 indicates a metabolic acidosis or respiratory alkalosis. A HCO_3 <15 is usually due to metabolic acidosis. An elevated HCO_3 of >45 occurs most commonly with metabolic alkalosis. Use of the formulas in Table 8-1 assumes adequate time has elapsed to allow full compensation. The nomogram in Figure 8-2 can also be used in place of the equations in Table 8-1.

Table 8-3 Common Causes of Mixed Acid-Base Disorders

Acid-Base Disorder	Etiology	Clinical
Metabolic acidosis/respiratory acidosis	Cardiopulmonary arrest Severe pulmonary edema Poisonings	Lactic acidosis with decreased ventilation Lactic acidosis or specific metabolite (e.g., methanol) with respiratory depression
Metabolic acidosis/respiratory alkalosis	Salicylate intoxication Sepsis Severe liver disease Major burns Acetate hemodialysis	Elevated anion gap acidosis and central respiratory stimulation Lactic acidosis with respiratory stimulation
Metabolic acidosis/metabolic alkalosis	Renal failure with vomiting Alcoholic or diabetic ketoacidosis with vomiting Critically ill patients on gastric suction	Sepsis, renal failure, or diabetic keto-acidosis accompanied by gastric suction
Metabolic alkalosis/respiratory acidosis	Chronic obstructive pulmonary disease with vomiting Chronic obstructive pulmonary disease with diuretics Adult respiratory distress syndrome with gastric suction	Often due to theophylline toxicity Found in patients with cor pulmonale Can be exacerbated with chloride depletion from low NaCl diets
Metabolic alkalosis/respiratory alkalosis	Sepsis with vomiting or gastric suction Inappropriate mechanical ventilation with gastric suction Severe liver disease with vomiting Pregnancy with vomiting or diuretics	Respiratory stimulation with volume contraction Frequently seen in intensive care units Pregnancy normally induces a chronic respiratory alkalosis

The most common clinical settings for mixed acid-base disorders appear in Table 8-3. A severe acidemia can result from a combined metabolic and respiratory acidosis. Even though pCO_2 and bicarbonate may not be severely changed, the pH will be <7.35 and the pCO_2 >45 mm Hg.

In metabolic acidosis and respiratory alkalosis the bicarbonate and pCO_2 are both low, but the pCO_2 will be lower than predicted for the respiratory compensation of the metabolic acidosis.

A mixed metabolic acidosis and metabolic alkalosis can be difficult to diagnose because both disorders affect the serum bicarbonate primarily. The pH and bicarbonate can be high, low, or normal. An elevated anion gap with a high or normal bicarbonate suggests this diagnosis. Many of the causes of metabolic acidosis are accompanied by vomiting so this mixed disorder occurs frequently.

A combined metabolic alkalosis and respiratory acidosis is characterized by a high bicarbonate and high pCO_2. Using the formulas in Table 8-1 the bicarbonate elevation will be greater than predicted for compensation to respiratory acidosis if this is the primary disorder.

Severe alkalemia can result from a combined metabolic and respiratory alkalosis. A mixed alkalosis would be present if a respiratory alkalosis is not accompanied by the appropriate decrease in bicarbonate, or a metabolic alkalosis is not accompanied by the appropriate increase in pCO_2. This combination occurs frequently in critically ill patients due to excessive mechanical ventilation and diuretic use.

Finally, a triple acid-base disturbance can exist. This is due to combined metabolic acidosis and metabolic alkalosis accompanied by either respiratory acidosis or respiratory alkalosis. It frequently occurs in an alcoholic or diabetic patient with vomiting (metabolic alkalosis), lactic or keto acidosis (metabolic acidosis), and a respiratory alkalosis due to sepsis or liver disease.

SUGGESTED READING

Adrogue AJ, Basilver J, Cohen JJ. Influence of steady-state alterations in acid-base equilibrium on the fate of administered bicarbonate in the dog. J Clin Invest 1983;71:867-883.

Emmett M, Narins R. Clinical use of the anion gap. Medicine 1977; 56:38-54.

Galla JH, Luke RG. Pathophysiology of metabolic alkalosis. Hosp Prac 1987;22:95-118.

Hodgkin JE, Soeprone FF, Char DM. Incidence of metabolic alkalemia in hospitalized patients. Crit Care Med 1988;8:725-728.

Narins R, Emmett M. Simple and mixed acid-base disorders: a practical approach. Medicine 1980;59:161-187.

Schrier R. Renal and electrolyte disorders, 3rd ed. 1986;141-206.

Chapter 9

Renal Tubular Acidosis

Charles S. Wingo
Nancy G. Ahlstrom

DEFINITION

Renal tubular acidosis (RTA) is a hyperchloremic, normal anion gap, metabolic acidosis caused by inability of the kidney to excrete the daily acid load. Most of the acid load must be buffered by phosphate, which is the predominant ionic component of titratable acid (TA), or by ammonia (NH_3) to form ammonium (NH_4). **Net urinary (U) acid excretion** is, therefore, ($TA + NH_4 - HCO_3$).

The **fractional excretion of bicarbonate is:**

$$\frac{U_{HCO_3^-}}{P_{HCO_3^-}} \times \frac{P_{creatinine}}{U_{creatinine}}$$

This is normally less than 5%.

Type I RTA was originally described by Albright in 1946 and is also referred to as **classic distal RTA**. Urine pH is always above 5.5.

Type II RTA or **proximal RTA** describes a condition in which there is excessive bicarbonaturia in the absence of severe acidosis, but the urine can become maximally acid during acidosis.

Type III RTA describes a rare childhood disease with severe acidemia, urinary bicarbonate wastage, and failure to decrease the urine pH in the face of acidosis. It is a variant of type I RTA and, therefore, will not be discussed further.

Type IV RTA or **hyperkalemic RTA** describes disorders with modest renal insufficiency, hyperkalemia, and metabolic acidosis.

ETIOLOGY

The most common causes of each of these syndromes are listed in the following display.

Common Causes of RTA

<u>Distal RTA (type I)</u>[1]

- Primary
  Mendelian dominant inheritance
- Secondary
  Autoimmune (Sjögren's, systemic lupus erythematosus)
  Genetic disorders (Sickle cell anemia)
- Disorders causing nephrocalcinosis
  Idiopathic hypercalciuria
  Primary hyperparathyroidism
  Hyperthyroidism
  Medullary sponge kidney
- Toxin-induced nephropathy
  Amphotericin B
  Lithium

<u>Proximal RTA (type II)</u>[1]

- Isolated proximal tubular defect
  Drugs (acetazolamide)
  Genetic
- With Fanconi's Syndrome
  Mendelian recessive error of metabolism (cystinosis)
  As a metabolic consequence of:
    Chronic hypocalcemia and secondary hyperpara-
      thyroidism
    Malabsorption syndromes
    Drugs or toxins (e.g., lead)
- After renal injury from:
  Medullary cystic disease
  Multiple myeloma
  Postrenal transplant
  Nephrotic syndrome

<u>Hyperkalemic RTA (type IV)</u>[2]

- Aldosterone Deficiency
  Addison's disease
  Chronic heparin administration
- Drugs
  Spironolactone
  Amiloride
  Triamterene

- Generalized collecting duct dysfunction frequently associated
  with renal insufficiency
     Lupus nephritis
     Obstructive uropathy
     Chronic pyelonephritis
     Renal transplantation
     Chronic glomerulonephritis

---

[1] Modified from McSherry E. Renal tubular acidosis in childhood.
Kidney Int 1981;20:799-809.
[2] Modified from Brenner BM, Rector FC Jr, eds. The kidney.
Philadelphia: Saunders, 1986; 534.

PATHOPHYSIOLOGY

Several defects have been implicated in the cause of distal RTA.
A common factor is a low excretion of ammonium. This can be assessed
indirectly by the urine anion gap, $U_{Cl} - (U_{Na} + U_K)$. A negative value
implies little ammonium is in the urine. Damage to a proton pump in
the collecting duct or lack of aldosterone stimulation of this pump
could be responsible. Incomplete forms of distal RTA are common and
produce less severe acidosis.

Proximal RTA is the result of impaired reabsorption of bicarbonate in the proximal tubule. Normally, 85% of the filtered load of bicarbonate is reabsorbed in the proximal tubule and 15% is reclaimed by
the distal tubule. The plasma bicarbonate concentration decreases because of increased fractional bicarbonate excretion (FE_{HCO_3}). Eventually, the plasma bicarbonate falls sufficiently to limit the amount
presented to the distal tubule to within its capacity to reabsorb bicarbonate, thus permitting a low urine pH. Therefore, patients with
proximal RTA have only a mild to moderate acidosis (plasma bicarbonate
approximately 15 mEq/l).

CLINICAL PRESENTATION AND DIAGNOSIS

Distal RTA (type I) presents in half of the patients as musculoskeletal complaints (weakness or pain) and in the other half as recurrent nephrolithiasis. Nephrocalcinosis may be seen by X-ray. Because
of the progressive, severe metabolic acidosis seen in "complete"
forms, distal RTA may present in children as a medical emergency with
acute hypokalemic paralysis, coma, shock, or even death if the plasma
bicarbonate is below 3 mEq/l. In type I (distal) RTA, the serum
potassium concentration (S_K) is low or normal, and the urine pH is
always greater than 5.5.

Proximal RTA (type II) generally presents in children as failure
to thrive, growth retardation, vomiting, volume depletion, and
lethargy. X-rays may document rickets in children and osteopenia in
adults. Stone disease is not a clinical feature. The S_K is low or
normal, while the plasma bicarbonate concentration is rarely below 15

mEq/l. The urine pH may be less than 5.5 if the metabolic acidosis is severe, but the FE_{HCO_3} is always greater than 15% if the plasma bicarbonate concentration is > 20 mEq/l.

Hyperkalemic RTA (type IV) is characterized by a mild to moderate metabolic acidosis and hyperkalemia out of proportion to the degree of renal insufficiency. With the complete form of this disorder, the S_K is invariably above 5.5 mEq/l. Most patients will have a history of diabetes mellitus or interstitial nephritis and a creatinine clearance below 45 ml/min. The urine pH may be less than 5.5 in the face of acidosis. Table 9-1 summarizes this information.

If the urine anion gap, $U_{Cl} - (U_{Na} + U_K)$, is positive, U_{NH_4} concentration is probably high and the differential diagnosis includes:

- Proximal RTA
- Gastrointestinal bicarbonate loss
- Renal excretion of ketoacids (diabetic ketoacidosis)
- Increased ingestion of acids (usually iatrogenic--NH_4Cl or $CaCl_2$)

If the urine anion gap is negative, urinary U_{NH_4} is probably decreased and a defect in distal urine acidification exists implicating classic distal or hyperkalemic RTA. If the S_K is greater than 5.5 mEq/l, the patient has hyperkalemic RTA. To further diagnose the cause of hyperkalemic RTA, follow the steps in Figure 9-1.

THERAPY

Therapy for classic **distal RTA (type I)** requires sufficient bicarbonate administration to correct the acidosis. In adults, this is accomplished by oral bicarbonate ingestion at a dose of 1.0 to 2.0 mEq/kg/24 hr. In many patients who also have nephrolithiasis, the stones will resolve with this therapy alone. Others may require potassium citrate or a combination of sodium citrate and potassium citrate. Alkali therapy will generally correct the hypokalemia.

Proximal RTA (type II) is much harder to control. Doses of bicarbonate required for correction range from 10-25 mEq/kg/24 hr due to the increased FE_{HCO_3} as the plasma bicarbonate concentration rises. The increased distal delivery of HCO_3 promotes the secretion of K and can lead to severe hypokalemia. Osteomalacia may require vitamin D and calcium supplements, whereas rickets will be corrected with vitamin D and 1.6 g/day of sodium phosphate.

Table 9-1 Renal Tubular Acidosis -- Distinguishing Features

Type	Clinical Presentation	Serum K	U_{Cl^-} $(U_{Na} + U_K)$	Urine pH in Metabolic Acidosis	Alkali Dose
Classic distal (type I)	Stones, musculo-skeletal complaints	Normal or low	Negative	> 5.5	1.0 - 2.0 mEq/kg/24 hr
Proximal (type II)	Vomiting, volume depletion, growth retardation, failure to thrive, bone disease	Normal or low	Positive	< 5.5 if acidosis is severe	10 - 25 mEq/kg/24 hr
Hyperkalemic (type IV)	Fatigue, weakness, hypotension, nausea, vomiting	> 5.5 mEq/l	Negative	< 5.5 in aldosterone deficiency	1.0 to 2.0 mEq/kg/24 hr
	Edema, hypertension, renal insufficiency, nausea, vomiting			> 5.5 in other conditions	

Figure 9-1 Hyperchloremic Acidosis With Hyperkalemia*

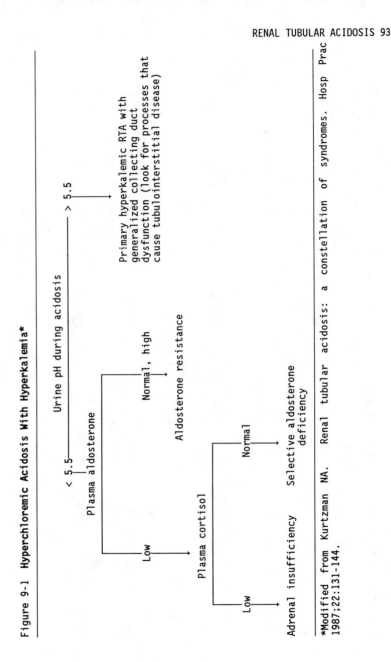

*Modified from Kurtzman NA. Renal tubular acidosis: a constellation of syndromes. Hosp Prac 1987;22:131-144.

Table 9-2 Orally Administered Preparations for Alkali Therapy*

Drug	How Supplied		Dosage Equivalent
Bicitra	Solution	5 ml = sodium citrate, 500 mg; citric acid, 300 mg	1 ml = 1 mEq base
Calcium carbonate	Tablet	420 or 650 mg	
	Powder	1000 mg/½teaspoon	1000 mg = 22.3 mEq base
Polycitra	Solution	5 ml = potassium citrate, 550 mg; sodium citrate, 500 mg; citric acid, 334 mg	1 ml = 2 mEq base and 1 mEq potassium
Polycitra-K	Solution	5 ml = potassium citrate, 1100 mg; citric acid, 334 mg	1 ml = 2 mEq base and 2 mEq potassium
Sodium bicarbonate	Tablet	325 or 650 mg	325 mg = 4 mEq base
	Solution	1 ml = 1 mEq base	650 mg = 8 mEq base
Shohl solution	Solution	1000 ml = citric acid, 140 g; hydrated crystalline sodium citrate, 90 g	1 ml = 1 mEq base

*Modified from Chan JC. Renal tubular acidosis. J Pediatr 1983;102:327-340.

In **hyperkalemic RTA (type IV)**, correction of mineralocorticoid deficiency can be accomplished with fludrocortisone. Glucocorticoid replacement will also be required if adrenal insufficiency is present. However, in many cases a combination of restriction of dietary potassium, use of loop diuretics, and modest alkali therapy (1-2 mEq/kg/24 hr) may be necessary. See Table 9-2 for use of common bicarbonate-containing medications.

SUGGESTED READING

Battle DC, Hiton M, Cohen E, Gutterman C, Gupta K. The use of the urinary anion gap in the diagnosis of hyperchloremic metabolic acidosis. N Engl J Med 1988;318:594-599.

Brenner RJ, Spring DB, Sebastian A, et al. Incidence of radiographically evident bone disease, nephrocalcinosis, and nephrolithiasis in various types of renal tubular acidosis. N Engl J Med 1982;307:217-221.

Chan JC. Renal tubular acidosis. J. Pediatr 1983;102:327-340.

Halperin ML, Goldstein MB, Richardson RMA, Stinebaugh BJ. Distal renal tubular acidosis syndrome: a pathological approach. Am J Nephrol 1985;5:1-8.

Harrington T, Bunch TW, Van Den Berg CJ. Renal tubular acidosis: a new look at treatment of musculoskeletal and renal disease. Mayo Clin Proc 1983;58:354-360.

Kurtzman NA. Renal tubular acidosis: a constellation of syndromes. Hosp Prac 1987;22:131-144.

McSherry E. Renal tubular acidosis in childhood. Kidney Int 1981;20:799-809.

Oster JR, Perez GO, Vaamonde CA. Drug-induced impairment of renal acidification. Clin Update Nephrol 1984;1:1-12.

Richardson RMA, Halperin ML. The urine pH: a potentially misleading diagnostic test in patients with hyperchloremic metabolic acidosis. Am J Kid Dis 1987;10:140-143.

Chapter 10

Calcium, Phosphorus, and Magnesium Disorders

John C. Peterson

CALCIUM

MEASUREMENT OF CALCIUM IN THE BLOOD

Total serum calcium concentration (S_{Ca}) normally is 8.8 to 10.4 mg/dl (2.2 to 2.6 mmol/l). It consists of three portions: 1) protein-bound calcium (~40%); 2) complexed calcium (~15%), which is bound to several anions--citrate, sulfate, lactate, phosphate; and 3) ionized calcium (~45%), which is the biologically active component. Ionized calcium can be measured anaerobically on freshly drawn serum with ion exchange electrodes and ranges from 4.0 to 4.8 mg/dl (1.0 to 1.2 mmol/l).

Factors Altering Total Calcium Concentration

Serum albumin. A decrease of 1 g/dl in serum albumin decreases total S_{Ca} by 0.8 mg/dl.

Tourniquet. Transudation of plasma water (but **not** plasma protein) into the tissues elevates the total S_{Ca}.

Factors Causing Change in Ionized Calcium Without Total S_{Ca} Change

pH. The binding of Ca to protein increases with pH. A change of 0.1 pH units causes a change of 0.12 mg/dl of the ionized calcium in the opposite direction.

Parathyroid hormone (PTH). PTH increases ionized calcium at the expense of protein-bound calcium. All patients with hyperparathyroidism (in the absence of a confounding clinical problem such as renal failure or severe vitamin D deficiency) have elevated ionized calcium.

Serum phosphate. At high concentrations this first lowers ionized calcium, then lowers total S_{Ca} as the calcium phosphate crystals are deposited in bone. In end-stage renal disease a serum phosphate that is twice normal can lower an elevated ionized S_{Ca} to normal.

Because of the previously described relationships, serum albumin and phosphate should always be measured with S_{Ca}.

CALCIUM HOMEOSTASIS

PTH and/or 1,25-D_3 increases S_{Ca}, whereas calcitonin and/or 24,25-D_3 can reduce S_{Ca}.

PTH

Osteoclastic bone resorption is stimulated by PTH. It also enhances distal tubular reabsorption of calcium and stimulates formation of 1,25-D_3, thus increasing gastrointestinal (GI) absorption of calcium and increases fractional excretion of phosphorus.

1,25-D_3

This form of D_3 stimulates both osteoclastic resorption of bone and GI absorption of calcium and augments renal tubular reabsorption of calcium.

Calcitonin

Calcitonin inhibits osteoclastic reabsorption of bone and enhances renal excretion of calcium but does not change **normal** calcium levels.

24,25-D_3

This form of D_3 stimulates bone matrix synthesis and mineralization by osteoblasts and augments GI absorption of calcium (much less potent than 1,25-D_3).

HYPERCALCEMIA

DEFINITION

Hypercalcemia is defined by total S_{Ca} >10.5 mg/dl (2.63 mmol/l) or an ionized calcium of >4.8 mg/dl (1.2 mmol/l).

INCIDENCE AND PREVALENCE

The prevalence in the general population ranges from 0.05 to 0.6%. Malignancy and primary hyperparathyroidism account for 70-80% of all causes of hypercalcemia.

PATHOPHYSIOLOGY

Following a calcium infusion, S_{Ca} returns to normal when only 10-15% of the infused load has been excreted. Thus, the skeleton has a remarkable ability to buffer changes in S_{Ca}. Hypercalcemia is a perturbation of the dynamic equilibrium between osteolytic and osteoblastic factors.

Figure 10-1 Evaluation of Hypercalcemia

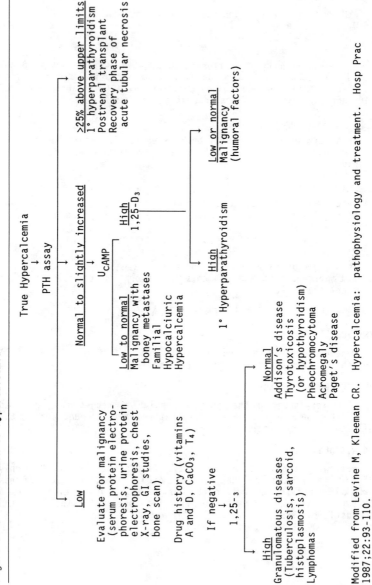

Modified from Levine M, Kleeman CR. Hypercalcemia: pathophysiology and treatment. Hosp Prac 1987;22:93-110.

CAUSES AND PATHOGENESIS OF HYPERCALCEMIA

Overall, 90% of cases of hypercalcemia are due to primary hyperparathyroidism (most common cause), malignancy, or granulomatous diseases.

Primary Hyperparathyroidism

The hypercalcemia is due to increased bone resorption, increased absorption of calcium caused indirectly through PTH stimulation of $1,25-D_3$, and increased renal reabsorption of calcium. Asymptomatic hypercalcemia is now the major presentation.

Primary hyperparathyroidism occurs more frequently in women, especially after the menopause, reflecting the efficacy of estrogens as inhibitors of PTH-mediated osteolysis.

Approximately 75% of patients with primary hyperparathyroidism have single adenomas, while 25% have multiglandular adenomatosis or hyperplasia. Parathyroid carcinoma is found in only 1-2% of patients.

Malignancy

The incidence of hypercalcemia in patients with neoplasms is 10-20%. The most common primaries are breast and lung cancer and multiple myeloma. Malignant hypercalcemia is mediated via three mechanisms:

- Local destruction of bone by metastatic lesions.
- Recruitment of osteoclasts by tumor-produced humoral factors.
- Very rarely, the tumor may secrete an ectopic PTH.

Granulomatous Disorders

Sarcoidosis, tuberculosis, and histoplasmosis all produce elevation of $1,25-D_3$ levels from activated monocytes.

Thyroid Disease

Thyroid hormone accelerates osteolysis, and 10-20% of thyrotoxic patients have hypercalcemia and suppressed PTH levels. Hypothyroidism can also cause hypercalcemia presumably by reducing bone turnover.

Vitamin D Intoxication

This condition is seen most commonly in dialysis patients or women undergoing treatment for osteomalacia. The half-life of the 25-hydroxylated analogue is from 10-20 days, whereas that of $1,25-D_3$ is much less.

Immobilization

Immobilization inhibits bone accretion but does not produce hypercalcemia unless bone turnover is accelerated (e.g., an adolescent or an elderly patient with Paget's disease).

End-Stage Renal Disease

These patients (especially dialysis patients) are at risk for hypercalcemia due to vitamin D toxicity, phosphate depletion (overvigorous use of phosphate binders resulting in increased osteolysis), conversion of secondary hyperparathyroidism to an autonomous condition (so-called "tertiary hyperparathyroidism"), or aluminum toxicity which inhibits bone mineralization.

Postrenal Transplant

Hypercalcemia may be caused by parathyroid gland hyperplasia that developed during renal insufficiency; it usually abates within 6 months.

Acute Renal Failure

Hypercalcemia can occur in the polyuric recovery phase. It is due to elevated PTH and 1,25-D$_3$ levels and dissolution of ectopic (usually muscle) calcium phosphate deposits.

Milk-Alkai Syndrome

This condition is caused by ingestion of large amounts of calcium (>5 g/day) and alkali. The alkalosis increases protein binding of calcium and stimulates tubular Ca reabsorption, thus preventing renal excretion of the calcium load.

Thiazide Diuretics

Thiazides can worsen hypercalcemia in patients with primary hyperparathyroidism, whereas normal individuals have only a mild or transient hypercalcemia. Thiazides increase Ca reabsorption in the proximal and early distal tubule.

CLINICAL PRESENTATION

Signs and Symptoms Associated with Hypercalcemia

- Anorexia, nausea, and vomiting
- Constipation
- Polyuria and polydipsia
- Hypertension
- Confusion, stupor, and coma
- Nephrolithiasis
- Decreased renal function
- Peptic ulcer disease
- Metastatic calcification
- Electrocardiogram changes (shortened conduction intervals)

DIAGNOSTIC TESTS

PTH Assay

The primary metabolism of PTH produces two fragments--the carboxy-terminus (C-terminal) which is inactive, and the amino-terminus (N-terminal) which contains the active portion. The intact hormone assay most accurately reflects the time-integrated level of PTH secretion and is the preferred assay but it is not widely available. The N-terminal fragment has an extremely short turnover time. Thus, it reflects the secretion of PTH and is more useful in research. The C-terminal fragment is a good estimate of the steady-state secretory rate of PTH but is metabolized by the kidney and cannot be used in patients with impaired renal function.

Urinary Cyclic AMP (cAMP)

Since the urinary cAMP is a result of the renal actions of PTH, it represents the minute-to-minute activity of PTH on the renal tubule. Excretion of cAMP depends on the number of responding tubules. Correction for this can be performed by dividing the absolute value of urinary cAMP by the creatinine clearance. The great majority of patients with primary hyperparathyroidism will have massively elevated values even in the presence of mild renal insufficiency (up to creatinine <3 mg/dl). A carefully timed 1- or 2-hr urine collection will suffice.

DIFFERENTIAL DIAGNOSIS

Certain signs and symptoms related to specific entities causing hypercalcemia are discussed below.

Signs and Symptoms Associated with Specific Diseases

- Hyperparathyroidism - nephrolithiasis, hyperchloremic acidosis, hypophosphatemia, pseudogout, osteitis fibrosa cystica on bone X-rays
- Sarcoidosis - hilar adenopathy on chest X-ray, rash, lymphadenopathy, conduction abnormalities on ECG
- Malignancy - S_{Ca} above 15 mg/dl (3.75 mmol/l), anorexia, weight loss
- Thyrotoxicosis - hyperreflexia, systolic hypertension

The PTH levels in patients with hypercalcemia of malignancy are normal or low, whereas levels in patients with primary hyperparathyroidism are generally 25% above the upper limit of normal.

Table 10-1 lists in order of preference the major agents used to treat hypercalcemia. Etidronate is investigational.

Table 10-1 Treatment for Hypercalcemia

Agent	Mechanism of Action	Initial Dose/Route	Onset of Action	Complications/ Limitations
Saline	Increased urinary calcium excretion	Load with 2 liters/1 hr, then replace urine volume with saline	4 hr	Volume overload
Furosemide	Increased urinary calcium excretion	40-80 mg intravenously every 2-4 hr	4-8 hr	Volume, Mg and K depletion
Calcitonin	Decreased bone resorption	4 IU/kg every 12 hr subcutaneously or intramuscularly	6-24 hr	Nausea, tachyphylaxis
Mithramycin	PTH or Vitamin D antagonsim	25 μg/kg intravenously via slow infusion (3-6 hr)	12-36 hr	Bleeding disorders
Corticosteroids	Vitamin D antagonism	40-100 mg by mouth every day with rapid taper	3-6 days	Hypercorticism
Oral phosphate	Deposition of calcium in bone	By mouth-1.5 g phosphorus/ day in divided doses	2-4 days	Diarrhea
Etidronate disodium	Inhibition of osteoclasts	7.5 mg/kg intravenously every day	1-2 days	None reported (Am J Med 82:Supplement 2A, 1987)
Hemodialysis	Removal of calcium	Standard 4 hr treatment - use low calcium bath!	4-8 hr	General complications of dialysis

TREATMENT OF HYPERCALCEMIA

Treatment of Hypercalcemia

- Volume repletion; correction of associated hypokalemia or hypomagnesemia.
- Discontinuance of drugs contributing to hypercalcemia (vitamins D and A, thiazide diuretics, lithium, theophylline).
- Regulation of digitalis dose; hypercalcemia accentuates its toxicity.
- Early mobilization diminishes hypercalcemia.

The safest acute therapy is saline and a furosemide diuresis as outlined below.

Forced Diuresis for Treatment of Hypercalcemia

- Priming dose of 1-2 liters of isotonic saline intravenously (IV) over 1 hr.
- Furosemide, 40-80 mg IV, every 2-3 hr.
- Measure urine volume hourly and urine Na, K, Mg every 4-6 hr.
- Replace urinary losses with isotonic saline and KCl.
- If diuresis is to be continued over 24-48 hr, replace Mg losses with intermittent doses of 1 g $MgSO_4$ added to IV fluids.

Hypercalcemia requires immediate therapy when:

- Central nervous system symptoms are present.
- Total S_{Ca} is >13 mg/dl (3.25 mmol/l).
- Calcium times the phosphorus product exceeds 80 (risk of metastatic calcification is high).

HYPOCALCEMIA

DEFINITION

Total S_{Ca} below 8.5 mg/dl (2.13 mmol/l) with a normal albumin concentration.

ETIOLOGY

Hypoalbuminemia (Pseudohypocalcemia)

Hypomagnesemia

- Secretion of PTH and resistance to PTH action on bone

Acute Respiratory Alkalosis

- Increase in pH results in increased protein binding of Ca with decreased ionized Ca.

Vitamin D Deficiency (↓ GI absorption of Ca)

- Nutritional (decreased intake or malabsorption).
- Decreased production of 25-OH D_3 (liver disease) or 1,25-D_3 (chronic renal failure).
- Accelerated loss of 25-OH D_3 (nephrotic syndrome, abnormalities of enterohepatic circulation).

PTH Deficiency

- Absence of tissue (surgical, tumor, amyloid infiltration, or idiopathic).
- Pseudohypoparathyroidism (end-organ resistance to effects of PTH associated with short stature, mental retardation, round face, obesity and foreshortened fourth metacarpals and metatarsals).

"Chemical" Removal of Calcium from the Serum

- Hyperphosphatemia (end-stage renal disease, laxatives, phosphate enemas, tumor lysis syndromes, rhabdomyolysis).
- Osteoblastic metastases (prostatic carcinoma).
- Pancreatitis (retroperitoneal saponification).
- "Hungry bone syndrome" - (patients with severe secondary hyperparathyroidism after parathyroidectomy).

CLINICAL PRESENTATION

Manifestations include tetany, muscle spasms, cramps, carpopedal spasm, and seizures. Latent tetany can be detected by a light tap over the facial nerve resulting in an ipsilateral facial twitch (Chvostek's sign) or by inflation of a sphygmomanometer above the systolic pressure for more than 3 minutes resulting in carpal spasm (Trousseau's sign).

Hypocalcemia can cause congestive heart failure, hypotension, prolongation of the Q-T interval, ventricular conduction abnormalities, and resistance to digitalis.

DIFFERENTIAL DIAGNOSIS

The first step is verification of true hypocalcemia, i.e., reduction of ionized calcium. Serum albumin and pH must be measured to exclude pseudohypocalcemia and acute respiratory alkalosis. The next step is to exclude hypomagnesemia. The third step is to evaluate the PTH and, if necessary, the vitamin D axis as indicated in Figure 10-2.

Figure 10-2 Evaluation of Hypocalcemia

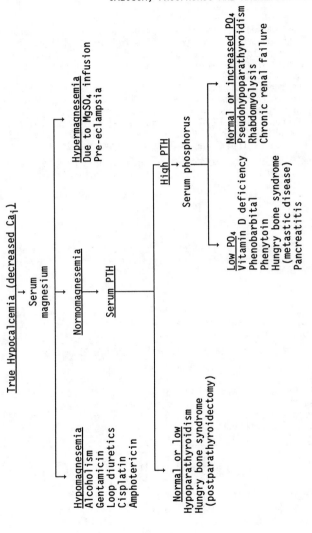

True Hypocalcemia (decreased Ca_i)
→ Serum magnesium

Hypomagnesemia
Alcoholism
Gentamicin
Loop diuretics
Cisplatin
Amphotericin

Normomagnesemia
→ Serum PTH

Hypermagnesemia
Due to $MgSO_4$ infusion
Pre-eclampsia

Normal or low
Hypoparathyroidism
Hungry bone syndrome
(postparathyroidectomy)

High PTH
→ Serum phosphorus

Low PO_4
Vitamin D deficiency
Phenobarbital
Phenytoin
Hungry bone syndrome
(metastic disease)
Pancreatitis

Normal or increased PO_4
Pseudohypoparathyroidism
Rhabdomyolysis
Chronic renal failure

TREATMENT

Acute symptomatic hypocalcemia requires immediate therapy with 10-15 mEq (200-300 mg) of intravenous Ca to forestall laryngeal spasm and/or seizures. This can be supplied by one 10-ml ampule of $CaCl_2$ (272 mg Ca per 10-ml vial) or preferably by 10-20 ml of calcium gluconate (90 mg Ca per 10-ml ampule), which is less irritating. The infusion rate should not exceed 2 ml/min. Patients on digoxin require ECG monitoring. Intravenous Ca should not be mixed with any solution containing bicarbonate because $CaCO_3$ will precipitate. In severe hypocalcemia, continuous IV infusion of Ca may be necessary, i.e., 15-20 mg/kg body weight over 4 to 8 hr (30-40 ml of 10% Ca gluconate in 500-1000 ml of 5% Dextrose over 4-8 hr) to prevent tetany.

Thereafter start oral calcium supplements (and vitamin D if indicated) as $CaCO_3$ and Ca lactate (1.0 - 2.0 g of calcium three times a day by mouth.)

PHOSPHORUS

INTRODUCTION

The normal concentration of serum phosphorus in adults is 2.8-4.5 mg/dl (0.9 - 1.6 mmol/l). It exists mainly as a free ion; only 15% is protein-bound.

PHOSPHORUS BALANCE

The major influence on phosphorus balance is renal; 85-90% of the filtered load is reabsorbed in the proximal tubule and the final ~10% in the distal nephron.

Factors Known to Increase Urinary Phosphate Excretion

• PTH (inhibits proximal and distal phosphate reabsorption)
• Cortisol
• Vitamin D - increased tubular phosphate reabsorption acutely, but chronically phosphaturia may occur secondary to an increased filtered load.
• Lack of growth hormone
• High dietary phosphorus intake

HYPOPHOSPHATEMIA

INCIDENCE

In hospitalized patients, 10-15% develop moderate hypophosphatemia (1.0-2.5 mg/dl).

ETIOLOGY

Hypophosphatemia is caused by external losses (GI or renal) or redistribution of extracellular phosphorus into cells. Inadequate dietary intake does not cause severe hypophosphatemia.

Organ Systems Affected by Hypophosphatemia

- Red blood cells - decreased deformability causes hemolysis; also reduced 2, 3-DPG content thereby decreasing O_2 delivery.
- White blood cells - decreased phagocytic and chemotactic responses predisposing to bacterial and fungal infections.
- Muscle - skeletal myopathy (elevated creatine phosphokinase) can cause respiratory failure; cardiomyopathy is frequent.
- Bone - osteolysis can progress to osteomalacia.
- Central nervous system - metabolic encephalopathy with diffuse slowing on electroencephalogram.

CLINICAL PRESENTATION

Symptoms rarely result until the serum phosphorus falls below 1.0 mg/dl.

Causes of Hypophosphatemia

Excessive External Losses
- Decreased GI absorption
  Prolonged malnutrition
  Malabsorption
  Vitamin D deficiency (vitamin D-dependent rickets)
  Chronic diarrhea
  Aluminum-containing antacids
- Primary renal losses
  Primary hyperparathyroidism
  Secondary hyperparathyroidism (including postrenal transplantation)
  Extracellular fluid (ECF) expansion
  Diuretics (acetazolamide)
  Fanconi's syndrome
  Postobstructive diuresis
  Diuretic phase of recovery from acute tubular necrosis
  Glycosuria (especially with chronic diabetic keto-acidosis)

Redistribution
- Respiratory alkalosis
- Recovery from malnutrition
- Alcohol withdrawal
- Severe burns
- Parenteral hyperalimentation

DIFFERENTIAL DIAGNOSIS

The key to diagnosis is the urinary phosphorus excretion. Values below 100 mg/day imply GI losses or redistribution. If urinary phosphorus exceeds 100 mg/day, tubular defects (glycosuria, amino-aciduria, or bicarbonaturia) associated with Fanconi's syndrome should be considered. If these are absent, a S_{Ca} will discriminate between primary hyperparathyroidism (elevated calcium), secondary hyperparathyroidism, or vitamin D-resistant rickets (low calcium).

TREATMENT

The goal of therapy is to provide a daily intake of approximately 1000 mg (32 mmols) of elemental phosphorus.

Phosphorus Repletion

Oral Compounds

Compound	Phosphorus Content
Skim milk	1000 mg/qt
Whole milk	850 mg/qt
Neutra-Phos-K-capsules*	250 mg/capsule
Neutra-Phos solution	128 mg/ml solution

*Contain 1.90 mEq/ml when given in solution form.

Intravenous Compounds

Compound	Phosphorus Content (mmol/ml)	Na (mEq/ml)	K (mEq/ml)
K phosphate	3.0	0	4.4
Na phosphate	3.0	4.0	0
Neutral Na, K phosphate	1.1	0.2	0.02

If given along with hyperalimentation, 450 mg of elemental phosphorus should be given with each 1000 Kcal infused. The dose of intravenous phosphorus should not exceed 2 mg elemental phosphorus/kg body weight per 6-hr period to prevent metastatic calcium phosphate crystallization. Serial treatments should be given to restore the serum phosphorus to 2.5 mg/dl.

HYPERPHOSPHATEMIA

DEFINITION

Serum phosphorus level exceeds 5 mg/dl (1.6 mEq/l).

CAUSES

- Decreased glomerular filtration rate - usually <20 ml/min.

- Increased tubular reabsorption
    Hypoparathyroidism (including pseudohypoparathyroidism)
    Acromegaly
    Thyrotoxicosis
    EHDP (ethane-1-hydroxy-1, 1-diphosphanate) - a potent
    stimulator of phosphorus reabsorption which is approved
    for use in Paget's disease of bone.

- Massive release of phosphorus into the ECF

- Massive release of phosphorus into the ECF
    Endogenous
        Tumor lysis (cytotoxic therapy)
        Rhabdomyolysis
    Exogenous
        Vitamin D administration - especially use of $1,25-D_3$
        in patients with chronic renal failure
        Phosphate enemas

CLINICAL PRESENTATION

The main symptoms of hyperphosphatemia are due to hypocalcemia caused by precipitation of insoluble complexes of calcium phosphate. In addition, phosphate decreases renal conversion of $25-D_3$ to $1,25-D_3$ and thereby decreases GI absorption of calcium.

TREATMENT

Because phosphorus is ubiquitous in food, dietary restriction is impractical and phosphate binders are required to decrease GI absorption. Aluminum-containing antacids have been associated with aluminum toxicity in patients with chronic renal failure. Combined use of $CaCO_3$ and $Al(OH)_3$ reduces the amount of aluminum exposure. The goal is to maintain the serum phosphorus below 4.5 mg/dl.

For **acute hyperphosphatemia**, saline infusion will increase renal clearance. The addition of 1 ampule of D_{50} combined with 10 units of regular insulin can be given intermittently or as a continuous infusion to partition phosphorus into cells. Hemo- or peritoneal dialysis can remove large quantities of inorganic phosphorus.

MAGNESIUM

SERUM MAGNESIUM

The serum magnesium concentration (S_{Mg}) is maintained between 1.8 and 2.3 mg/dl (0.75-0.95 mmol/l). Only 15% is protein bound.

PATHOPHYSIOLOGY

With a normal daily intake of 300 mg (12.5 mmol) of magnesium per day, 30-40% is absorbed. Renal excretion of magnesium is generally about 5% of the filtered load (100 mg/day) but can be greatly reduced (0.5%) by hypomagnesemia or increased (40-80%) by hypermagnesemia. The thick ascending limb of the loop of Henle is responsible for the bulk of magnesium reabsorption.

HYPERMAGNESEMIA

DEFINITION

Hypermagnesemia is defined as serum magnesium above 2.3 mg/dl (1.9 mEq/l).

ETIOLOGY

- Chronic renal failure
- Acute renal failure
- $MgSO_4$ administration (toxemia of pregnancy)
- Mg-containing antacids or enemas (especially in setting of renal insufficiency or failure)

Hypermagnesemia is rare in patients with normal renal function unless massive loads of magnesium are given.

SIGNS AND SYMPTOMS

Hypermagnesemia blocks neuromuscular transmission, cardiac conduction, and CNS function. Tendon reflexes decrease at a S_{Mg} above 5-6 mg/dl (2.1-2.5 mmol/l). Higher levels cause confusion, lethargy, hypotension, respiratory and cardiac depression, and ultimately death.

TREATMENT

All effects of hypermagnesemia are antagonized by intravenous calcium. This should be used only as a temporary measure before removal of excess magnesium by hemodialysis.

HYPOMAGNESEMIA

DEFINITION

Hypomagnesemia is defined as serum magnesium below 1.8 mg/dl (0.75 mmol/l).

ETIOLOGY

- Decreased intake
    Chronic alcoholism
    Starvation or enteral feeding without Mg
- Decreased GI absorption
    Prolonged nasogastric suction
    Malabsorption
- Increased renal losses
    Chronic alcoholism
    Diuretic therapy (especially loop diuretics)
    Postobstructive diuresis
    Polyuric phase of recovery from ATN
    Diabetic ketoacidosis
    Hypercalcemia
    Primary hyperaldosteronism
    Drugs (aminoglycosides, cis-platin, cyclosporine)
    Bartter's syndrome

PATHOPHYSIOLOGY

Chronic alcoholism is the most common cause of hypomagnesemia. Acute intake of alcohol increases urinary excretion of magnesium and when this is compounded by poor dietary intake of magnesium-containing foods (green, leafy vegetables), hypomagnesemia results.

Hypomagnesemia can produce hypokalemia and hypocalcemia. Magnesium depletion causes excessive urinary losses of K which are correctable only with Mg replacement.

Patients with severe hypomagnesemia may have muscular fasciculations and positive Chvostek and Trousseau signs. Electrocardiographic changes may mimic those of hypokalemia (prolonged QT and broadening and flattening of T waves with U wave formation). Clearly, Ca and K should always be measured when hypomagnesia is suspected. Digitalis toxicity is markedly potentiated by hypomagnesemia.

TREATMENT

Hypomagnesemic tetany requires IV $MgSO_4$ (each gram of $MgSO_4$ contains 8.12 mEq or 98 mg of Mg). With normal renal function, mix 6 g (24 mmol) of $MgSO_4$ in 1000 ml D_5W and infuse continuously over 6 hr. Thereafter, adjust the infusion to the serum Mg.

For prolonged oral supplement, MgO (1 g contains 600 mg Mg), 250-500 mg by mouth four times daily is well tolerated.

SUGGESTED READING

Editronate disodium: a new therapy for hypercalcemia of malignancy (proceedings of a symposium). Am J Med 1987;82 (Suppl 24).

Levine MM, Kleeman CR. Hypercalcemia: pathophysiology and treatment. Hosp Prac 1987;22:93-110.

Mundy GR. Hypercalcemia of malignancy revisited. J Clin Invest 1988;82:1-6.

Slatopolsky E, Klahr S. Disorders of calcium, phosphorus and magnesium metabolism. In: Schrier RS, Gottschalk CW, eds. Diseases of the kidney. 4th ed. Boston: Little, Brown, and Company, 1988;2865-2921.

Chapter 11

Renal Stone Disease

Joel T. Van Sickler
John C. Peterson

INTRODUCTION

Renal stone disease affects 4% of the general population. After an initial episode, the risk of recurrence ranges from 20 to 50% during the following 10 years. Prompt diagnosis and therapy are required to prevent complications such as infection, obstructive uropathy, and bleeding.

Table 11-1 **Classification of Kidney Stones**

Types of Stones	Incidence %	Predisposing Factors
Calcium salts	70	
Calcium oxalate Calcium oxalate and hydroxyapatite	67	Hypercalciuria, hyperoxaluria, hyperuricosuria
Brushite and hydroxyapatite	3	Renal tubular acidosis, alkaline urine
Struvite	20	Alkaline urine due to urea-splitting organisms
Uric acid	5	Gout, hyperuricosuria, acidic urine
Cystine	3	Cystinuria, acidic urine
Insoluble organic compounds	2	Triamterene

PATHOPHYSIOLOGY

Stone formation is preceded by crystallization within the tubules or collecting system. The salts which precipitate to form renal stones are present in urinary concentrations above their solubility limits (supersaturated) in both normal individuals and those with stone disease. Thus, there is potential for developing a solid phase (nucleation) (Fig. 11-1). A transient rise in supersaturation or the addition of urinary debris can initiate nucleation.

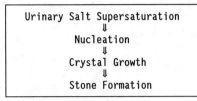

Urinary Salt Supersaturation
⇓
Nucleation
⇓
Crystal Growth
⇓
Stone Formation

Figure 11-1 **Events in Stone Formation**

Therefore, supersaturation of urinary salts, which is the primary pathogenetic mechanism, can be due to:

- Low urinary volumes (e.g., hot climates).

- High excretory concentrations of ionic substances (e.g., calcium, uric acid, or oxalate).

- Abnormal urinary pH (e.g., uric acid and cystine are less soluble in acid urine, while struvite and calcium phosphate are less soluble in alkaline urine).

- A urinary nidus for crystal precipitation (e.g., uric acid crystallization promotes calcium oxalate stone formation).

- Deficiency of inhibitors of stone formation (e.g., citrate, magnesium, pyrophosphate, and glycoproteins).

CLINICAL PRESENTATION

Stones (except struvite) form on the surfaces of renal papillae. While they may remain asymptomatic, there are several clinical sequelae to stone formation:

- *Hematuria* may occur from stone erosion into the renal pelvis.

- *Nephrocalcinosis* can be the presenting feature (e.g., patients with distal renal tubular acidosis).

- *Dislodgement of a stone* may cause flank pain (intense, steady pain radiating to the groin associated with nausea and vomiting), distal obstruction, and/or hematuria.

- *Renal damage* may result from urinary tract obstruction, infection, or nephrocalcinosis.

- *Staghorn calculi* (struvite, uric acid, or cystine stones which grow in the renal pelvis and branch into the calices) may result in obstruction, recurrent urinary tract infections, and renal failure.

DIAGNOSIS

The following points are essential for an accurate diagnosis:

- *History* with emphasis on diet, drug ingestion, familial disorders.

- *Urinalysis* usually reveals either gross or microscopic hematuria. If pyuria is present, infection should be excluded by a urine culture. Crystalluria may permit a presumptive identification of stone type (see Fig. 11-2).

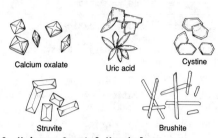

Calcium oxalate   Uric acid   Cystine

Struvite   Brushite

Figure 11-2 **Urinary Crystal Morphology**

- *Plain abdominal X-ray* may show a radiopaque stone (85% of all stones) containing either calcium, struvite, or cystine but may miss small and radiolucent stones (e.g., uric acid). An intravenous pyelogram can determine whether an opacity seen on plain X-ray is within the collecting system and may disclose radiolucent stones.

- *Ultrasonography* can also be used to identify radiolucent stones and obstructive uropathy.

- *Furosemide renogram* can define obstruction and quantify plasma flow to each kidney.

- *Crystallographic stone analysis* is critical to establish the chemical nature of a stone and to plan suitable therapy. The yield is increased if the urine is sieved by the patient.

Table 11-2 **Laboratory Tests to Evaluate Nephrolithiasis***

Serum (Fasting)	Frequency	Urine (24-hr)	Frequency
Calcium	2	Calcium	2
Uric acid	2	Uric acid	2
Phosphate	1	Oxalate	2
Creatinine	2	Creatinine	2
Sodium	1	Sodium	1
Carbon dioxide	1	Cystine (random)	1
Chloride	1	Urinalysis (random)	1
Potassium	1	pH (fasting)	1

* Patients should ingest their regular diet.

- Screening for appropriate metabolic disorders. There is sufficient variation in urine and plasma measurements (due to diet, etc.) that a metabolic cause for recurrent nephrolithiasis cannot be excluded without repeated measurements (Tables 11-2 and 11-3).

Table 11-3 **Urinary Excretion Rates of Salts**

Substance	Upper Limits of Normal	
	Men	Women
Calcium, mg/24 hr	300	250
mg/kg/24 hr	4	
mg/mg creatinine	0.14	
Oxalate, mg/24 hr	50	50
Uric acid, mg/24 hr	800	750

CHARACTERISTICS OF DIFFERENT FORMS OF NEPHROLITHIASIS

CALCIUM STONES

Hypercalciuria is detected in 50% of patients with calcium stones and is usually idiopathic (42% of patients) or secondary to a metabolic disorder.

Idiopathic hypercalciuria is frequently due to intestinal calcium hyperabsorption (absorptive hypercalciuria). This leads to transient hypercalcemia which suppresses parathyroid hormone (PTH) secretion and thereby decreases renal tubular calcium reabsorption and, thus, restores the serum calcium. Other patients have a primary abnormality in renal tubular reabsorption of calcium (renal hypercalciuria) and a normal serum PTH. The mechanism is unclear.

A variety of metabolic disorders can result in hypercalciuria predisposing to stone formation. Primary hyperparathyroidism causes hypercalcemia which increases the filtered load of calcium to cause hypercalciuria and accounts for 11% of calcium stones.

Major Metabolic Causes of Hypercalciuria

- Primary hyperparathyroidism
- Sarcoidosis
- Distal renal tubular acidosis
- Excess vitamin D and calcium intake
- Immobilization
- Milk-alkali syndrome

Approximately 10% of the normal population are hypercalciuric, yet less than half develop renal stone disease. Deficiency of endogenous inhibitors of calcium crystal formation (citrate, pyrophosphate, glycoproteins, and magnesium) are likely involved.

Calcium phosphate stones occur in patients with persistently alkaline urine. Ingestion of excessive alkali, infections, and distal renal tubular acidosis are predisposing factors.

Finally, approximately 50% of patients with calcium stones have no identifiable abnormality.

Hyperoxaluria (>60 mg/day) may be more important in predisposing patients to calcium oxalate stones than hypercalciuria. Primary hyperoxaluria is a rare, autosomal recessive inborn error of metabolism that leads to recurrent stone formation and renal failure in childhood. It is treated with phosphates and pyridoxine. Secondary hyperoxaluria is more common (see display below). In patients with fat malabsorption, calcium is bound by fatty acids instead of oxalate, leaving excessive oxalate for colonic absorption. Also unabsorbed fatty acids and bile salts may injure colonic mucosa, permitting increased oxalate absorption.

Secondary Causes of Hyperoxaluria

- Gastrointestinal Disorders
    Bacterial overgrowth
    Jejunoileal bypass
    Ileal resection
    Chronic pancreatitis
    Biliary disorders
    Inflammatory bowel disease

- Other Causes
    Dietary excesses of oxalate
    Ascorbic acid ingestion
    Pyridoxine deficiency
    Ethylene glycol intoxication
    Methoxyflurane

Hyperuricosuria is due mainly to excessive ingestion of purines. It also predisposes patients to calcium oxalate stones. The uric acid crystal probably acts as a nidus on which calcium oxalate crystals build.

STRUVITE (MAGNESIUM AMMONIUM PHOSPHATE) STONES

Urinary tract infections by urea-splitting bacteria (i.e., Proteus, Pseudomonas, Klebsiella, rarely Escherichia coli, and Staphylococcus) are a requirement for the development of struvite stones. Ammonia excretion is elevated in the face of an alkaline urine. Since about 50% of struvite stones develop on a nidus composed of another crystal (usually calcium oxalate), causes for calcium and uric acid stones must be sought. Stones can develop rapidly forming staghorn calculi that can cause obstruction and urosepsis.

URIC ACID STONES

These stones form when there is hyperuricosuria, persistence of an acidic urine, and/or reduction of urine volume (from dehydration). Most patients have normal uric acid levels in blood and urine. However, hyperuricosuria, especially >1 g/day, predisposes to stone formation. Myeloproliferative syndromes, chemotherapeutic treatment of malignant tumors, and Lesch-Nyhan syndrome cause profound hyperuricosuria and can result in stones or urate nephropathy (see Chapter 20).

CYSTINE STONES

Cystinuria results from an inherited tubular defect in the transport of cystine as well as ornithine, arginine, and lysine. Patients typically develop nephrolithiasis between the ages of 20 and 30 years. Cystine is poorly soluble, especially in acid urine. Cystine excretion in these patients is >1 g/day. Urinalysis will reveal the characteristic hexagonal crystals in 50% of affected patients. The urinary nitroprusside screening test is positive with 75-175 mg cystine/g of creatinine. Confirmation is made by measurement of cystine excretion (in a 24-hr urine) which normally exceeds 40 to 60 mg/g creatinine.

MANAGEMENT OF STONE DISEASE

ACUTE THERAPY

Initial therapy should be directed at providing pain relief, which usually requires narcotic administration. Intravenous fluid administration is warranted in patients who have dehydration from vomiting and fluid also increases urinary flow facilitating stone passage. Potential indications for hospitalization include:

- Inability to control pain
- Severe vomiting
- Severe urinary tract infection or sepsis
- Complete urinary tract obstruction
- Partial obstruction in a solitary kidney

Approximately 80% of stones will pass spontaneously. The single most predictive factor of stone passage is size; 93% <4 mm will pass, while stones >8 mm rarely pass. Extracorporeal shock-wave lithotripsy (ESWL) is an effective treatment of renal stone disease. Advantages include lower morbidity, fewer hospital days, and lower cost than surgery.

GENERAL APPROACH

Smith has categorized stone disease into 4 groups.

- Surgically active - obstruction, colic, or infection is present.
- Metabolically active - continuous stone formation while on therapy during the first year.
- Metabolically inactive - neither 1 or 2 is present for 3 years.
- Disease of indeterminate metabolic activity - no stone has passed and prior studies for comparison are lacking.

Patients with metabolically active stone disease require a full evaluation and specific long-term therapy. Patients with inactive disease are treated with a high fluid intake and close follow-up. Patients in the indeterminate group are placed on a high fluid intake plus specific dietary restrictions. They require regular follow-up with periodic X-rays (e.g., plain abdominal X-ray).

CALCIUM STONES

<u>Dietary Considerations</u>

- Increase urine output to 3 l daily.
- Reduce dietary intake of calcium when excessive (e.g., decrease dairy products and avoid calcium-containing antacids). If hyperoxaluria is present, calcium intake should not be restricted (oxalate absorption will increase).
- Restrict dietary intake of spinach, cranberries, tea, cocoa, and nuts if hyperoxaluria is present.
- In presence of hypercalciuria restrict NaCl to 6 g/day (increased sodium excretion is associated with increased calcium excretion).
- In presence of hyperuricosuria restrict meat intake to 8-10 oz or 225-300 g/day.

<u>Drug Therapy of Hypercalciuric Patients</u>

- **Thiazide diuretics** including hydrochlorothiazide (25-50 mg twice a day) can decrease calcium excretion 40-60% and lower urinary excretion of oxalate. Dietary salt must be restricted. Furosemide which increases calcium excretion is contra-indicated.
- **Cellulose sodium phosphate**, which binds to intestinal calcium and decreases absorption, is useful in absorptive hypercalci-uria. Hyperoxaluria and hypomagnesiuria can occur. Therefore,

dietary oxalate restriction and magnesium supplements are needed. Side effects include gastrointestinal (GI) discomfort and arthralgias.

- **Neutral sodium phosphate** (500 mg of phosphate four times a day) increases pyrophosphate excretion and decreases calcium excretion. The primary side effect is diarrhea.

- **Thiazide and allopurinol** are useful in patients with both hypercalciuria and hyperuricosuria. Hyperuricosuric patients can benefit from allopurinol (200 mg/day), which will inhibit urate synthesis and decrease urinary saturation of monosodium urate. Side effects of allopurinol include: skin rash (especially if there is renal insufficiency), GI disturbances, and occasionally interstitial nephritis.

- **Thiazides and phosphate therapy** decrease stone formation in patients who are neither hypercalciuric nor hyperuricosuric.

STRUVITE STONES

- Eliminate any metabolic predisposition to stone formation.
- Sterilize the urine with an appropriate antimicrobial agent.
- Consider surgical intervention or ESWL for symptomatic stone.

URIC ACID STONES

- Increase urine output to 3 l/day.
- Alkalinize the urine to decrease uric acid precipitation ($NaHCO_3$, K-citrate, or Shohls solution, 1-3 mEq/kg/day in 4 doses).
- Avoid purine-rich foods.
- Use allopurinol when hyperuricosuria occurs (>1 g/day).

CYSTINE STONES

- A large fluid output of up to 4 l/day is required to keep urinary cystine <250 mg/l. Nighttime fluid intake is needed.
- Alkalinization of the urine can be tried. However, alkali administration to achieve a urinary pH above 7.5 is difficult (requires 15-25 g/day of $NaHCO_3$).
- Dietary restriction of methionine will decrease cystine excretion, but compliance is difficult.
- D-Penicillamine forms soluble mixed disulfides. It is used when other measures fail (in patients excreting >1 g of cystine/day). Side effects are common and include: proteinuria, leukopenia, skin rash, arthritis, hypogeusia, and, rarely, a vasculitis.

FOLLOW-UP

The effect of therapy on identified metabolic abnormalities must be monitored by measurement of urinary and plasma chemistries 1-2 months after initiating treatment, and then yearly. In addition, yearly X-rays should be obtained to identify new stones and assess the success of therapy.

SUGGESTED READING

REVIEWS

Andriani RT, Carson CC. Urolithiasis. Clin Symp 1986;38:3.

Coe FL, Favus MJ. Disorders of stone formation. In: Brenner BM, Rector FC Jr, eds. The kidney. Philadelphia: WB Saunders Co, 1986;1403-1442.

PATHOGENESIS

Coe FL, Parks JH. Pathophysiology of kidney stones and strategies for treatment. Hosp Prac 1988;23:145-168.

Coe FL, Strauss AL, Tembe V, Dun SL. Uric acid saturation in calcium nephrolithiasis. Kidney Int 1980;17:662-668.

DIAGNOSIS

Muldowney FP. Diagnostic approach to hypercalciuria. Kidney Int 1979;16:637-648.

Smith LH. Medical evaluation of urolithiasis. Etiologic aspects and diagnostic evaluation. Urol Clin North Am 1974;1:241-260.

THERAPY

Finlayson B, Thomas WC Jr. Extracorporeal shock-wave lithotripsy. Ann Intern Med 1984;101:387-389.

Pak CYC, Fullner C. Idiopathic hypocitraturic calcium-oxalate nephrolithiasis successfully treated with potassium citrate. Ann Intern Med 1986;104:33-37.

Chapter 12

Urinary Tract Obstruction

Charles S. Wingo

DEFINITION

Urinary tract obstruction can affect the urethra, bladder, or one or both ureters. It is caused by an extrinsic lesion (tumor, fibrosis), an intrinsic lesion (stone, tumor, blood clot), or functional impairment of the bladder (neurogenic bladder) or ureter.

INCIDENCE

The incidence of urinary tract obstruction varies with age and sex. In infants and children, posterior urethral valves are the most frequent cause of bladder or urinary tract obstruction. Less frequent causes of obstruction include ureteral valves, a ureterocele, or congenital stenosis at the ureteropelvic junction. All of these causes are more frequent in males. In men after age 55, prostatic hyperplasia is the main cause of obstruction.

ETIOLOGY

Common causes of obstruction are listed in the display on page 122.

PATHOPHYSIOLOGY

RENAL HEMODYNAMIC CHANGES

Obstruction of the ureter results in a prompt increase in ureteral, renal parenchymal, and intratubular pressure. The ureteral pressure gradually returns toward normal. Ureteral obstruction produces biphasic changes in renal blood flow (RBF). An **increase** in RBF to 40-50% above normal occurs within 15 minutes of ureteral occlusion and is due to a decrease in renal vascular resistance. Over the next few days, RBF **decreases** sharply below normal. These changes are related to an early generation of vasodilatory prostaglandins (e.g., prostacyclin) followed by generation of the vasoconstrictor prostaglandin, thromboxane.

Common Causes of Obstruction

Renal Pelvis

- Congenital stenosis
- Calculus
- Papillary necrosis
- Clotted blood
- Vascular compression

Ureter

- Intrinsic
  Congenital stricture
  Carcinoma
  Calculus and clotted blood
  Papillary necrosis
- Extrinsic
  Ureterocele
  Retroperitoneal fibrosis
  Inflammatory bowel disease
  Surgical complication
- Functional
  Pregnancy

Bladder and Urethra

- Anatomic
  Prostatic hyperplasia
  Carcinoma of the prostate or bladder
  Urethral valves and stenosis
  Calculus and clotted blood
- Functional
  Neurogenic bladder

GLOMERULAR FILTRATION RATE (GFR) AND RENAL FAILURE

GFR decreases because of the increase in intraluminal pressure and later, renal vasoconstriction. If the obstruction is bilateral, progressive reduction in GFR occurs. The chance for recovery diminishes as the duration of obstruction increases. Normal renal function can be restored if obstruction is corrected within 1 week. Relief of complete urinary tract obstruction of 1-4 weeks duration usually produces some permanent loss of renal function, but GFR may still return to a significant fraction of normal. Relief after more than 6 weeks of complete obstruction usually produces only small increases in GFR (10-20 ml/min). Most of this improvement occurs within the first week after relief of the obstruction. Although significant functional recovery is unlikely after 12 weeks of **complete** obstruction, the degree of recovery from **partial** obstruction of even longer duration can be gratifying.

TUBULAR DEFECTS

Both nephrogenic diabetes insipidus (decreased renal concentrating ability) and renal tubular acidosis are complications of chronic urinary tract obstruction. Some improvement in these tubular defects may occur after relief of obstruction.

INFECTION

Obstruction increases the incidence of infection, in part by impairing the normal defenses for elimination of bacterial contamination in the urine. Lower urinary tract infection is usually manifest by symptoms of dysuria, frequency, pyuria, and hematuria. Symptoms of upper urinary tract infection and pyelonephritis include flank pain, nausea, vomiting, and fever. The urinalysis of a patient with pyelonephritis may show white cell casts in addition to pyuria and bacteriuria. Repeated urinary tract infections can lead to papillary necrosis.

HYPERTENSION

Acute unilateral ureteral obstruction can cause a renin-dependent hypertension similar to unilateral renal artery stenosis. With chronic unilateral or bilateral obstruction, hypertension is quite common. The hypertension seen in bilateral ureteral obstruction is usually secondary to renal failure and extracellular fluid volume expansion. Relief of the obstruction may restore the blood pressure to normal.

POSTOBSTRUCTIVE DIURESIS

A brisk diuresis frequently follows relief of obstruction. Where the obstruction is bilateral, the postobstructive diuresis can be related to an expanded extracellular fluid volume and an osmotic diuresis as the retained solutes are eliminated. However, obstruction also impairs tubular function directly; this contributes to sodium and phosphate wasting and to the development of a nephrogenic diabetes insipidus, renal tubular acidosis, and abnormal tubular transport of potassium.

CLINICAL PRESENTATION

Symptoms of urinary tract obstruction are related to the **rate of development** of obstruction, the **cause of obstruction**, and the **site of obstruction**. Processes that produce gradual stenosis will generally produce fewer symptoms than acute obstruction; for example, obstruction due to retroperitoneal fibrosis frequently does not produce pain unless infection supervenes. Symptoms are frequently related to the cause of the obstruction. Clotted blood or a renal calculus causes ureteral irritation and ureteral colic, whereas extrinsic compression from a vessel or tumor is frequently asymptomatic. Symptoms also depend on the location of the obstruction. Lower urinary tract obstruction due to prostatic hyperplasia may result in difficulty controlling micturition. Some patients remain asymptomatic and present with signs of uremia.

INVESTIGATIONS

RENAL ULTRASOUND

Renal ultrasound is frequently employed in the initial examination to evaluate possible obstruction. While this test has a reported sensitivity of approximately 95% compared to an intravenous pyelogram, it may not detect obstruction in the presence of nephrolithiasis. If a flatplate of the abdomen reveals no calcifications and the ultrasound examination is technically satisfactory, this effectively excludes hydronephrosis. The causes of a false-positive ultrasound test are listed in the following display.

Causes of Nonobstructive Dilatation of the Renal Pelvis

- Corrected obstruction
- Reflux
- Infection
- Diuresis
- Distended bladder
- Large extrarenal pelvis
- Papillary necrosis with sloughed papilla

INTRAVENOUS PYELOGRAPHY (IVP)

When there is doubt and renal function is not severely impaired (serum creatinine less than 2.5 mg/dl), the IVP remains the preferred method for determining the presence of obstruction. It can demonstrate renal size as well as the degree of dilatation of the renal pelvis, ureter, and bladder. However, the procedure is not without risk for acute renal failure. Caution should be exercised in the diabetic, particularly with azotemia. The presence of dehydration and multiple myeloma also predisposes patients to dye-induced acute tubular necrosis. More recently, nonionic dyes have been developed that are reported to have a lower incidence of nephrotoxicity. Although their use cannot be justified routinely, in selected high risk groups these agents may be preferred for visualizing the urinary tract.

CT SCAN

A computed tomography (CT) scan with or without radiocontrast dye is valuable to diagnose obstruction. It is particularly helpful in defining lesions extrinsic to the collecting system.

RETROGRADE PYELOGRAPHY

An IVP provides poor visualization in patients with little renal function. In such patients, where renal ultrasound and CT scan are equivocal, a retrograde pyelogram may be the only accurate way to determine the presence of obstruction.

FUROSEMIDE RENOGRAM

This test may distinguish between ureteral obstruction and a nonobstructed but dilated ureter. However, normal values that exclude the possibility of obstruction have not been clearly defined.

DIFFERENTIAL DIAGNOSIS

Certain clinical settings deserve particular attention. The older man with abdominal pain should be evaluated for obstruction due to prostatic hyperplasia or malignancy. Recent lower abdominal or pelvic surgery should raise the possibility of iatrogenic obstruction. A history of diabetes mellitus or extensive use of analgesics should alert one to the possibility of papillary necrosis. The diabetic and individuals with spinal trauma or spinal cord disease may have functional obstruction due to a neurogenic bladder. Recurrent urinary tract infections suggest partial obstruction. Chronic inflammatory bowel disease, pelvic inflammatory disease, malignant bowel tumors, and occasionally endometriosis can produce urinary tract obstruction by extrinsic compression. In the patient with lymphoma, retroperitoneal nodal involvement may lead to obstruction.

The drug history should be reviewed carefully. Patients with lymphoma may develop uric acid nephropathy after receiving chemotherapy. Methysergide is associated with retroperitoneal fibrosis although this syndrome is frequently idiopathic. Theophylline and atropine-like drugs can precipitate obstruction in a patient with prostatic hyperplasia.

The amount of urine output cannot be used to diagnose the presence or absence of obstruction or its location. Although complete obstruction is associated with anuria, partial obstruction is frequently associated with increased urinary output because of the impaired renal concentrating ability. Conversely, the absence of urine output does not necessarily mean that the obstruction is bilateral. Anuria may also result from ureteral obstruction to a single functioning kidney. During the physical examination the lower abdomen should be carefully inspected for signs of a distended bladder. The pelvic or rectal examination may detect a mass.

MANAGEMENT

In most patients the evaluation of obstruction should begin with catheterization of the bladder. A Coude catheter may be used in place of a Foley in the elderly man with an enlarged prostate. It should be emphasized, however, that the rapid decompression of the bladder can result in bladder hemorrhage or circulatory collapse. In the patient with a grossly distended bladder it is wise to remove no more than 500-1000 ml of urine from the bladder acutely and the remainder over several hours. Obstruction of the upper urinary tract is generally managed by a urologist.

The choice of therapy depends on whether the obstruction is contributing to renal insufficiency and **the risk of the obstruction to the individual**. Relief of the obstruction is imperative in individuals with sepsis and infection proximal to the obstruction. In other patients, for example, those with only partial obstruction of one ureter due to congenital causes, it may be preferable first to evaluate the need for corrective surgery.

The major causes of obstruction of the upper urinary tract in adults are related to calculi and neoplasms. In cases of neoplastic involvement, the decision to operate must take into consideration the degree of intrinsic function of the obstructed kidney. If the kidney is small and the estimated creatinine clearance is less than 5 ml/min, the benefit from relief of the obstruction will be small.

In the patient with progressive nonresponsive malignancy and bilateral ureteral obstruction or unilateral obstruction of a single functioning kidney, the overall benefit to the patient must be weighed against the potential complications. In general, diversion is worthwhile when disease is localized and confined to the original organ.

After relief of obstruction to both kidneys a postobstructive diuresis may develop. Urine losses should be only partially replaced since they reflect retention of extracellular salt and water as well as an osmotic diuresis. Complete intravenous replacement may result in a persistent diuresis. If frank hypotension or orthostatic symptoms occur, replacement therapy should be increased.

SUGGESTED READING

Holden S, McPhee M, Grabstald H. The rationale of urinary diversion in cancer patients. J Urol 1979:121;153-156.

Kalika V, Bard RH, Iloreta A, Freeman LM, Heller S, Blaufox MD. Prediction of renal functional recovery after relief of upper urinary tract obstruction. J Urol 1981;126:301-305.

Wennberg JE, Mulley AG Jr, Hanley D, et al. An assessment of prostatectomy for benign urinary tract obstruction. JAMA 1988;259:3027-3030.

Whitaker RH, Buxton-Thomas MS. A comparison of pressure flow studies and renography in equivocal upper urinary tract obstruction. J Urol 1984;131:446-449.

Chapter 13

Urinary Tract Infection

Paul B. Lim
John C. Peterson

DEFINITION

Urinary tract infections (UTIs) are among the most common problems in clinical practice. Traditionally they have been subdivided into upper (pyelonephritis) and lower (cystitis, urethritis, prostatitis) tract infections. Recurrent infection by the same organism within 2 weeks of therapy is termed a "relapse," implying incomplete eradication of the initial infection, while recurrence with a different pathogen or beyond 2 weeks is considered a "reinfection." The diagnosis of "acute urethral syndrome" in women refers to a presentation of dysuria, often with a lower urinary tract infection.

INCIDENCE

Male infants have a higher rate of UTI because of a greater frequency of congenital urological anomalies, and men beyond age 50 have a high incidence of UTI due to the development of prostatism. Between these age ranges, the female:male ratio varies from 10:1 to 50:1. About 10-20% of all women will have an episode of UTI during their lifetime and among sexually active women the annual incidence of UTI varies from 3 to 10%. Approximately 33% of women with dysuria have the acute urethral syndrome. The incidence of UTI doubles during pregnancy and is higher in pregnant women with a childhood history of UTI.

ETIOLOGY

Overall, *Escherichia coli* accounts for 80-90% of uncomplicated acute UTI in the ambulatory patient. Organisms such as Proteus, Klebsiella, Enterobacter, Pseudomonas, Enterococci, Serratia, and Staphylococcus assume more importance in hospitalized patients with recurrent infection, obstruction, calculi, immunosuppression, or following urinary tract instrumentation. *Staphylococcus sapropyticus* is responsible for 10-15% of acute UTI in young women. *Staphylococcus aureus* bacteriuria is uncommon and usually indicates the presence of an extrarenal source of infection (endocarditis, osteomyelitis, skin abscess) leading to hematogenous renal involvement. *Mycobacterium tuberculosis* and *Candida albicans* are other uncommon causes of hematogenous UTI.

Most women with the acute urethral syndrome have dysuria, pyuria, and bacteriuria with the usual uropathogens but in smaller numbers than the traditional criteria of 10^5 organisms/ml of urine. Some have dysuria and pyuria but sterile urine, while others have urethritis associated with *Chlamydia trachomatis, Herpes simplex, Neisseria gonorrheae, Trichomonas vaginalis,* or bacterial vaginosis. A final group in this category may have dysuria alone, without pyuria or bacteriuria. Although the cause is obscure, some may have mechanical or chemical irritation of the urethra. They do not respond to antibiotic therapy.

PATHOPHYSIOLOGY

The vast majority of UTI episodes arise as an ascending infection. In females, endogenous enteric bacteria initially colonize the perineum, vagina, and urethra and are readily introduced retrograde into the bladder, perhaps during coitus. The use of a contraceptive diaphragm appears to enhance the risk of vaginal colonization and subsequent UTI in susceptible women. Once in the bladder, whether a bacterial inoculum leads to established bacteriuria, local infection, or involvement of the upper tract depends on the interplay between microbial virulence and host defense.

In the normal host, a number of potential defense mechanisms mitigate against ascending bacterial invasion of the urinary tract.

- The normal nonpathogenic flora of the periurethral region resist colonization by bowel uropathogens.
- Rapid turnover and shedding of epithelial cells promote clearance of mucosally adherent bacteria.
- Micturition mechanically flushes bacteria from the bladder.
- The transitional epithelium of the bladder secretes a hydrophilic glycosaminoglycan layer which retards mucosal adherence by uropathogens.
- Urinary Tamm-Horsfall protein, produced by renal tubules, is rich in mannose residues and may protect uroepithelium by competitive binding of type 1 fimbriae.
- Some intrinsic urinary factors inhibit bacterial growth (very high or low osmolality, high urea concentration, high organic acid concentration, low pH).
- In males, prostatic secretions have an antibacterial effect.
- Polymorphonuclear leukocytes possess a receptor for type 1 fimbriae that mediates nonimmune phagocytosis, and mucosal leukocytes may contribute to local defense against infection.

However, many circumstances can allow pathogens to breach this impressive array of host defenses and predispose to UTI.

- Obstructive lesions which cause urine stasis.
- The presence of calculi or foreign objects.
- Vesicoureteral reflux.
- Incomplete bladder emptying due to mechanical or neurogenic causes.
- Instrumentation of the urinary tract.
- Use of broad spectrum antibiotics that reduce the density of perineal nonpathogens and facilitate colonization by virulent coliform bacteria.
- Pregnancy in susceptible women.

PATHOLOGY OF PYELONEPHRITIS

Ascending renal infection develops in discrete foci and spreads in a wedge distribution from renal pelvis to the medulla to the overlying cortex. The kidney is grossly edematous and small subcapsular abscesses may be present. Microscopically, there is an acute focal inflammatory cell infiltration of the interstitium and tubules, interspersed with regions of normal histology. White cell casts may be present within the tubules.

In chronic pyelonephritis, there are asymmetric areas of cortical scarring and caliceal dilatation. Intervening normal renal parenchyma may undergo hypertrophy, giving rise to a mass appearance or "pseudotumor." On microscopic examination, one finds lymphocytes, plasma cells, and eosinophils in the interstitium along with tubular atrophy and interstitial fibrosis. This pathologic appearance is characteristic of interstitial nephritis from any cause and is not specific for an infectious etiology (see Chapter 14).

BACTERIOLOGIC AND RADIOGRAPHIC EVALUATION

Ideally, urinalysis and quantitative urine culture with antibiotic sensitivities should be obtained in all cases to confirm infection and guide therapy. In the otherwise healthy ambulatory patient with community-acquired clinically uncomplicated lower urinary tract infection who can be reliably followed, initial empiric therapy without culture is acceptable.

The finding of bacteria by high power field in an uncentrifuged urine sample correlates well with $\geq 10^5$ organisms/ml of urine on culture. This is a useful rapid screening test for high grade bacteriuria but will not detect bacteriuria in low counts. To detect bacteriuria the Griess test for urine nitrates and the leukocyte esterase test is available as a combined dipstick, with a sensitivity of 70-95% and specificity of 65-85%.

Significant bacteriuria is defined by the isolation of $\geq 10^5$ of a single uropathogen/ml of urine collected by a clean catch technique, or by recovery of 10^2 organisms/ml of urine obtained by sterile urethral catheterization or suprapubic needle aspiration of the bladder. Recovery of low counts ($<10^3$ organisms/ml) by clean catch or the presence of polymicrobial flora may imply an improper collection technique. True polymicrobial bacteriuria, however, can occur with chronic indwelling catheters, neurogenic bladder, or enteric fistulae to the urinary tract. Follow-up urine cultures should be obtained 2 weeks after completion of antibiotic therapy to look for "relapsed" UTI.

The antibody-coated bacteria assay has been proposed to differentiate upper tract from lower tract infection. It is subject to a host of confounding factors resulting in a high rate of false positives and false negatives and is not currently recommended for routine clinical use.

The majority of otherwise healthy women with recurrent UTI have "reinfections" by uropathogenic bacteria from the endogenous fecal flora. In this population, less than 1% of patients will have structural abnormalities detected by IVP, voiding cystourethrography, and cystoscopy. On the other hand, urologic studies are integral to the evaluation of UTI in men, and in selected women with a history of "relapsing" UTI, recurrent symptomatic pyelonephritis, stone disease, or whenever there is suspicion of obstruction or renal abscess. Renal imaging with intravenous pyelography, ultrasonography, or computed tomography is helpful in the management of complicated upper tract infections. Table 13-1 lists the findings in a variety of conditions.

CLINICAL PRESENTATION AND MANAGEMENT OF SPECIFIC UTI SYNDROMES

ASYMPTOMATIC BACTERIURIA

Patients with true asymptomatic bacteriuria should have this documented by several urine cultures growing $\geq 10^5$ colonies of a single organism/ml of urine. In most adult or elderly patients who do not have abnormalities of the urinary tract, immunocompromised host status, or a history of pyelonephritis and bacteremia, asymptomatic bacteriuria has a benign prognosis and may not require specific treatment. An important exception are pregnant women with asymptomatic bacteriuria of whom 20-30% will subsequently develop symptomatic pyelonephritis. The greater susceptibility to upper tract infection during pregnancy is attributed to functional impairment of ureteral tone and peristalsis, a "physiologic" hydroureter particularly prominent on the right, and an enlarged bladder capacity, all of which tends to allow reflux of urine into the upper tract.

In the nonpregnant adult with asymptomatic bacteriuria, initial therapy with a single dose or a conventional short course (3-7 days) of appropriate antibiotics can be tried. If bacteriuria persists or recurs and the patient is at low risk for symptomatic pyelonephritis or bacteremia, no further therapy is indicated. In immunocompromised hosts, long-term suppressive antibiotics may be required.

Asymptomatic bacteriuria in the pregnant patient should be treated and monitored for recurrence. Tetracyclines, trimethoprim, and chloramphenicol should not be used in pregnancy; sulfonamides should be avoided in the third trimester.

Table 13-1 Findings by Renal Imaging in Complicated Urinary Tract Infections

	Intravenous Pyelography	Ultrasonography	Computed Tomography
Acute pyelonephritis uncomplicated	Normal in 75% ↑ renal size *Prolonged nephrogram Delayed excretion of contrast agent	↑ renal size Variable parenchymal echogenicity No hydronephrosis	↑ renal size ↓ corticomedullary definition ↓ function
Chronic pyelonephritis	↓ cortical width ↓ function Focal scarring and caliectasis	↓ renal size Lobar hypertrophy with "pseudo tumor"	↓ renal size ↓ function "Pseudo tumor"
Renal/perinephric abscess	Mass effect Distortion of renal contour and calices Absent psoas margin	Thick-walled cystic mass with external echoes	Thick-walled cystic mass ↓ attenuation of contents
UTI with obstruction	↓ function Mass effect	Dilated collecting system with echogenic debris	Dilated collecting system ↓ function Contents of variable density
Renal tuberculosis	Punctate calcifications Caliceal deformity Autoamputation		Scattered areas of decreased attenuation or caseation
Chronic prostatitis	Evidence of bladder outlet obstruction	Gland enlargement Numerous echogenic areas of fibrosis Abscess appears echolucent	

* ↓ function = prolonged nephrogram and delayed excretion of contrast agent.

Modified from Benson M, LiPuma JP, Resick MI. Urol Clin North Am 1986;13:605-625

ACUTE URETHRAL SYNDROME

Most women with the acute urethral syndrome have pyuria, but only 10^2-10^4 colonies/ml of urine. These women with dysuria, pyuria, and bacteriuria should receive empiric single dose or short course anti-biotic therapy for cystitis.

Some women with acute dysuria and pyuria will have negative urine cultures and may respond to doxycycline, 100 mg orally twice daily for 14 days. They should be evaluated for the presence of sexually transmitted diseases with secondary urethritis or underlying gynecologic disorders. Women who have dysuria alone, without pyuria or bacteriuria, do not respond to antibiotics and are usually treated with urinary analgesics.

CYSTITIS AND PYELONEPHRITIS

The following findings are suggestive of acute cystitis:

- Dysuria
- Frequency
- Pelvic pain
- No systemic symptoms
- Pyuria without white cell casts
- Bacteriuria $\geq 10^5$ pathogens/ml of urine
- Hematuria

In contrast to the above, the following constellation suggests upper tract involvement:

- Symptomatic cystitis
- Flank pain and tenderness
- High fevers and rigors
- Nausea and vomiting
- Prostration
- Tachycardia
- Hypotension
- Leukocytosis
- Pyuria with white cell casts
- Bacteriuria $>10^5$ pathogens/ml of urine

Although the separation of urinary tract infections into lower tract or upper tract infection is conceptually attractive, in the individual patient this distinction may occasionally be difficult to make on clinical grounds. Some 30-50% of women presenting with symptomatic cystitis and $>10^5$ colonies/ml of urine bacteriuria can be found to have concomitant silent upper tract infection.

In general, lower urinary tract infections respond readily to either single dose or short (3-7 days) courses of appropriate anti-biotics, while upper tract infections often require longer (>2 weeks) courses of therapy. Early "relapsing" infection following treatment directed at the lower urinary tract should prompt a search for silent upper tract disease, the presence of a resistant pathogen, or complicating host factors such as calculi, obstruction, vesicoureteral reflux, or prostatitis. Lower urinary tract "reinfections," on the other hand, can be treated episodically or by long-term prophylaxis without further investigation.

Single dose regimens for acute cystitis have the advantages of convenience, lower cost, high compliance, and less tendency to select for yeast or resistant pathogens. Conversely, it is usually ineffective for treatment of silent pyelonephritis and does not eradicate periurethral colonizing coliforms. Patients who are not suitable candidates for initial empiric single dose antibiotic therapy include males, patients with indwelling urinary catheters, those with structural abnormalities of the urinary tract or nephrolithiasis, those with evidence of upper tract disease, or individuals who may not be available for follow-up evaluation.

Single dose regimens:

	Dose	Cure rate
• Trimethoprim, 160 mg/ sulfamethoxazole, 800 mg	2 tablets	76-95%
• Amoxicillin	3 g	50-85%

Patients who do not respond to single dose therapy should have quantitative urine culture performed and treatment with 3-7 days of appropriate antibiotics. Patients who relapse following a short course should be treated for an additional 2-6 weeks and investigated for underlying factors predisposing to UTI. Patients who are successfully cured but who subsequently develop frequent reinfections could be treated with prophylactic or intermittent therapy regimens:

- Nitrofurantoin, 50-100 mg orally every night.
- Trimethoprim, 80 mg/sulfamethoxazole, 200 mg orally every night.
- Trimethoprim, 40 mg, sulfamethoxazole, 200 mg orally 3x/week.
- Cephalexin, 250 mg orally every night.
- Patient-initiated single dose therapy at onset of acute dysuria or postcoitus

Patients with acute pyelonephritis often require hospitalization and parenteral antibiotics until they have been afebrile for 24-48 hr, then are treated with oral antibiotics for at least 2 weeks. Relapse should be treated with an additional 6-week course. Therapy is guided by susceptibility testing. Posttreatment urine cultures should be obtained at 2 weeks to detect relapse, and again between 6-12 weeks to screen for reinfection.

Recurrent pyelonephritis in early childhood (under 5 years) may result in parenchymal scarring and atrophy, particularly when associated with vesicoureteral reflux. Radiographic evidence of renal scarring in an adult, therefore, may imply previous childhood disease. Acute pyelonephritis in adults usually does not lead to progressive renal impairment unless superimposed on reflux, obstruction, or chronic interstitial nephritis when parenchymal destruction can be markedly accelerated.

Patients with pyelonephritis who do not respond to appropriate therapy within a few days or patients who present with Gram-negative sepsis and shock should undergo prompt renal imaging to rule out the presence of complicating obstructive uropathy (see Chapter 12), infected renal calculi (see Chapter 11), and intrarenal or perinephric abscess.

COMPLICATIONS OF PYELONEPHRITIS

Intrarenal abscess may complicate UTI; less commonly it may arise following hematogenous infection with *S. aureus*, *M. tuberculosis*, or Candida species. Patients with obstructive abnormalities of the urinary tract, vesicoureteral reflux, renal calculi, and diabetes mellitus are at particular risk. An intrarenal abscess may rupture through the renal capsule to create a perinephric abscess which itself may dissect into the peritoneal cavity, colon, chest, or overlying skin. The mortality of perinephric abscess is 20-50%.

The clinical findings of intrarenal or perirenal abscess may be those of pyelonephritis only, although a palpable tender flank or abdominal mass may be present. Urinalysis often reveals pyuria, proteinuria, hematuria, and bacteriuria but may be normal in a third of these patients. Diagnosis requires timely investigation with ultrasonography, IVP, or computed tomography. Appropriate antibiotic therapy can successfully resolve most cases of intrarenal abscess, although patients with very large abscesses may require percutaneous needle aspiration or nephrostomy drainage. Immediate surgical drainage, in addition to antibiotic therapy, is always required for a perinephric abscess. Xanthogranulomatous pyelonephritis is a rare type of chronic renal infection in association with calculi, obstructive uropathy, abscess formation, and fibrosis that may mimic a renal neoplasm. It does not respond to antibiotics and often requires partial or total nephrectomy.

TUBERCULOUS UTI

Genitourinary tract tuberculosis represents hematogenous spread from a pulmonary source and is the most commonly encountered form of extrapulmonary infection. Caseating granulomata in the cortex and medulla cavitate into the calices to initiate a descending infection of the ureters and bladder. Pathologically, there is cavitary destruction of renal parenchyma, papillary necrosis, calcification, fibrosis, and stenosis of the collecting system with segmental obstructive uropathy and bladder contracture.

Presentation may be insidious and nonspecific; constitutional symptoms are found in fewer than 20% of patients. Tuberculous epididymitis, orchitis, or prostatitis may be the first manifestation of advanced disease. The degree of renal dysfunction due to chronic interstitial nephritis, hydronephrosis, nephrolithiasis, and secondary bacterial UTI is highly variable. Tuberculosis should always be suspected in patients with "sterile pyuria" and hematuria. Early morning urine specimens obtained for acid-fast bacilli culture are positive in 80-90% of patients. IVP may demonstrate renal calcifications, papillary necrosis, caliceal scarring, mucosal irregularities, strictures of the renal pelvis and ureter, and a small contracted bladder.

CATHETER-RELATED UTI

Chronic indwelling urinary catheters inevitably lead to bacteriuria, frequently with antibiotic-resistant strains. The usual ascending route of infection may occur through breaks in a closed collection system or by colonization of the periurethral mucous sheath along the outer surface of the catheter. Often such episodes of bacteriuria quickly resolve with removal of the catheter. However, catheter-related UTI is the most common cause of Gram-negative bacteremia in hospitalized patients. This has been associated with a 3-fold increase in mortality.

Indwelling bladder catheters should be used only when absolutely necessary and removed as soon as possible. They should be inserted under aseptic conditions and drained into a closed collection system, draining away from the patient at all times. There is no benefit to prophylactic antibiotic bladder irrigation, periurethral topical antibiotics or antiseptics, or instillation of disinfectant solutions into the collection bag. When bacteriuria or complicating prostatitis/epididymitis develops, the catheter should be removed. Intermittent catheterization or suprapubic catheterization are alternatives if the patient cannot void spontaneously. If a chronic indwelling suprapubic or ureteral catheter must be left in place, antibiotic therapy should be reserved for episodes of symptomatic invasive renal infection. Nonsymptomatic bacteriuria should not be treated as long-term suppressive therapy will tend to select out multiple-resistant pathogens which are more difficult to eradicate.

PROSTATITIS SYNDROMES

Acute bacterial prostatitis may complicate UTI or the use of urinary catheters. Patients manifest fever, chills, dysuria, urgency, frequency, low back and perineal pain, and obstructive symptoms. On examination, the prostate is often swollen and tender. Urinalysis reveals pyuria and bacteriuria. Typical uropathogens are found on urine culture. Antibiotics used for UTI, such as trimethoprim, 160 mg/sulfamethoxazole, 800 mg orally twice daily, can be given for a 30-day course. Urethral instrumentation should be avoided.

Chronic bacterial prostatitis is an important cause of recurrent UTI in males. The symptoms may be nonspecific unless there is concurrent cystitis. Inflammatory cells and bacteria are found in expressed prostatic fluid. Currently available therapy is poor. Trimethoprim, 160 mg/sulfamethoxazole, 800 mg orally twice daily, can be given for 4-16 weeks, with an expected 30-40% cure rate. Other agents used include carbenicillin indanyl sodium, 764 mg four times daily, ciprofloxacin, 500 mg twice daily, and doxycycline, 100 mg twice daily. Refractory cases may require long-term antibiotic suppression or, in selected patients, total prostatovesiculectomy.

Most men with symptomatic prostatitis and pyuria will have sterile urine and prostatic fluid cultures. They may have a sexually transmitted urethritis or a "nonbacterial prostatitis" possibly related to *Ureaplasma urealyticum* or *C. trachomatis*. A trial of minocycline or erythromycin may be warranted.

UTI IN CHRONIC RENAL DISEASE

In the setting of chronic renal insufficiency, nephrotoxic drugs such as aminoglycosides should be avoided whenever possible. Nitrofurantoin is contraindicated in the presence of renal failure as it is both ineffective and may cause a peripheral neuropathy. Tetracycline, sulfonamides, and methenamine mandelate should not be used in renal failure (see Chapters 21 and 22).

When renal disease is unilateral, the contralateral normal kidney may excrete sufficient antibiotic to sterilize bladder urine, resulting in apparent bacteriologic cure despite a persisting focus of infection in the affected kidney which will subsequently give rise to recurrent UTI.

Patients with infected single renal cysts may be treated as for intrarenal abscess. Patients with infected polycystic kidneys may require long-term antibiotic therapy with drugs such as trimethoprim, clindamycin, or chloramphenicol which penetrate into cyst fluid. Instrumentation of the urinary tract is a major instigator of UTI in polycystic kidney disease and should be avoided when possible.

Dialysis patients with anuric end-stage renal failure may still accumulate a reservoir of urine in the bladder that can become infected. In the evaluation of such a patient with a febrile illness, a single diagnostic bladder catheterization to exclude UTI should not be overlooked.

INTERSTITIAL CYSTITIS

Interstitial cystitis is a poorly understood entity primarily affecting young women and clinically defined by the following features:

- Frequency, urgency, suprapubic pain relieved by voiding, and dyspareunia. Dysuria, however, is uncommon and differentiates this condition from the acute urethral syndrome.
- Physical examination may reveal bladder tenderness to palpation. Urinalysis, urine culture, urine cytology, and radiographic studies of the urinary tract are normal.
- At cystoscopy under general anesthesia, pinpoint mucosal hemorrhages are seen after hydrodistension of the bladder. This finding alone, however, is nonspecific and may also occur following infectious, toxic, or radiation cystitis.

Bladder biopsy reveals nonspecific chronic inflammation. No infectious bacterial, fungal, or viral etiologic agent has been demonstrated, and these patients do not respond to antibiotics. There is no effective therapy.

SUGGESTED READING

Benson M, LiPuma JP, Resnick MI. The role of imaging studies in urinary tract infection. Urol Clin North Am 1986;13:605-625.

Fowler JE, Pulaski ET. Excretory urography, cystography, and cystoscopy in the evaluation of women with urinary tract infection: a prospective study. N Engl J Med 1981;304:462-465.

Krieger JN. Complications and treatment of urinary tract infections during pregnancy. Urol Clin North Am 1986;13:685-693.

Kunin CM. Genitourinary infections in the patient at risk: extrinsic risk factors. Am J Med 1984;76:131-139.

Parsons CL. Pathogenesis of urinary tract infections: bacterial adherence, bladder defense mechanism. Urol Clin North Am 1986;13:563-568.

Schaeffer AJ. Catheter associated bacteria. Urol Clin North Am 1986;13:735-747.

Stamey TA. Recurrent urinary tract infections in female patients: an overview of management and treatment. Rev Inf Dis 1987;9(Suppl 2):S195-S210.

Stamm WE, Running K, McKevitt M, Counts GW, Turck M, Holmes KK. Treatment of the acute urethral syndrome. N Engl J Med 1981;304:956-958.

Tolkoff-Rubin N, Rubin RH. New approaches to the treatment of urinary tract infection. Am J Med 1987;82(Suppl 4A):270-277.

Wilhelm MP, Edson RS. Antimicrobial agents in urinary tract infections. Mayo Clin Proc 1987;62:1025-1031.

Chapter 14

Tubulointerstitial Nephritis

Nicolas J. Guzman

DEFINITION

Tubulointerstitial nephritis (TIN) is an inflammatory disorder of the renal interstitium which is commonly accompanied by tubular inflammation. Occasionally, inflammation of the renal tubules may be the primary process with involvement of the interstitium occurring as a secondary event. TIN that accompanies primary glomerular or vascular diseases and allograft rejection will not be discussed here.

INCIDENCE

In autopsy series the incidence of acute TIN (excluding pyelonephritis) and chronic TIN was 1.7 and 0.2%, respectively. In biopsy series acute TIN was found in 1.1-3.4% of patients with approximately one-half of them having a drug-related etiology. TIN is responsible for 11-14% of the cases of acute renal failure, while chronic TIN is an infrequent cause of end-stage renal disease.

ETIOLOGY

According to the clinical presentation, TIN can be divided into acute and chronic forms as shown in the list that follows:

Acute and Chronic Tubulointerstitial Nephritis

INFECTIONS

Acute
- Bacterial
    Acute pyelonephritis
    Leptospirosis
    Rocky Mountain spotted fever
- Viral
    Cytomegalovirus

Chronic
- Bacterial
    Chronic obstructive pyelonephritis
    Reflux-associated chronic pyelonephritis
    Tuberculosis
- Fungal
    Histoplasmosis

- Parasitic
    Schistosomiasis
    Malaria (*Plasmodium falciparum*)
- Xanthogranulomatous pyelonephritis
- Malakoplakia

TIN Without Direct Kidney Infection (Reactive)
- Bacterial (e.g., streptococcus, *Legionella pneumophilia*, *Mycoplasma pneumoniae*)
- Viral [e.g., rubeola (measles), Kawasaki disease]
- Parasites (e.g., *Toxoplasma gondii*)

DRUGS

Acute (Hypersensitivity) TIN (see display on page 142)

Chronic
- Analgesic nephropathy
- Lithium nephropathy

METABOLIC CAUSES

- Hypokalemic nephropathy
- Hypercalcemic nephropathy
- Urate nephropathy
- Oxalate nephropathy

MISCELLANEOUS

- Heavy metals
- Reflux nephropathy
- Obstructive uropathy
- Neoplastic diseases
    Plasma cell dyscrasias
        Myeloma kidney
        Light chain deposition disease
    Lymphoproliferative diseases
    Leukemia
- Granulomatous sarcoid nephropathy

CLINICAL MANIFESTATIONS

With the exception of the acute diffuse forms of TIN (e.g., drug hypersensitivity), the early stages of the disease are characterized by a normal or mildly decreased glomerular filtration rate (GFR) and proteinuria of less than 2 g/24 hr. The urinary sediment usually contains white blood cells, red blood cells, and occasionally white blood cell casts. Eosinophils may be seen on Wright's or Hansel's stain of the urinary sediment in patients with drug-induced hypersensitivity TIN. Peripheral eosinophilia is, however, a more consistent finding. As inflammation progresses, the glomeruli may also be involved, resulting in progressive renal insufficiency, worsening proteinuria and hematuria, oliguria, and hypertension. At these more advanced stages of the disease, the clinical picture is very difficult to differentiate from that of a primary glomerular disease, and the diagnosis will often have to be made by kidney biopsy.

Three characteristic patterns of renal dysfunction can be seen in the early stages of TIN.

Proximal Tubular Dysfunction

This is manifested clinically as proximal renal tubular acidosis (type II RTA) with or without Fanconi syndrome.

Distal Tubular Dysfunction

This is manifested as distal renal tubular acidosis (type I RTA), salt wasting or hyperkalemia, or both (usually out of proportion to the degree of azotemia).

Renal Medullary Dysfunction

There is decreased concentrating ability manifested as polyuria and nocturia.

ACUTE TUBULOINTERSTITIAL NEPHRITIS

The two most common causes of acute TIN are acute bacterial pyelonephritis (see Chapter 13) and acute drug-induced hypersensitivity TIN. Other forms of acute TIN such as TIN associated with systemic infections (reactive TIN) and acute idiopathic TIN are seen less commonly and will not be discussed here.

ACUTE DRUG-INDUCED HYPERSENSITIVITY (TIN)

The number of drugs reported to cause acute TIN is large and continues to increase (see page 142). Drugs implicated more frequently include the beta-lactam antibiotics, particularly methicillin, and the nonsteroidal anti-inflammatory drugs. These drugs appear to have particular pharmacological characteristics that make them more prone to cause TIN. For example, among the beta-lactam antibiotics, methicillin has been reported to cause acute TIN in up to 15-20% of patients, whereas the incidence in patients receiving other penicillins or cephalosporins for the same indications is much less. The risk of developing acute TIN increases with prolonged therapy. The mean duration of therapy before the onset of methicillin-induced TIN is 15 days, but it has been seen as early as 2 days and as late as 44 days. The absence of prior penicillin allergy is no protection against the development of TIN.

Pathophysiology

Drug-induced acute TIN occurs as a result of both humoral and cell-mediated hypersensitivity reactions mounted against a hapten (drug or drug metabolite)-endogenous protein complex. The response is idiosyncratic, not dose related, and recurs rapidly after drug rechallenge. Within a class of related drugs, structural similarity can lead to immunological cross-reactivity. For example, the presence of a sulfa group in both furosemide and bumetanide precludes their use in patients who have demonstrated hypersensitivity to either drug. Ethacrynic acid is the loop diuretic of choice in these patients.

Histologically, the majority of patients will present with the "classic" form of acute TIN, similar to that originally described with methicillin. Light microscopy reveals a focal interstitial infiltrate of mononuclear cells, predominantly lymphocytes, usually localized to the corticomedullary junction. This is accompanied by edema and variable numbers of eosinophils. There is commonly some degree of tubular necrosis, but the medulla, glomeruli, and vessels are usually spared. A smaller number of patients will present with one or more of three described variations: a) a granulomatous response usually associated with allopurinol, thiazides, sulfonamides, oxacillin, and polymixin; b) minimal change nephrotic syndrome associated with nonsteroidal anti-inflammatory drugs; and c) a predominant tubular injury as in rifampin-induced TIN.

Clinical Manifestations

Acute drug-induced TIN presents with signs and symptoms characteristic of an allergic reaction. The most common presenting features are listed below:

Signs and Symptoms	Laboratory Findings
• Fever (85-100%) • Maculopapular rash (25-50%) • Arthralgias • Uremic symptoms	• Hematuria (95%) • Eosinophilia (80%) • Sterile pyuria • Low grade proteinuria • Eosinophiluria • White blood cell casts

Blood eosinophilia is usually transient, lasting only 1 to 2 days. Although eosinophiluria is a common finding in acute TIN, it is also frequently seen in other kidney diseases. Acute renal failure occurs in 20-50% of patients and is seen more frequently in the elderly. Even in the absence of all of the above clinical features, acute drug-induced TIN should be suspected in all patients with acute renal failure of unknown etiology.

Investigations

Since acute drug-induced TIN commonly presents as rapidly progressive acute renal failure, the differential diagnosis includes diseases such as rapidly progressive glomerulonephritis and acute tubular necrosis secondary to ischemia and nephrotoxic drugs. A detailed history of drug intake and previous allergic reactions should be obtained. Careful examination of the urinary sediment, looking for the findings described above and for evidence of glomerulonephritis (e.g., red blood cell casts), is essential in the differential diagnosis. Radioactive gallium scanning during acute TIN shows intense uptake of the isotope by the kidneys. Although this test is also positive in other inflammatory kidney diseases, it is reported to be very useful in differentiating acute TIN from acute tubular necrosis in which gallium uptake by the kidneys is not increased. A kidney biopsy should be performed in those patients in whom the diagnosis is unclear.

Treatment and Prognosis

Treatment for acute drug-induced TIN consists of discontinuation of the offending agent since, if it is not discontinued, progressive renal insufficiency will ensue. Acute dialysis therapy is necessary in up to 35% of patients. Although corticosteroids have been reported to be beneficial in a number of patients, controlled clinical trials are not available to support these claims.

Most patients will have complete recovery of renal function within a year, and only a few will have permanent functional impairment. Prolonged acute renal failure of more than 3 weeks duration and advanced age at onset are adverse prognostic indicators.

Specific Drugs

Drugs Commonly Associated with Acute Hypersensitivity TIN

- Antibiotics
  Beta-lactam antibiotics (penicillins, cephalosporins)
  Sulfonamides
  Trimethoprim-sulfamethoxazole
  Rifampin
  Ethambutol
  Tetracyclines
  Vancomycin
  Erythromycin

- Nonsteroidal anti-inflammatory drugs
  Indomethacin
  Fenoprofen
  Ibuprofen
  Naproxen
  Phenylbutazone
  Mefenamic acid
  Aspirin
  Tolmetin

- Diuretics
  Furosemide
  Bumetanide
  Thiazides

- Others
  Cimetidine
  Phenytoin
  Alpha-methyl-dopa
  Carbamazepine

___

Nonsteroidal Anti-Inflammatory Drugs (NSAIDs). The NSAID can cause a variety of adverse effects on the kidney including sodium retention, hyporeninemic hypoaldosteronism with hyperkalemia, acute renal failure, nephrotic syndrome, and acute TIN. The pathology of the NSAID-induced TIN is similar to that of classic drug-induced TIN. Patients with this entity tend to be older and generally have taken the drugs for a prolonged period of time (1 to 2 years). Some patients will present with signs and symptoms characteristic of a hypersensitivity reaction. Others, however, will not demonstrate any evidence of hypersensitivity. This is particularly true in patients who have associated NSAID-induced minimal change nephrotic syndrome. The pathogenesis of these syndromes is unclear, but both conditions are rapidly reversed upon discontinuation of the offending drug.

Rifampin. This drug can cause three different patterns of renal injury: a) classic acute TIN; b) direct proximal tubular injury with little interstitial involvement (probably due to a toxic mechanism); and c) minimal change nephrotic syndrome.

The clinical pattern of rifampin-induced TIN is unique with the abrupt onset of renal failure occurring upon rechallenge with the drug. Most cases have occurred during intermittent therapy (2 to 3 times a week) or after resumption of therapy following a drug-free interval. The clinical presentation is highly suggestive of a hypersensitivity reaction with fever, chills, myalgias, arthralgias, skin rashes, eosinophilia, eosinophiluria, and oliguric acute renal failure. The toxic form of rifampin-induced renal injury presents as a more gradual decline in renal function associated with granular casts. In either case, renal function improves over several weeks once the drug is discontinued.

CHRONIC TUBULOINTERSTITIAL NEPHRITIS

CHRONIC DRUG-INDUCED TIN

The most common form of chronic drug-induced TIN is analgesic nephropathy. The ingestion of large amounts of analgesic compounds over prolonged periods can lead to the development of both chronic TIN and papillary necrosis. Analgesic nephropathy is one of the most common causes of end-stage renal disease in certain geographic areas such as Australia and Switzerland.

Incidence

The incidence of analgesic nephropathy in the United States varies significantly among different geographic areas. An estimated 13-38% of patients with interstitial nephritis have been found to have analgesic nephropathy. Studies on patients with end-stage renal disease in Washington DC and Philadelphia showed an incidence of analgesic abuse of 2.8 and 1.7%, respectively. In North Carolina, however, where there was a high incidence of the use of over-the-counter phenacetin-containing powders, analgesic nephropathy was found in up to 13% of patients with end-stage renal disease. Thus, despite being an uncommon cause of renal failure in the United States overall, analgesic nephropathy constitutes a real and important problem in certain geographic areas.

Pathophysiology

Analgesic nephropathy can occur after prolonged high intake of a number of analgesic combinations. It was initially thought that phenacetin, which is metabolized to acetaminophen, was solely responsible for the renal injury. Epidemiological studies, however, have demonstrated that although papillary necrosis is seen most commonly after ingestion of mixtures of aspirin and phenacetin (particularly in the presence of water depletion), TIN can occur with prolonged use of mixtures containing combinations of aspirin and phenacetin, aspirin and acetaminophen, aminopyrine and phenacetin, phenazone and phenacetin, and aspirin and salicylamide. Renal injury occurs in a dose-dependent fashion. The average cumulative analgesic intake in patients with nephropathy is around 10 kg over a mean period of 13 years. The accepted criteria for the diagnosis of analgesic nephropathy in a patient with TIN is a cumulative analgesic intake of 3 kg or more or ingestion of 1 g/day for 3 years. Phenacetin metabolites (e.g., acetaminophen) and aspirin are concentrated in the kidney, particularly in the papillae, where dehydration further increases their concentration. Acetaminophen is metabolized in the renal papillae to reactive metabolites which may cause toxic injury by covalently binding to macromolecules or by lipid peroxidation.

On pathological examination, the early stages of analgesic nephropathy are characterized by patchy necrosis of interstitial cells, loops of Henle, and capillaries of the inner medulla. As the disease progresses, there is necrosis of the tip of the papillae and outer medulla and early focal atrophy of cortical tubules. Later stages are characterized by total necrosis of the inner medulla and papillae and cortical atrophy.

Clinical Manifestations

Analgesic nephropathy occurs most frequently in women with a history of chronic headaches, arthritis, or muscular pain. When questioned about analgesic use, they will usually deny or underestimate the actual intake. Nocturia due to the inability to concentrate urine is a common early symptom. Gross hematuria, sometimes associated with sloughed papillary fragments in the urine and renal colic, is an occasional presenting symptom. Patients with analgesic nephropathy commonly present with moderate hypertension and anemia. The latter is usually compounded by occult gastrointestinal blood loss from analgesic-induced gastritis or peptic ulcer, and it is characteristically out of proportion to the degree of renal insufficiency. Both persistent sterile pyuria and bouts of bacterial pyelonephritis occur frequently. Therefore, urinary tract infection should be excluded in all patients presenting with pyuria. Proteinuria (<1 g/24 hr) and renal tubular acidosis of variable severity are common. Occasionally, the renal tubular defect in association with diminished citrate secretion may lead to nephrocalcinosis. As the disease progresses, renal insufficiency develops, resulting eventually in end-stage renal disease.

Investigations

Most patients (90%) with analgesic nephropathy will have an abnormality on the IVP. Initially, the calices will appear widened and incipient papillary detachment may lead to leakage of contrast material into the renal parenchyma. Papillary necrosis, followed by detachment of the necrotic papillae, will result in cavity formation. Blunting of the calices and reduction in kidney size occur in advanced disease.

Treatment

Cessation of analgesic abuse, control of the hypertension, and treatment of urinary tract infections are essential. Early diagnosis and treatment of obstructive episodes are also critical to avoid progressive renal insufficiency. The prognosis in patients treated early is usually good and renal function can stabilize or improve with time. Persistent analgesic abuse invariably leads to chronic renal insufficiency and end-stage renal disease.

SUGGESTED READING

Cotran RS. Tubulointerstitial nephropathies. Hosp Prac 1982;17:79-92.

Kleinknecht D, Vanhille PH, Morel-Maroger L, et al. Acute interstitial nephritis due to drug hypersensitivity. Adv Nephrol 1983;12:277-308.

Linton AL, Clark WF, Driedger AA, et al. Acute interstitial nephritis due to drugs. Ann Intern Med 1980;93:735-741.

Murray T, Goldberg M. Analgesic-associated nephropathy in the USA. Kidney Int 1978;13:64-71.

Murray T, Goldberg M. Chronic interstitial nephritis. Etiologic factors. Ann Intern Med 1975;82:453-459.

Chapter 15

Renal Cystic Disease

Christopher S. Wilcox

DEFINITIONS

Renal cysts are fluid-filled cavities with epithelial lining that develop from renal tubules. Simple renal cysts are of little clinical importance. In contrast, three cystic diseases that occur in adults cause significant complications: autosomal dominant polycystic kidney disease (adult type) (ADPKD), medullary sponge kidney, and medullary cystic kidney disease. Their major clinical features are shown below. Additionally, an autosomal recessive polycystic kidney disease is encountered predominantly in children in which cases it presents with renal failure usually in infancy.

Clinical Features of the Major Renal Cyst Diseases

	Simple Renal Cyst(s)	*Autosomal Dominant Polycystic Kidney Disease*	*Medullary Sponge Kidney*	*Medullary Cystic Kidney Disease*
Incidence	1:10	1:600	1:5000	Rare
Median age at onset	Variable	20-40	40-60	Variable
Inheritance	None	Autosomal dominant	None	Mainly autosomal dominant
Cyst location	Variable	Proximal and distal tubules	Collecting ducts	Cortico-medullary junction
Flank pain or hematuria	Rare	Frequent	With stones or infection	None
Major complications	Rare	Hypertension UTIs Renal stones Aneurysms	UTIs Renal stones	Salt-wasting Polyuria
Renal failure	Absent	Frequent	Rare	Inevitable

ETIOLOGY

Renal cysts develop from tubules with .which they retain continuity. Therefore, they usually increase slowly in size due to accumulation of glomerular filtrate or secreted solutes and fluid. The etiology of renal cysts is unclear but may involve tubular obstruction elevating luminal pressure, increased elasticity of the tubular basement membrane, or proliferation of epithelial cells with production of excessive basement membrane.

AUTOSOMAL DOMINANT POLYCYSTIC KIDNEY DISEASE

CLINICAL PRESENTATION

Inheritance by an autosomal-dominant trait with nearly complete penetrance implies that each patient should have one affected parent and that the disease will be present on average in half of the siblings. However, there is considerable variability of expression and some patients die before the disease becomes manifest. Moreover, approximately one in four cases appears to arise **de novo**, presumably by a mutation. The mutant gene is closely linked to the alpha-globulin gene locus on the short arm of chromosome sixteen.

When fully developed, the disease is easy to diagnose. A family history consistent with ADPKD can be obtained in 75%. Most patients have episodes of abdominal or flank pain, often associated with gross or microscopic hematuria. More than half have hypertension and many have urinary tract infections or renal stone disease. Both kidneys are usually enlarged with irregular surfaces which can often be appreciated by abdominal palpation. Some 20% have hepatic cysts which may also be palpable. Urinalysis typically shows modest proteinuria (<200 mg/day). The hematocrit may be higher than expected for the degree of renal failure, presumably because of increased erythropoietin secretion.

The diagnosis can be confirmed by ultrasonography which shows many echolucent areas scattered throughout both kidneys. The most sensitive test is computed axial tomography (CAT) scanning.

DIAGNOSIS

The diagnosis rests on a typical spectrum of clinical findings.

Diagnostic Criteria for ADPKD

- Primary criteria
  Inumerable fluid-filled cysts scattered diffusely
  throughout the renal cortex and medulla.
  Definite history of polycystic kidney disease in
  genetically related family members.
- Secondary criteria
  Polycystic liver.
  Aneurysms of cerebral arteries.
  Cysts of pancreas.
  Renal insufficiency.

THERAPY OF COMPLICATIONS

Pain

Many patients have episodes of disabling abdominal or flank pain related to rupture of a blood vessel into a cyst or around the kidney. It usually responds to bed rest and analgesics.

Hematuria

This can be caused by rupture of a cyst into the pelvis or by renal stones, cyst infection, or malignant transformation. Hematuria should prompt a search to determine the cause.

Renal Infection

Bacterial cyst infection is difficult to irradicate. The urinalysis may be normal since cyst fluid does not communicate directly with the urine. Helpful signs include pain, fever, diaphoresis, bacteremia, and leukocystosis. Infected cysts may have an increased wall thickness by CAT scanning and occasionally show accumulation of radioactive gallium or indium by nuclear imaging techniques. Infecting organisms include *Escherichia coli*, Staphylococcae, and Bacteriodes. Some infected cysts respond to high-dose, relatively prolonged (2-3 weeks) therapy with a conventional antibiotic regimen such as a broad-spectrum penicillin or cephalosporin with an aminoglycoside. However, other infected cysts are quite impenetrable except by lipid-soluble antibiotics such as trimethoprim-sulfamethoxazole, ciprofloxacin, clindamycin, or chloramphenicol; occasionally, patients may respond to erythromycin or tetracycline.

Hypertension

Most patients eventually develop hypertension. The pathophysiology is not clearly linked to the renin-angiotensin system or to salt retention, although both are implicated with the development of chronic renal insufficiency. Dietary salt restriction and diuretics should be undertaken only with care since some patients have a salt-losing nephropathy and develop prerenal azotemia. Usually, the hypertension responds to alpha- or beta-blockers, angiotensin-converting enzyme (ACE) inhibition, or calcium antagonists.

Cerebral Aneurysms

About 15% of patients have a cerebral aneurysm. Where the diameter is below 1 cm, rupture is unusual. In contrast, larger aneurysms can produce intracerebral or subarachnoid hemorrhage. Currently, arteriography or CAT scans to diagnose cerebral aneurysms are not universally recommended in the absence of symptoms.

Nephrolithiasis

Some 10-20% of patients have nephrocalcinosis and/or nephrolithiasis. Renal stones are typically calcium oxalate. Patients should be advised to maintain a high fluid intake sufficient to produce 2 liters of urine daily. Established renal stone disease requires careful evaluation and treatment as discussed in Chapter 11, since it can accentuate the decline in renal function and predisposes to infection.

Renal Insufficiency

Renal failure eventually develops in most patients although occasionally this may be delayed into old age. Once renal failure is established (serum creatinine >2 mg/dl), there is characteristically a persistent loss of a fixed amount of creatinine clearance over time. Therefore, it is helpful to plot the reciprocal of plasma creatinine concentration (1/Scr) against time. This can predict the approximate date for dialysis or transplantation while a steepening of the slope of the line may indicate the need for more aggressive treatment of hypertension or a search for a complication such as an unrecognized renal stone or nephrocalcinosis. General measures which may delay progression of renal failure include meticulous treatment of hypertension, use of an angiotensin-converting enzyme inhibitor for antihypertensive therapy, and prescription of a low-protein intake. However, the specific value of these treatments has not been assessed in these patients.

Patients with ADPKD respond well to **chronic hemodialysis**. **Peritoneal dialysis** is less satisfactory because the enlarged kidneys may limit the abdominal space available for fluids. **Renal transplantation** is used routinely. It is critical to evaluate living related donors very carefully to ensure that they do not have an early form of the disease.

COUNSELING

Once a patient with autosomal-dominant polycystic kidney disease has been identified, the help of a nephrologist should be sought to plan a counseling service and, where indicated, a screening of potentially affected family members. Currently, CAT scanning with contrast is the most sensitive method for detecting early forms of the disease.

PROGNOSIS

The expression of the disease cannot be predicted from the presentation of other family members. Typically, the creatinine clearance halves (i.e., the serum creatinine doubles) about every 36 months once renal failure has developed. No therapy has yet been shown to prolong renal function.

MEDULLARY SPONGE KIDNEY

PATHOLOGY

Although probably present at birth, manifestations are usually delayed until ages 40-60. There is marked enlargement of the medullary and papillary portions of the collecting ducts, which may affect one or more papillae and is usually bilateral. Unless there are complications from stone disease or infection, renal function is well maintained and cortical structure is preserved.

CLINICAL PRESENTATION

The disease usually presents with hematuria (gross or microscopic), recurrent urinary tract infections, or nephrolithiasis. There is a defective urinary concentrating ability, a distal-type renal tubular acidosis with a reduced ability to lower urinary pH below 5.5, and a variable degree of nephrocalcinosis. Diagnosis is by intravenous pyelography, which demonstrates the dilated terminal collecting ducts.

THERAPY

Renal tubular acidosis may require alkali therapy. Nephrolithiasis is frequent; these patients typically have hypercalciuria which, with the renal tubular acidosis, accounts for the high incidence of stone disease. Asymptomatic patients should be encouraged to drink sufficiently to excrete 2 liters of urine daily. Hypercalciuric patients respond to thiazide therapy.

MEDULLARY CYSTIC DISEASE

PATHOLOGY

Multiple small cysts develop predominantly at the corticomedullary junction. The kidneys are small, the cortex is reduced, and the glomeruli are sclerotic.

CLINICAL PRESENTATION

Progressive renal failure may be seen in childhood, but can present in the adult. Patients often have a history of urinary concentrating defects, polyuria and polydipsia, and sometimes a remarkable degree of sodium wasting. There is no specific therapy, although the free water and sodium-losing condition require careful management. The disease progresses relentlessly to end stage. Definitive diagnosis is by open biopsy.

ACQUIRED POLYCYSTIC KIDNEY DISEASE

About half of the patients receiving prolonged dialysis develop multiple cysts in their remnant kidneys which may contribute to erythrocystosis or hypertension. These cysts can contain neoplastic nodules arising from the cyst lining which resemble a renal adenoma or adenocarcinoma.

The diagnosis is usually made by ultrasound or CAT scanning. Fortunately, the neoplastic potential of these cysts is not usually expressed by invasion or metastasis, although this can definitely occur. Cystic kidneys can be removed surgically, or ablated radiologically using intra-arterial alcohol or concentrated radiocontrast media. Cysts, once detected, can be identified by regular CAT scanning with contrast, and any change suggestive of neoplasia should trigger consideration of nephrectomy or renal ablation.

SUGGESTED READING

Gardener KD. Cystic kidneys. Kidney Int 1988;33:610-621.

Gehring JJ, Gottheiner TI, Swenson RS. Acquired cystic disease of the end-stage kidney. Am J Med 1985;79:609-620.

Sklar AH, Caruana RJ, Lammers JE, Strauser GD. Renal infections in autosomal-dominant polycystic kidney disease. Am J Kidney Dis 1987;10:81-88.

Welling LW, Grantham JJ. Cystic and developmental diseases of the kidney. In: Brenner BM, Rector FC, eds. The kidney. 3rd ed. Philadelphia: WB Saunders Co, 1986:1341-1376.

Welling LW, Grantham JJ. Cystic diseases of the kidney. In: Tisher CC, Brenner BM, eds. Renal pathology with clinical and functional correlations. 1st ed. Philadelphia: JB Lippincott, 1989:1233-1277.

Chapter 16

AIDS and Kidney Disease
C. Craig Tisher

INTRODUCTION

Although the kidney is not usually the major organ involved in the acquired immune deficiency syndrome (AIDS), acute and chronic renal failure is observed in affected patients and often requires intervention by a nephrologist. The magnitude of the problem is difficult to assess because detailed epidemiologic data are limited. Most of the experience has been reported from three major areas in the United States including Miami, San Francisco, and metropolitan New York. It is clear, however, that the number of patients with human immunodeficiency virus (HIV) seropositivity, AIDS-related complex (ARC), and full blown AIDS is increasing and, hence, the number of individuals who develop renal failure will increase in parallel.

The renal involvement falls into three categories: 1) acute renal failure (ARF); 2) chronic renal failure (CRF), most often associated with proteinuria and histologic lesions of focal and segmental glomerulosclerosis (FSGS); and 3) patients with CRF on maintenance hemodialysis who subsequently develop AIDS. In addition, patients with AIDS often manifest complicated fluid and electrolyte disorders during the course of their illness.

ACUTE RENAL FAILURE

ARF is observed frequently in patients with AIDS. Diagnosis is essentially the same as in any patient who manifests a rising blood urea nitrogen (BUN) or plasma creatinine (see Chapter 21).

Although clinical experience is limited, Rao, Friedman, and Nicastri found that sepsis with hypotension and drug nephrotoxicity secondary to pentamidine, antibiotics, and radiocontrast agents explained the ARF in the majority of their patients. Other potentially nephrotoxic agents commonly employed to treat many of the infectious complications of AIDS include rifampin, dapsone, trimethoprim-sulfamethoxazole, and amphotericin B. Occasionally, ARF may be secondary to hyperuricemia resulting from the use of certain chemotherapeutic agents in the treatment of AIDS-related malignancies.

There is little doubt that ARF contributes to the mortality and morbidity in these patients, although sepsis remains the leading cause of death. If these patients are hemodynamically stable, hemodialysis can be beneficial, and the decision to treat should be made using the same clinical criteria as in non-AIDS patients.

CHRONIC RENAL FAILURE

It has been proposed that there is a specific AIDS-related nephropathy with nephrotic range proteinuria, rapidly advancing renal failure, and histologic lesions of focal and segmental glomerulosclerosis. However, this form of CRF is encountered as a complication of prolonged heroin abuse in the absence of AIDS. This form of CRF has been seen most commonly in AIDS patients treated in Miami and the greater New York area where most are black and the risk factors include homosexuality, intravenous drug abuse, and a Haitian background. However, even in this population FSGS appears to be uncommon in those patients in whom homosexuality is the sole AIDS risk factor. In San Francisco where the majority of patients are white and homosexuality is the major risk factor, renal failure with nephrotic range proteinuria and FSGS is uncommon. Despite strong arguments to the contrary, evidence still appears insufficient to permit identification of a specific AIDS-related nephropathy.

The results of chronic dialysis treatment in patients with end-stage renal disease (ESRD) complicating AIDS generally has been dismal. Most are too debilitated to be treated as outpatients, and they die of other complications of their illness within a few months. Rao, Friedman, and Nicastri observed that many of their patients on maintenance hemodialysis became cachectic despite intensive nutritional support and all died of a combination of uremia, malnutrition, and infections. Although the decision to treat in this group of patients must be individualized, there is growing evidence that maintenance hemodialysis is not effective in prolonging survival.

In contrast to the experience in patients with AIDS and ESRD, those patients with CRF who have ARC or are seropositive for HIV appear to have a better prognosis with maintenance dialysis. Although the experience is limited to small numbers of patients, both continuous ambulatory peritoneal dialysis (CAPD) and hemodialysis, including self-dialysis at home, have met with some success. Again, treatment decisions must be individualized.

Another group of patients has been described who develop AIDS after becoming uremic and beginning dialysis. The typical patient has a history of intravenous drug abuse which often contributed to the CRF initially. While intravenous drug addicts maintained on chronic hemodialysis exhibit a relatively stable course, the additional complication of AIDS is generally fatal within a few weeks.

TRANSPLANTATION

Patients with AIDS and CRF are not candidates for renal transplantation. The requirement for use of immune suppressive drugs simply precludes serious consideration.

There are now several reported instances in which an organ donor has served as a source for transmission of an HIV infection. The recipients who have contracted AIDS via a graft or through contaminated blood products have generally experienced a rapid downhill course. Therefore, prospective donors with positive enzyme-linked immunosorbent assay (ELISA) screens are excluded in most transplant centers, regardless of the results of the Western blot. In addition, organ donation is avoided in certain high risk groups for AIDS including hemophiliacs, intravenous drug addicts, and homosexuals.

DIALYSIS PROCEDURES IN AIDS PATIENTS

Because of the potential lethal nature of HIV infections, there has been great concern among health care workers regarding the establishment of necessary and proper precautions for dialysis of patients who are known to be HIV positive. At present the Centers for Disease Control recommend that those procedures currently employed in dialysis units to prevent hepatitis B transmission are adequate to prevent transmission of the human immunodeficiency virus. These include: blood precautions, restriction of nondisposable supplies to a single patient unless the items are sterilized between uses, and cleaning and disinfection of dialysis machine and surrounding surfaces. It has also been suggested that to minimize blood spray from a dislodged needle, a transparent plastic bag should be placed over the patient's arm during dialysis. Although disagreement exists, we recommend that HIV-positive patients be separated from noninfected patients within the dialysis unit.

Protection of the staff is critically important. Even though the current limited experience with HIV-infected patients suggests that the risk of the infection to medical workers exposed to AIDS is very low, the lethal nature of the disease dictates extreme caution. Therefore, the policies developed by San Francisco General Hospital (Humphreys MH, Schonfeld PY. The kidney (NY) 1987;20:7-12.) for their personnel are quite appropriate.

Precautions When Caring for HIV-Infected Patients

- Dispose of needles and syringes in puncture-resistant containers without breaking or recapping the needle. Dispose of needles immediately after use. Do not throw needles into regular trash. Home dialysis patients should be provided with containers which are brought to the hospital for disposal with other contaminated waste.
- Wear gloves for contact with blood or body substances.
- Wear gloves to cover cuts, abrasions, ulcers, rash, or skin infections on your hands while working.
- Wash hands as soon as possible after contact with blood or body substances or after touching objects which have been in contact with blood or body substances.
- Wear protective eyewear when you are performing procedures which may result in splashes to the face (e.g., operative procedures, venous catheter placement, dialyzer reuse, endoscopies, etc.).
- Wear a mask when the patient is coughing and the diagnosis of tuberculosis has not been excluded or when performing a procedure which may result in splashes of blood or body fluids to the face and mucous membranes. Wear a mask when specified for communicable diseases which require respiratory precautions.
- Wear a gown when you expect spills of blood or body fluids onto your uniform or clothing or when in contact with wounds or infected sites.
- Contact your supervisor when you have had a needle stick or other exposure or splash.

DETECTION OF ANTI-HIV IN ESRD PATIENTS

Considerable controversy exists regarding the value of routine screening for AIDS virus antibodies in patients with ESRD, especially for those not in the high risk categories. It is argued that the low transmission rate of the AIDS virus in dialysis units and the apparent success of current precautions to prevent transmission of viral infections render routine screening unnecessary. In many states, routine screening is not permitted without the consent of the patient.

As noted in an earlier section on transplantation, where permitted, all prospective transplant donors should be tested. Otherwise, routine screening in patients who fall outside the high risk categories is not advocated. Results of recent voluntary testing for HIV seropositivity in inner city chronic hemodialysis patients reveals that in high risk patients the prevalence of seropositivity is high (30-40%), whereas in patients without such risk factors (intravenous drug abuse, male homosexuality, Haitian background, blood transfusion) the risk is negligible. The findings provide additional evidence that transmission of HIV in chronic hemodialysis units must be a rare event. Another survey of voluntary testing involving several dialysis centers that included far fewer patients in high risk categories for AIDS reported an HIV-seropositive rate of 0.77%, which is somewhat higher than in blood donors.

SUGGESTED READING

Berlyne GM, Rubin J. Adler AJ. Dialysis in AIDS patients. Nephron 1986;44:265-266.

Centers for Disease Control, DHHS. Recommendations for providing dialysis treatment to patients infected with human T-lymphotropic virus type III/lymphadenopathy-associated virus. Ann Intern Med 1986;105:558-559.

Chirgwin K, Rao TKS, Landesman SH, Friedman EA. Seroprevalence of antibody to human immunodeficiency virus (HIV) in patients treated by maintenance hemodialysis (MH). Kidney Int 1989;35:242.

Favero MS. Recommended precautions for patients undergoing hemodialysis who have AIDS or non-A, non-B hepatitis. Infection Control 1985;6:301-305.

Humphreys MH, Schoenfeld PY. AIDS and renal disease. The kidney (NY) 1987;20:7-12.

Humphreys MH, Schoenfeld PY. Renal complications in patients with the acquired immune deficiency syndrome (AIDS). Am J Nephrol 1987;7:1-7.

Kumar P, Pearson JE, Martin HD, et al. Transmission of human immunodeficiency virus by transplantation of a renal allograft, with development of the acquired immunodeficiency syndrome. Ann Intern Med 1987;106:244-245.

Marcus R, Solomon SL, Favero MS, et al. Human immunodeficiency virus (HIV) antibody in patients undergoing chronic hemodialysis. Kidney Int 1989;35:255.

Rao TK, Friedman EA, Nicastri AD. The types of renal disease in the acquired immunodeficiency syndrome. N Engl J Med 1987;316:1062-1068.

Chapter 17

Approach to the Hypertensive Patient

Christopher S. Wilcox

DEFINITIONS

HYPERTENSION

Hypertension is a level of blood pressure (BP) sufficiently high to increase the risk of stroke or renal or cardiovascular system (CVS) disease. In practice BP which is persistently above 140/90 mmHg in a young adult, 150/95 mmHg in middle age, or 160/95 mmHg in the elderly is often considered abnormal. However, the degree of risk may rise with BP even within the "normal" range.

The following definitions affect the urgency, prognosis, and response to therapy. Therefore, each patient should be assigned within these subgroups:

Severity

- Borderline: diastolic blood pressure (DBP) 90-94 mmHg
- Mild: DBP 95-104 mmHg
- Moderate: DBP 105-114 mmHg
- Severe: DBP above 115 mmHg

Treatment of mild hypertension is not urgent, whereas moderate hypertension requires treatment within a few weeks and severe hypertension within hours or, at most, days.

Systolic/Diastolic

Systolic BP may be an even greater risk factor than DBP. Systolic hypertension in the young is due to a high cardiac output and rapid left ventricular ejection with a normal or reduced peripheral resistance. In the elderly, it is due to loss of baroreflex control or elasticity in the distributing arteries, and implies advanced atherosclerosis of the large vessels. It is not surprising, therefore, that it carries an unfavorable prognosis for stroke and CVS events in the elderly.

INCIDENCE

Approximately 5% of young adults have a BP above 140/90 mmHg; this increases to 20% by age 60 and 50% by age 80. The incidence is higher in blacks than whites and increases strikingly in patients with diabetes mellitus, renal insufficiency, or vasculitis.

RISKS

Hypertension increases the risk of the following:

- Myocardial infarction
- Cardiac failure
- Stroke
- Renal failure (notably nephrosclerosis)
- Arterial aneurysm
- Peripheral vascular disease

The degree of risk is increased by the following factors:

- Age (elderly have worse prognosis)
- Organ damage (e.g., previous stroke or myocardial infarction)
- Coincident arterial disease (e.g., atherosclerosis, aneurysm, arterial calcification, or high-grade funduscopic changes)
- Race (black subjects have a worse prognosis than white)
- Presence of compensatory mechanisms [e.g., left ventricular hypertrophy (LVH)]

Hypertension accelerates damage caused by other diseases affecting the heart and kidneys. Thus, the decline in renal function in diabetic nephropathy is greater in untreated hypertension. Hypertension is at least additive with other risk factors for myocardial infarction or stroke. These include smoking, hypercholesterolemia, diabetes mellitus, LVH, and decreased physical activity. Therefore, these other factors must also be addressed in hypertensive subjects.

CLASSIFICATION

Each patient with hypertension must be firmly classified according to the pathologic type (benign or malignant) and the major cause (essential or secondary).

BENIGN HYPERTENSION

Benign hypertension is usually asymptomatic and progresses slowly over many years. The pathologic changes in the large and small arteries are concentric medial hypertrophy without necrosis. The end organs show hypertrophy (heart) or fibrosis and sclerosis (kidney).

MALIGNANT HYPERTENSION

Malignant hypertension accounts for less than 1% of all hypertension. The BP usually exceeds 200/120 mmHg and is accompanied by papilledema, usually with retinal hemorrhages and exudates. Patients almost always have headache and fluctuating neurologic signs due to increased intracranial pressure and patchy cerebral ischemia and edema; this can progress to seizures, fixed neurologic deficits, coma, and death. Most patients have proteinuria and a rapidly progressive decline in renal function. Some have a microangiopathic hemolytic anemia. There can be visual disturbance; blindness can occur from retinal or vitreous hemorrhage. The pathologic changes in the arterioles are fibrinoid necrosis, proliferation of the intima, and narrowing or obliteration of the lumen. The end organs show ischemia or necrosis.

Hypertension can be malignant at presentation or this may develop abruptly in a patient with long-standing benign hypertension. A high proportion of patients with malignant hypertension have a secondary cause, often renovascular.

The life expectancy for patients with untreated malignant hypertension is 3-4 months. Renal function deteriorates rapidly, and often irreversibly, and there is a high risk of serious damage to the brain and other vital organs. Therefore, treatment of malignant hypertension is a medical emergency (see Chapter 20).

ESSENTIAL HYPERTENSION

This encompasses the majority (90-98%) of patients with hypertension in whom no discernible cause is apparent. Most (60%) have a family history of hypertension which typically presents between 20 and 55 years of age.

SECONDARY HYPERTENSION

Renal and Renovascular Diseases

- Renovascular disease (usually atherosclerosis or fibromuscular dysplasia of the renal vessels or a renal infarct)
- Systemic sclerosis or vasculitis
- Constrictive renal capsulitis (Page kidney)
- Renal parenchymal disease (any cause of chronic renal failure).
- Obstructive uropathy

Endocrine Diseases

- Hyperaldosteronism (adrenal adenoma or Conn's syndrome, bilateral adrenal hyperplasia, dexamethasone-suppressible hyperaldosteronism, adrenal enzyme defects)
- Pheochromocytoma
- Cushing's syndrome
- Acromegaly
- Hyperthyroidism
- Diabetes mellitus
- Hyperparathyroidism

Other

- Toxemia of pregnancy
- Coarctation of the aorta
- Obesity and Pickwickian syndrome
- Drugs (alcoholism; cocaine abuse; birth control pill or estrogen; nonsteroidal anti-inflammatory agents; monoamine oxidase inhibitors; sympathomimetic amines; licorice; mineralocorticosteroids; glucocorticosteroids)
- Raised intracranial pressure
- Polycythemia (Gaisböck's syndrome)

These conditions are considered in Chapter 18.

CAUSES OF ESSENTIAL HYPERTENSION

During the development of hypertension, the cardiac output may be increased, but with established hypertension, raised BP is due generally to a raised peripheral vascular resistance especially in the elderly. Raised peripheral resistance is due in part to increased basal resistance (vessel wall hypertrophy) and to vasoconstriction (angiotensin II, catecholamines, heightened sympathetic tone, and unidentified mediators).

The ultimate cause of these hemodynamic changes is unclear. One theory ascribes hypertension to an inappropriate salt intake and renal salt retention. The ensuing increase in blood volume and venous return raises cardiac output. However, organ blood flow is governed by the metabolic requirements of the tissues (i.e., flow is autoregulated). Thus, the increased organ flow is eventually countered by increased peripheral vascular resistance. A second theory ascribes the increased peripheral resistance to vascular hypertrophy in response to repeated transient increases in cardiac output or BP (caused by anxiety, renin release, etc.). The two theories are not mutually exclusive.

Certain etiologic factors have been defined in essential hypertension.

GENETIC

The risk of hypertension is increased 6-fold if one parent is hypertensive and 10-fold if an identical twin is hypertensive. The expression of the genetic factor may include a membrane transport defect leading to subtle renal salt retention or increased intracellular calcium concentration in vascular tissues.

DIET

Excessive intake of the following dietary constituents is associated with increased BP: sodium chloride, unsaturated fats, caffeine, and alcohol (>2 drinks per day). Lower BP is associated with high intakes of calcium, potassium, and fish oils.

RENIN-ANGIOTENSIN-ALDOSTERONE AXIS

There is an abnormal spread of renin values in hypertensive patients. About 40% are in the low-renin category. These patients, including many blacks and elderly hypertensives, often have salt-sensitive hypertension. About 10% are in the high-renin category but do not have renovascular hypertension; they are often young. Even among the normal-renin category, about one-half have abnormal regulation of aldosterone secretion, renal blood flow, sodium balance, and BP by angiotensin II. Thus, the renin axis is intimately involved in the etiology of hypertension, but its role is subtle, incompletely understood, and expressed differently in various subgroups of patients.

SYMPATHETIC NERVOUS SYSTEM

Plasma levels of norepinephrine and epinephrine are normal or mildly elevated in most hypertensives. However, vascular responsiveness to these neurotransmitters can be increased. Baroreceptor function is impaired in hypertension, which permits greater fluctuations of BP. Some patients, especially during the developing phase of hypertension, clearly have increased sympathetic tone (hyperdynamic circulation, raised heart rate, elevated catecholamine levels).

RENAL FUNCTION

Early in the development of hypertension, renal blood flow is reduced while glomerular filtration rate (GFR) is maintained. The ensuing rise in filtration fraction promotes renal salt retention. In poorly controlled hypertension, renal function deteriorates, further creating a vicious cycle whereby declining renal function impairs salt excretion and raises BP, which leads to future renal damage.

LIFESTYLE

BP is increased by emotional stress, fear, or anxiety. Repeated emotional episodes may lead to established hypertension. Obesity and smoking raise BP, whereas regular exercise lowers it.

CLINICAL PRESENTATION

There are no specific symptoms of hypertension. Hypertensive headaches occur in severe hypertension and are usually occipital, throbbing, and present on awakening in the morning.

Examination of all hypertensive patients should include measurement of the BP and pulse while lying and after 2 minutes of standing. An orthostatic fall in BP implies blocked cardiovascular reflexes (e.g., drugs, autonomic neuropathy, pheochromocytoma) or volume depletion (heart rate will rise with standing). Initially, measure BP in both arms (marked differences suggest aortic atherosclerosis or coarctation) and compare radial and femoral pulses for delay (suggests coarctation). In patients who become hypertensive in childhood or adolescence, measure the BP in the leg to exclude coarctation of the aorta. Examine and palpate the brachial artery; a tortuous, stiff vessel (locomotor brachialis) implies severe atherosclerosis. Examine the fundi for evidence of hypertensive and atherosclerotic changes. More severe changes imply prolonged duration of disease and a poor prognosis. Grade IV retinal changes are seen in malignant hypertension (see Table 17-1).

The following questions need to be answered in the routine history and examination of each patient suspected of hypertension.

- **Does the patient have hypertension?** More than one measurement of BP is necessary since patients are often anxious at the first visit. Patients can usually be trained to record their own BP at home, but the patient's self-recorded BP should be checked against a clinic measurement. Ambulatory 24-hr BP monitoring may provide the best estimate of the overall level of BP and its control during therapy. The following can cause a serious overestimation of BP: fear, pain and anxiety, a rigid arterial wall (checked by palpation at wrist during BP measurement), a large arm (use a large cuff).

- **Is the BP stable, labile, or accelerated?** Labile hypertension is seen in the prehypertensive phase and in the elderly. An accelerated course implies rapid progression of hypertension or rapid increase in drug requirements. It often heralds the onset of malignant hypertension or an underlying secondary cause (e.g., renal failure, renovascular hypertension).

- **Has there been organ damage?** Assess impact on **heart** (heart failure, hypertrophy, ischemia, extra heart sounds, pulmonary rales, a raised jugular venous pressure); **kidney** (proteinuria, microscopy of urine sediment); **vessels** (peripheral pulses and bruits, abdominal aneurysms); and **fundi** (see Table 17-1).

- **Is there a secondary cause?** Most patients with essential hypertension have a positive family history and present between the ages of 20 and 55 years. Therefore, the absence of these factors suggests a secondary cause. For further discussion see Chapter 18.

- **Are there dietary factors contributing to hypertension?** Assess the level of Na intake from measurements of 24-hr renal Na excretion; measure creatinine excretion on the same sample to ensure the adequacy of collection. Patients on a "no added salt" diet should achieve daily Na excretion of 120 mmol (equals 120 mEq) or less. Alcohol intake (greater than two drinks per day) is a major contributor to hypertension. Calcium supplementation can produce a small fall in BP.

- **What are the coincident risk factors?** These include hyperlipemia, smoking, glucose intolerance, electrocardiogram (ECG) abnormalities, and obesity.

Table 17-1 Classification of Retinopathy

Class	A:V Ratio*	Focal Arteriolar Spasm†	Hemorrhages and Exudates	Papilledema	Arteriolar Light Reflex	AV Crossing Defects††
Normal	3:4	1:1	0	0	Fine yellow line, blood column seen	0
Grade I	1:2	1:1	0	0	Broad yellow line, blood column seen	Mild venous depression
Grade II	1:3	2:3	0	0	Broad "copper wiring" line, no blood column seen	Obvious venous depression
Grade III	1:4	1:3	+	0	Broad "silver wire" line, no blood column seen	Right angle crossing; V disappears under A and is dilated distally
Grade IV	Fine	Obliteration	+	+	Fibrous cords, no blood column seen	Right angle crossing; V disappears under A and is dilated distally

* Ratio of arterial to venous diameters.
† Ratio of diameters of regions of spasm to more proximal segments.
†† Tortuosity increases with severity.

LABORATORY TESTS

The following tests are normally required in patients with significant hypertension:

- Urinalysis (protein, glucose, and blood; microscopy)
- Electrolytes, blood urea nitrogen, and creatinine
- Blood sugar, cholesterol, and triglycerides
- ECG
- 24-hr urine Na excretion, creatinine clearance, and total protein excretion (important where proteinuria is detected on dipstick or the creatinine concentration is raised)
- Chest X-ray

Unfortunately, these routine tests will not identify some secondary causes, especially renovascular hypertension. Therefore, where clinical suspicion is present, some physicians will request a plasma renin activity (PRA) with coincident 24-hr Na excretion or a captopril challenge test (see Chapter 18).

SPECIAL INVESTIGATIONS

The following have value in selected patients.

INTRAVENOUS PYELOGRAM (IVP) OR COMPUTED TOMOGRAPHY (CT)

These are indicated where the kidneys are palpated on examination (suggesting polycystic kidney disease or tumor), or anatomical abnormalities of the collecting system are suspected, e.g., patients with recurrent urinary tract infection, unexplained pyuria or hematuria, symptoms of prostatism, or previous renal stone disease.

RADIONUCLIDE SCANNING

The [^{131}I]-Hippuran renogram traces renal plasma flow to the two kidneys, while the [^{99}Tc]-DTPA scan traces GFR. DTPA is convenient to image the kidneys with a gamma camera. These tests can be used in the work-up of suspected unilateral renal disease and renovascular hypertension (see Chapter 16) and prior to renal reconstructive surgery or nephrectomy to assess reserve in the residual kidney.

RENAL ULTRASOUND

Renal ultrasound is used to assess renal size (decreased in unilateral renal artery stenosis or renal parenchymal disease), to exclude obstructive uropathy, or to assess renal cyst disease.

RENAL ARTERIOGRAPHY

Aortography and selective renal arteriography are the definitive procedures for visualizing renal artery stenosis. They are also valuable in the work-up of polyarteritis nodosa (classic type for demonstration of renal aneurysms) and in the diagnosis of renal infarction or tumor. Arteriographic imaging without the need for arterial puncture can be provided by digital subtraction intravenous angiography, but the quality of the images is often poor and the dye-load is high. On the other hand, a digital-subtraction arteriogram (DSA) can decrease the dye-load. For DSA, a small quantity of dye is injected into the aorta or renal arteries and the images are enhanced by a computer. This is useful where the risk of contrast-induced renal failure is increased due to impaired renal function, volume depletion, diabetes mellitus, etc. In these circumstances, the patient should be well hydrated before and during the procedure (maintain urine flow at 1-2 ml/min or above) and receive mannitol (12.5-25 g) during the procedure. The use of the new nonionic contrast agents may reduce the risk of nephropathy further.

CARDIAC ECHO

This provides valuable information about ventricular wall thickness and function, and the ejection fraction. It also reveals diastolic dysfunction as seen in severe hypertension but is too expensive for routine screening at present.

SUGGESTED READING

Carmichael DJS, Mathias CJ, Snell ME, Peart WS. Detection and investigation of renal artery stenosis. Lancet 1986;1:667-670.

Genest J, Kuchel O, Hamet P, Canten M. Hypertension: physiology and treatment. 2nd ed. Minneapolis: McGraw-Hill, 1983.

Kaplan NM. Clinical hypertension. 4th ed. Baltimore: Williams & Wilkins, 1982.

NIH Blood Pressure Regulation and Aging: Proceedings from a Symposium. Horran MJ, Steinberg GM, Dunbar JB, Hadley EC, eds. New York: Biomedical Information Corp, 1986.

Smith MC, Dunn MJ. Renovascular and renal parenchymal hypertension. In: Brenner BM, Rector FC, eds. The kidney. 3rd ed. Philadelphia: WB Saunders, 1986:1221-1252.

The 1988 Report of the Joint National Committee on Detection, Evaluation, and Treatment of High Blood Pressure. Arch Intern Med 1988;148;1023-1038.

Vaughan ED. Renovascular hypertension. Kidney Int 1985;27:811-827.

Chapter 18

Secondary Forms of Hypertension

Edward D. Frederickson

INTRODUCTION AND GENERAL STRATEGY

Diagnosing a secondary cause for hypertension may lead to a cure or a more specific drug regimen. However, the low prevalence of secondary causes dictates judicious use of diagnostic tests.

Etiology	Approximate Incidence
• Renal parenchymal disease	3-5%
• Renovascular disease	1-4%
• Primary aldosteronism	0.3%
• Pheochromocytoma	0.1%
• Cushing syndrome	0.5%
• Drug related	0.5-1%
• Others	0.5-1%

Specific clinical clues and laboratory abnormalities should trigger screening tests. These must be highly sensitive to avoid removing patients prematurely from the diagnostic schema but also reasonably specific to prevent investigating large numbers of patients unnecessarily.

RENAL PARENCHYMAL DISEASE

PATHOPHYSIOLOGY

Any renal disease with decreased renal function can cause hypertension by volume overload. Other parenchymal diseases, despite maintained renal function, can also cause renin-dependent hypertension. Hypertension itself can cause nephrosclerosis, especially in black subjects in whom it accounts for 10% of end-stage renal disease. Moreover, hypertension accelerates the progression of most renal parenchymal diseases, especially diabetic nephropathy. With the development of advanced renal failure it may be impossible to differentiate between nephrosclerosis and a primary renal disease causing hypertension.

The management of patients with renal parenchymal disease is discussed in Chapters 2-5, 13-16, 21, and 22. As renal function deteriorates, blood pressure (BP) becomes increasingly responsive to volume depletion with dietary salt restriction and loop diuretics. However, overzealous natriuresis can compromise renal function; sometimes hypertension may only be controlled by dialysis.

RENOVASCULAR HYPERTENSION

DEFINITION

Renovascular hypertension (RVH) results from renal hypoperfusion.

ETIOLOGY

Intrinsic Lesions	Extrinsic Lesions
• Atherosclerosis	• Retroperitoneal tumors
• Fibromuscular dysplasia	• Retroperitoneal fibrosis
• Emboli	
• Vasculitis	
• Renal cysts	
• Trauma	
• Renal capsular hematoma - Page kidney	

PATHOPHYSIOLOGY

A reduction in renal perfusion pressure stimulates renin release. Renin catalyzes the formation of angiotensin I (AI) from substrate, while angiotensin-converting enzyme (ACE), located on vascular endothelium, further catalyzes the formation of angiotensin II (AII) from AI. AII is a powerful vasoconstrictor and potentiates renal salt retention, both by acting on the kidney and indirectly by stimulating aldosterone secretion. If only one kidney is hypoperfused, the sodium-retaining effects of increased AII and aldosterone are counterbalanced by a pressure natriuresis in the contralateral kidney. However, a fall in renal perfusion pressure causes avid sodium retention by that kidney. Therefore, where there is no normal kidney (e.g., patient with bilateral renal artery stenosis or stenosis of a transplanted, solitary, or dominant kidney), hypertension becomes primarily volume dependent and renin levels may be normal. The natural history of atherosclerotic disease is a progressive decrease in renal blood flow which results ultimately in complete loss of renal function. Bilateral renal artery stenosis is recognized increasingly frequently as a cause of end-stage renal disease.

CLINICAL FINDINGS

Clinical Findings That Suggest RVH

- New onset hypertension in females <30 or >50 or males >50
- Poor response to medication
- Accelerated or malignant hypertension
- History of smoking
- Atherosclerosis elsewhere
- Epigastric bruit - if it has a diastolic component, it is highly specific for renovascular hypertension
- Progressive decline in renal function
- Decreased renal function with ACE inhibitor

SCREENING TESTS

Captopril Stimulation Test

- All antihypertensive drugs, including diuretics, should be discontinued for the prior 7 days or replaced with the short-acting labetolol and/or nifedipine which should be withheld on the morning of the test.
- The patient should be seated for 30 min before and throughout the test.
- Blood should be drawn for plasma renin activity (PRA) initially and 60 min after captopril (50 mg ground up and suspended in water).
- The criteria for a positive test depends on the PRA assay used (see Muller et al. Am J Med 1986;80:633-644). With the clinical assay laboratory, a positive test is a postcaptopril PRA above 5.7 ng/ml/hr or a rise in PRA of 4.7.

DIAGNOSTIC TESTS

Renal Ultrasound with Measurement of Renal Size

A size differential of >1.5 cm between kidneys suggests unilateral renal parenchymal or renal vascular disease. A kidney of 7.5 cm or less in length can rarely be revascularized successfully.

Captopril Renogram

A poststenotic kidney shows a persistent cortical uptake of [^{131}I]-Hippuran with delayed excretion after captopril. Captopril also reduces the GFR of a poststenotic kidney as shown by a reduction in the [^{99}Tc]-DTPA renogram.

Renal Vein Renins

This requires measurements of PRA in both renal veins (RVs) and the infrarenal vena cava (IVC). The test results are magnified by acute captopril administration (50 mg given 1 hr before sampling). A positive result predicts a good response to intervention.

Interpretation of Renal Vein Renins

Step 1: Calculate the renal vein index (RVI) for each kidney

$$RVI = \frac{RV - IVC}{IVC}$$

Step 2: Calculate the renal vein PRA ratio with the side with the highest RVI as the numerator.

Normal	Unilateral RVH	Bilateral RVH
Both RVI <0.24	Ipsilateral RVI >0.24	Ipsilateral and
	Contralateral <0.24	Contralateral RVI >0.24
PRA ratio <0.5	PRA ratio >1.5	PRA ratio <1.5

Renal Arteriography

Normally narrowing of an artery must exceed 75% to cause renovascular hypertension. Views in at least two planes, sometimes with obliques, may be necessary to visualize the aortic ostia. Demonstration of an anatomical stenosis does not prove renin-dependent hypertension or improvement with angioplasty, surgery, or nephrectomy. The captopril renogram or renal vein renins help to predict which patients will benefit from these procedures.

TREATMENT

Percutaneous transluminal angioplasty (PCTA) is successful in 80% of nonosteal lesions. However, the long-term success rate of osteal lesions is less than 20%.

Surgical revascularization is now reserved for patients with osteal lesions, those who have failed PCTA, and those with concomitant disease of the abdominal aorta requiring surgery.

ACE inhibitors frequently cause a profound fall in BP in RVH, but there may be a fall in the GFR in the poststenotic kidney. In unilateral RVH this is often offset by a rise in GFR of the contralateral kidney. Thus, ACE inhibitors are potentially dangerous in bilateral RVH or unilateral RVH with a solitary kidney. Refractory bilateral RVH, which is not approachable by angioplasty or surgery, often requires furosemide in combination with a beta-blocker or a calcium-channel antagonist.

ADRENAL DISEASES CAUSING HYPERTENSION
PHEOCHROMOCYTOMA

Definition

A chromaffin-cell tumor secreting catecholamines.

Pathophysiology

Chromaffin cells are found in the adrenal medulla, sympathetic ganglia, and organ of Zuckerkandl (a remnant of chromaffin tissue located anterior to the bifurcation of the aorta). Although pheochromocytomas can form at any of these sites, 90% are found in the adrenal glands and 20% are bilateral. Extra-abdominal locations are rare (1-2%). Most adrenal pheochromocytomas secrete some epinephrine, whereas extra-adrenal tumors secrete only norepinephrine. About 6% of pheochromocytomas are inherited by a dominant gene; these usually present early and are often bilateral or extra-adrenal. Approximately 40% of familial pheochromocytomas have multiple endocrine neoplasia (MEN) type II (Sipple's syndrome) consisting of medullary carcinoma of the thyroid, pheochromocytoma, parathyroid hyperplasia or adenoma, and, infrequently, Cushing's syndrome.

Clinical Findings

The classical presentation of pheochromocytoma is paroxysms of hypertension accompanied by headaches, palpitations, and sweating. However, the hypertension is sometimes sustained. The patients may become highly anxious with a sense of impending doom. These symptoms can be mimicked by intense sympathetic stimulation experienced during an episode of hypoglycemia or a panic attack. The episodes can be brought on by exercise, urination, defecation, enemas, sexual intercourse, histamine or glucagon injections, IVP dye, anesthesia, opiates, smoking, or pregnancy.

Patients with a pheochromocytoma can develop many findings related to the prolonged high levels of circulating catecholamines. They may have a high metabolic rate with fever, sweating, and weight loss. Orthostatic hypotension secondary to a decrease in plasma volume and down-regulation of the sympathetic response is frequent. Symptoms of peripheral vascular disease may be seen with decreased pulses, cold extremities, and acrocyanosis. Some patients develop abdominal pain, nausea, and vomiting. Patients may have concentric cardiac hypertrophy and congestive heart failure secondary to the effects of catecholamines on the myocardium. Coronary ischemia is frequent.

Screening Tests

Total urinary metanephrines. These can be measured on a single voided urine ($\geq$1.18 μg/mg creatinine). This screening test has a sensitivity of 96% which can be improved by sampling immediately following a paroxysm or overnight. Sympathomimetics, nose drops, bronchodilators, labetolol, triamterene, and chloropromazine may cause false elevations; IVP dye may cause false reductions.

Urinary catecholamines are helpful as confirmation.

Vanillylmandelic acid (VMA) assay is not as accurate as the metanephrine assay.

Diagnostic Tests

Plasma-free catecholamine measurements. These provide a sensitive test but have false-positive results which can be minimized by having the patient lie quietly for 1 hr, placing a venous catheter in advance, and avoiding a tourniquet. Samples should be collected in cold, heparinized tubes and the separated plasma stored at -70°C. Free catecholamines, not conjugate, should be measured.

Clonidine suppression test. Clonidine reduces the central sympathetic outflow. Therefore, catecholamine levels are reduced in normal subjects and those with anxiety but remain elevated in patients with a tumor which secretes autonomously. The patient is kept supine and plasma for free catecholamines is drawn before and 3 hr after 0.3 mg of clonidine. Total catecholamine values should be below 500 pg/ml (sensitivity 97%, specificity 99%). Beta-blockers and diuretics may cause false-positive results. Concomitant antihypertensives should be avoided to prevent profound hypotension.

Localization Tests

Abdominal computed tomography (CT) scan. This requires care since contrast can occasionally induce a crisis. Slices of 0.5 cm should be taken through the adrenal region, the anterior aspect of the aortic bifurcation, and the superior aspect of the bladder. A tumor smaller than 1 cm may not be visualized.

Selective venous catecholamine sampling. Where the CT scan is negative yet there is biochemical evidence of a pheochromocytoma, localization can sometimes be accomplished by selective venous sampling for measurement of plasma norepinephrine concentration. Samples should be taken from both adrenal veins, both renal veins (proximal and distal), the inferior vena cava above the diaphragm and inferior to the renal veins, the azygous vein, and the right and left jugular veins. A simultaneous cortisol value on each sample is helpful to determine sampling location as catheterization of the adrenal veins may be technically difficult.

Management

Pheochromocytomas require surgical removal. However, there is a high operative mortality unless the patients are carefully prepared. Phenoxybenzamine or prazosin should be used for alpha-1 blockade. The contracted plasma volume should be expanded with normal saline over several days and a clear weight gain documented. Following complete alpha-blockade, a beta-blocker can be used to control tachycardia.

PRIMARY HYPERALDOSTERONISM

DEFINITION

Primary aldosteronism results from autonomous secretion of aldosterone from an adenoma or bilateral adrenal hyperplasia.

PATHOPHYSIOLOGY

Aldosterone-secreting adenomas are small tumors whose cells resemble those of the zona glomerulosa. Multiple adenomas occur in 10%. Aldosterone secretion is autonomous but can be stimulated further by ACTH although not usually by angiotensin.

Bilateral adrenal hyperplasia usually produces a milder syndrome. Aldosterone secretion is highly responsive to angiotensin.

Primary aldosteronism should be differentiated from secondary aldosteronism caused by excess renin or ACTH secretion. Pseudohypoaldosteronism can follow ingestion of licorice or chewing tobaccos.

CLINICAL FEATURES

Hypertension is present in almost all patients. Persistent hypokalemia is found in 75%; 10-15% develop hypokalemia during diuretic therapy or on a high salt intake, while a few have persistent normokalemia. The symptoms of hypokalemia include:

- Muscular weakness and a flaccid ascending paralysis
- Polyuria secondary to decreased renal concentrating ability
- Glucose intolerance with impaired insulin secretion
- Orthostatic hypotension from blunted postural reflexes
- Palpitations or cardiac arrhythmias

Hypomagnesemia can occur and promote renal K wasting. Most patients have a metabolic alkalosis and many have a modest elevation of the plasma sodium concentration.

SCREENING TESTS

The diagnosis should be considered in patients with hypokalemia or normokalemic patients who are very resistant to therapy and have suppressed PRA values. Potassium replacement must precede measurements of aldosterone or renin since hypokalemia stimulates renin and suppresses aldosterone secretion, even from adenomas. The total body K deficit may be large and requires several days or weeks of high dose K (40-120 mEq daily) to replace fully.

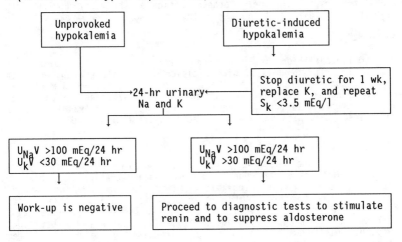

DIAGNOSTIC TESTS

Renin Stimulation Test

Administer 40 mg of furosemide at 1000, 1400, and 1800 hr followed by 2 hr of upright posture the next morning. A positive test (indicating a suppressed renin response) is a postdiuretic PRA below 2.5 ng/ml/hr.

Aldosterone Suppression Test

Infuse 2 liters of 0.9% NaCl over 4 hr. A positive test (indicating a failure to suppress aldosterone) is a postsaline value above 10 ng/dl.

TESTS TO DIFFERENTIATE AN ADENOMA FROM BILATERAL HYPERPLASIA

Overnight recumbent 18-hydroxycorticosterone (18-OHB). This is obtained supine prior to rising and repeated after 4 hr upright.

Adenoma	Hyperplasia
Basal 18-OHB >50 ng/dl	Basal 18-OHB <50 ng/dl
Supine > upright	Supine < upright

CT scan. This may fail to detect adenomas smaller than 1 cm.

Adrenal venous sampling. Measure cortisol, in addition to aldosterone, to confirm the sampling location. A high aldosterone:cortisol ratio with contralateral suppression implies unilateral aldosterone hypersecretion. Catheterization of the right adrenal vein is technically difficult and may be unsuccessful in 50% of patients.

MANAGEMENT

Differentiation of an adenoma from bilateral hyperplasia is essential since adenomas require excision while bilateral hyperplasia does not and requires medical therapy. BP may take up to 6 months to return to normal after excision of an adenoma. Treatment of bilateral adrenal hyperplasia usually requires large doses of spironolactone or amiloride. Many patients also require a thiazide or loop diuretic.

CUSHING'S SYNDROME

About 80% of patients with glucocorticoid excess are hypertensive. Most cases are due to steroid administration. Idiopathic disease results from hypothalamic-pituitary dysfunction and adrenocorticotrophic hormone (ACTH) over-secretion (70%), tumors with ectopic ACTH excretion (15%), or adrenal neoplasms (15%). The major features of Cushing's syndrome include: hypertension, bruising, myopathy, plethora, central obesity, hirsutism, glycosuria, and red striae. The best screening test is to administer 1 mg of dexamethasone at midnight and measure plasma cortisol at 8 a.m. This overnight dexamethasone-suppression test is 98% sensitive but only 80% specific. A 24-hr urinary free-cortisol measurement or a prolonged, 2-day dexamethasone-suppression test provides greater specificity. Ideally, Cushing's syndrome should be managed by removal of the source of excess glucocorticoid.

DRUG-INDUCED HYPERTENSION

Drugs That Cause Hypertension

- Agent

Estrogen	Amphetamine
Pseudoephedrine	Ergometrine
Neosynephrine	Cocaine
Phenylephrine	Ketamine
Monoamine oxidase (MAO) inhibitors	Cyclosporine
Phenylpropanolamine	Disulfiram
Methylphenidate	

- Hypertension After Withdrawal
    Ethanol
    Barbiturates
    Opiates
    Benzodiazepam
    Clonidine

OTHER CAUSES OF SECONDARY HYPERTENSION

Cause	Clinical Feature
• Coarctation of the aorta	Weakness in lower extremities
• Congenital adrenal hyperplasia	
1) 11-Hydroxylase deficiency	Virilization
2) 17-Hydroxylase deficiency	Abnormal sexual development
• Sleep apnea	Obesity, snoring, daytime somnolence
• Hypothyroidism	Sensation of cold, bradycardia, hair loss
• Hyperparathyroidism	Increased calcium
• Acromegaly	Growth
• Carcinoid	Diarrhea, flushing
• Burns	Significant 2nd or 3rd degree

SUGGESTED READING

GENERAL

Kaplan NM. Clinical hypertension. 4th ed. Baltimore: Williams & Wilkins, 1982.

RENOVASCULAR

Kuhlmann U, Greminger P, Grüntzig A, et al. Long-term experience in percutaneous transluminal dilatation of renal artery stenosis. Am J Med 1985;79:692-698.

Muller FB, Sealey JE, Case DB, et al. The captopril test for identifying renovascular disease in hypertensive patients. Am J Med 1986;80:633-644.

Vaughan ED Jr. Renovascular hypertension. Kidney Int 1985;27:811-827.

PRIMARY ALDOSTERONISM

Bravo EL, Tarazi RC, Dustan HP, et al. The changing clinical spectrum of primary aldosteronism. Am J Med 1983;74:641-651.

Kem DC, Tang K, Hanson CS, et al. The prediction of anatomical morphology of primary aldosteronism using serum 18-hydroxycorticosterone levels. J Clin Endocrinol Metab 1985;60:67-73.

PHEOCHROMOCYTOMA

Bravo EL, Gifford RW Jr. Pheochromocytoma: diagnosis, localization and management. N Engl J Med 1984;311:1298-1303.

Chapter 19

Treatment of Hypertension

Christopher S. Wilcox

AIM

The aim is to reduce the associated risk of stroke, cardiovascular system (CVS) and renal morbidity and mortality. Most physicians attempt to reduce blood pressure (BP) to 150/90 mmHg or less. Stricter reduction may be important in preventing progressive renal damage in patients with diabetic nephropathy. More gradual reduction is required in patients with decompensated neurological deficits (evolving stroke, subarachnoid hemorrhage), severe fixed vascular obstruction (e.g., claudication with pain at rest), or evolving myocardial infarction.

NONPHARMACOLOGIC THERAPY

Restriction of Dietary Salt Intake

Approximately two-thirds of subjects ("salt-sensitive") derive a 10-15 mmHg fall in diastolic blood pressure (DBP) with dietary salt restriction. Moreover, moderate salt restriction can reduce diuretic-induced K depletion. A "no added salt diet" in which salt is not used in cooking or added directly to food usually reduces daily Na intake to 100-120 mEq. The dietary salt intake can be assessed from 24-hr Na excretion providing the patient has not just started or stopped diuretic therapy.

Curtailing Alcohol Intake

Consumption of more than two drinks per day increases BP. Abrupt cessation of alcohol intake can precipitate delirium tremens. More gradual withdrawal leads to a reduction in BP.

Correction of Obesity-Underactivity

Loss of body weight and increased daily exercise reduce BP.

Other

Increased dietary intake of calcium, potassium, or fish oils can lower BP but are of a less clear benefit. Stress management and biofeedback can lower BP, but the effect is often transient.

PRINCIPLES OF DRUG THERAPY

INDIVIDUALIZE TREATMENT

There is no uniform way of treating hypertension. However, some factors can help to predict the best antihypertensive response. Thus, beta-blockers and angiotensin-converting enzyme (ACE) inhibitors are more effective in young, white patients and those with high renin levels. In contrast, calcium antagonists (CAs) and perhaps alpha-receptor blockers are more effective in elderly or black patients, and those with lower renin values. Diuretics are effective in most patients.

A low renin or black subject may become more responsive to drugs that are effective in higher renin states (beta-blockers, ACE inhibitors) when the renin system is stimulated by a diuretic.

Use of More Than One Class of Drug at Low Dose Is Preferable to a Single Drug at High Dose

Antihypertensive drugs have widely divergent mechanisms of action and adverse effects. Therefore, when one drug is not sufficient, addition of one from a different class may produce an additive fall in BP without precipitation of dose-dependent adverse effects. However, as the number of drugs prescribed increases, so does the likelihood of noncompliance.

Anticipate Adverse or Unwanted Effects

For example, unless there are compelling reasons do not use:

- Beta-blockers in athletes (limits maximal levels of cardiac output), asthmatics (precipitates bronchospasm), or patients with bradyrhythmias (reduces heart rate and atrioventricular (AV) nodal conduction).
- ACE inhibitors in patients with bilateral renal artery stenosis or stenosis of a single or dominant kidney (decreases renal function) or those with collagen vascular disease (increases incidence of blood dyscrasias).
- Thiazide diuretics in patients with hypokalemia, gout, hyperglycemia, or hyperlipidemia.
- Centrally acting agents in depressed or lethargic patients.
- Vasodilators in patients with angina (reflex increase in cardiac work).

Consider Cost and Convenience of Therapy

Drugs which are expensive and have to be given frequently are less likely to be taken.

Low Price (less than 25 cents daily)
- Thiazide diuretic with KCl supplements
- Reserpine

Medium Price (26 to 60 cents daily)
- Combined thiazide with K-sparing diuretic or aldosterone antagonist
- Beta-blocker
- Central agent
- ACE inhibitor

High Price (greater than 60 cents daily)
- Calcium antagonist
- Alpha 1-antagonist

The need for biochemical tests (e.g., diuretics) or high dosage increase the cost to the patient.

Patient Education is Required for Good Compliance

The patient must understand the risks of not complying with the treatment, the need for life-long treatment (in all but about 5-10% of patients), and that other drugs are available if the initial therapy is not satisfactory. Patients receiving clonidine and perhaps beta-blockers should be warned of the dangers of suddenly stopping these drugs.

Therapeutic Requirements Change with Time

Therefore, remember to arrange for continued follow-up.

Secondary Hypertension Requires Specific Therapy

Drugs are required during preparation for definitive therapy or in those unable to tolerate a curative procedure. The selection of therapy is important.

Renovascular hypertension. This responds well to beta-blockers and especially ACE inhibitors. However, the latter can cause a reversible fall in glomerular filtration rate (GFR) in patients with stenosis of a single kidney (e.g., renal transplant recipients) or bilateral renal artery stenosis. The fall in GFR, which is usually reversible, is due to the fall in BP and a decrease in glomerular capillary pressure produced by relaxation of the efferent arteriole.

Chronic renal failure. Hypertension responds well to extracellular volume depletion and often remits with the onset of dialysis. However, diuretics must be used carefully since they can reduce renal function further. Thiazides are ineffective when used alone in patients with a serum creatinine above 2-4 mg/dl. The following are significantly metabolized and relatively safe in renal failure:

- Short-acting beta-blockers (metoprolol, propranolol, labetolol, timolol)
- Central agents (clonidine, alpha-methyldopa)
- Prazosin
- Vasodilators (minoxidil is preferable to hydralazine whose metabolites may accumulate in renal failure)
- Calcium antagonists

Pheochromocytoma. The following must be avoided as they can precipitate a crisis:

- Beta-blockers (unopposed alpha-mediated vasoconstriction)
- Reserpine
- Sympatholytic agents, e.g., guanethidine
- Vasodilators

Preoperative management requires blockade of alpha-receptors with phenoxybenzamine (irreversible antagonist of alpha 1- and alpha 2-receptors, long duration) or prazosin (shorter-acting competitive antagonist of alpha 1-receptors). Beta-blockers are used to control tachycardia only after effective alpha-blockade. The contracted plasma volume must be expanded (liberal salt intake; stop diuretics) to prevent sharp falls in BP following removal of the tumor.

Hyperaldosteronism. Definitive therapy for adrenal adenoma is surgery but for bilateral adrenal hyperplasia is spironolactone. Dose requirements increase in proportion to the plasma aldosterone level (i.e., up to 600-800 mg/day). Distal K-sparing diuretics (e.g., amiloride) are an effective alternative.

Consider Step-Care Treatment

The report of the Joint National Committee on Detection, Evaluation, and Treatment of High Blood Pressure recommends a stepwise approach to treatment:

Step 1 Nonpharmacologic therapy. Consider Na and alcohol restriction, weight reduction, and control of other cardiovascular risk factors.

Step 2 Use a diuretic, a beta-blocker, a calcium antagonist, or an ACE inhibitor.

Step 3 Add a second drug of a different class, increase the dose of the first drug, or substitute another drug.

Step 4 Add a third drug of a different class or substitute a second drug.

Step 5 The patient needs to be further evaluated at a specialist unit, or a third or fourth drug can be added.

INDIVIDUAL DRUG CATEGORIES

The dose ranges given are generally those recommended in the 1988 Report of the Joint National Committee on the Detection, Evaluation, and Treatment of High Blood Pressure.

DIURETICS

Advantages

Diuretics with salt restriction are effective monotherapy for about two-thirds of hypertensives. They are inexpensive, convenient, well tolerated by most subjects, and are proven to reduce the risk of stroke in hypertension; they potentiate the antihypertensive actions of most other drugs; they can be given only once daily.

Disadvantages

Diuretics may not reverse the increased risk of death from myocardial infarction. There is a small incidence of drug allergy (fever, rash, interstitial nephritis) and impotence. They produce unwanted biochemical changes including hypokalemia, metabolic alkalosis, hypomagnesemia, hyperlipidemia, azotemia, hypercalcemia (thiazides), glucose intolerance, and hyperuricemia. These drugs are described in detail in Chapter 26.

Drugs and Doses

Hydrochlorothiazide (Hydrodiuril), 12.5-50 mg/day.

Furosemide (Lasix), 20-40 mg twice daily. Indicated in patients with renal insufficiency when the dose increases up to 400 mg/day in proportion to the reduction in creatinine clearance.

Bumetanide (Bumex), 1 mg twice daily.

Triamterene (Dyrenium), 50 mg twice or three times a day. Potassium-sparing diuretic.

Amiloride (Midamor), 5-10 mg daily. Potassium-sparing diuretic.

Spironolactone (Aldactone), 25-100 mg daily. Aldosterone antagonist with potassium-sparing actions.

Combinations. Hydrochlorothiazide + triamterene (Dyazide, Maxzide); hydrochlorothiazide + amiloride (Moduretic); spironolactone + hydrochlorothiazide (Aldactazide).

BETA-BLOCKERS

Their efficacy is increased by concurrent diuretic therapy.

Advantages

Beta-blockers are effective as single-agent therapy in about half of hypertensives; proven efficacy in secondary prevention of myocardial infarction; generally good patient acceptability; relatively low cost; and availability of drug with once or twice daily dosing regimes.

Table 19-1 **Choice of Beta-Blocker in Specific Categories of Patients.**

Beta-Blocker	Cardio-selective	ISA	Alpha-Blockade	Once daily Dosing	Dose Range (mg/day)
Propranolol (Inderal)					40-320
Nadolol (Corgard)				+	40-320
Metoprolol (Lopressor)	+			+	50-200
Atenolol (Tenormin)	+			+	25-150
Pindolol (Visken)		+			10-60
Acebutolol (Sectral)	+	+		+	200-1200
Labetolol (Trandate, Normodyne)	+		+		200-1800

+, present; acebutolol has significant hepatic metabolism but its active metabolites require renal excretion. Propranolol is available as a long-acting preparation that can be given once or twice daily. ISA, intrinsic sympathomimetic activity.

Disadvantages

These drugs often require a diuretic for effective antihypertensive action. They are not universally effective in primary prevention of myocardial infarction. They cause a spectrum of mild adverse effects which include: lethargy, malaise, sleep disturbance and vivid dreams, depression, impotence, decreased capacity for prolonged exercise, and gastrointestinal distress. Additional adverse effects occur in certain defined groups of patients.

Cardioselective drugs. These have less action on beta-receptors in the bronchioles than in the heart. However, this selectivity is reduced at higher doses.

Alpha-blockade. This additional action increases efficacy.

Hepatic metabolism. Shorter-acting drugs are safer in renal failure.

Heart failure, atrioventricular block, bradyrhythmias. Drugs with ISA are safer.

Bronchospasm. Cardioselective drugs (only at low dosage) or those with ISA are preferable.

Peripheral vascular disease or Raynaud's phenomenon. Nonselective and cardioselective beta-blockers can reduce skin blood flow. Drugs with ISA are safer.

Diabetes mellitus. Epinephrine released during insulin-induced hypoglycemia causes many of the warning symptoms and also helps to counter hypoglycemia. Cardioselective agents are probably safer.

Hypercholesterolemia. Drugs with ISA are preferable.

Black and elderly subjects. Labetolol, with its alpha 1-blocking action, is more effective.

Since all beta-blockers lower BP equivalently, the choice depends on cost, convenience, pharmacokinetics, and adverse effects.

ANGIOTENSIN-CONVERTING ENZYME INHIBITORS

These drugs (e.g., captopril, enalapril, lisinopril) lower BP by preventing generation of angiotensin II (AII) from angiotensin I (AI).

These ACE inhibitors not only increase the antihypertensive actions of diuretics but also diminish diuretic-induced hypokalemia (probably by diminishing aldosterone secretion).

Advantages

They are generally well tolerated. Usually these drugs do not impair exercise or sexual ability, lower cardiac output, or affect the central nervous system. Special indications are patients who have sustained such adverse effects from other drugs and those with diuretic-induced hypokalemia. Preliminary studies suggest that they may reduce proteinuria and perhaps diminish the progression of renal disease in patients with diabetic nephropathy. They are shown to increase life expectancy in patients with severe congestive heart failure.

Disadvantages

These drugs produce occasional severe adverse effects including drug allergy (rash, fever, eosinophilia), abnormal taste, and blood dyscrasias (agranulocytosis or pancytopenia). Occasionally they cause renal functional impairment (in patients with prerenal azotemia, bilateral renal artery stenosis, or renal artery stenosis in a single functioning kidney). All adverse effects are more common in patients with renal failure who, therefore, require careful monitoring. However, these adverse effects are quite uncommon. Most patients, especially those with mild renal parenchymal impairment (e.g., nephrosclerosis) actually have an **increase** in GFR and renal blood flow.

Adverse Drug Interactions

- Hyperkalemia can occasionally occur when combined with distal potassium-sparing diuretics or vigorous K replacement.
- Nonsteroidal anti-inflammatory agents (e.g., aspirin, indomethacin) can blunt the antihypertensive action.
- Beta-blockers inhibit renin secretion and normally should not be combined with ACE inhibitors.

Special Precautions

- Renal failure requires dosage adjustment.
- Bilateral renal artery stenosis or stenosis of a dominant kidney can have a severe but reversible reduction in GFR.
- Uncompensated cardiac failure or cirrhosis of the liver can cause prolonged hypotension.
- Collagen vascular disease, particularly scleroderma, is associated with a higher incidence of drug allergy and blood dyscrasias.

Drugs and Dosages

Captopril (Capoten^R), 12.5-100 mg twice or three times daily.

Enalapril (Vasotec^R), 2.5-40 mg daily.

Lisinopril (Zestril^R; Prinivil^R), 5-40 mg daily.

VASODILATORS

Advantages

These drugs have dose-dependent, powerful antihypertensive actions. Minoxidil is particularly effective in refractory renal parenchymal hypertension.

Disadvantages

Concurrent therapy is often required with diuretics and salt restriction (to prevent fluid retention) and beta-blockers (to prevent reflex cardiac stimulation). There is a high incidence of adverse effects including headaches, orthostatic hypotension, and impotence. Hydralazine can cause a lupuslike syndrome and minoxidil can cause pericardial effusion, particularly in patients with renal failure. Minoxidil causes hirsutism.

Special Precaution

These drugs are contraindicated in uncontrolled angina pectoris. The metabolic products of hydralazine accumulates in renal failure.

Drugs and Dosage

Hydralazine (Apresoline), 25-200 mg twice daily.

Minoxidil (Loniten), 2.5-40 mg twice daily.

ALPHA 1-RECEPTOR ANTAGONISTS

Advantages

They cause little reflex stimulation, salt retention, or impotence. They are particularly effective in the elderly and black patients with low-renin hypertension.

Disadvantages

They have rather poor patient acceptability. Adverse effects include orthostatic hypotension, fatigue, malaise, and gastrointestinal upsets. Their use is limited by cost, adverse effects, and need for frequent dosing.

Drugs and Dosage

Prazosin (Minipress), therapy should start with 1 mg of prazosin given at bedtime and a warning of possible orthostatic hypotension. Thereafter, the dose is increased slowly to a maximum of 20 mg given in three or four divided doses.

Terazosin (Hytrin), 1-20 mg daily.

CENTRAL AGENTS

Advantages

Effective in most hypertensives; little effect on renal hemodynamics; no reflex stimulation, salt retention, or increase in blood lipids.

Disadvantages

The main problems are the frequent, dose-related adverse effects which include sedation, depression, headache, weight gain, sleep disturbance, impotence, stuffy nose, dry mouth, weakness, lethargy, constipation, and orthostatic hypotension. Alpha-methyldopa causes a positive Coombs' test in 20% of patients, but hemolytic anemia in less than 1%; it can cause drug fever with rash and eosinophilia and occasionally hepatitis or cholestatic jaundice. A dangerous hypertensive crisis, associated with tachycardia, chest pain, nausea, and sweating, may occur on abrupt discontinuation of clonidine.

Drugs and Dosages

Alpha-methyldopa (Aldomet), 125-1000 mg twice daily.

Clonidine (Catapres), initially 0.1 mg twice daily; maximum dose, 1.2 mg daily. Clonidine can also be prescribed as a skin patch, but patients may develop a dermatitis.

Guanabenz (Wytensin), 4-32 mg twice daily.

Guanfacine (Tenex), 1-3 mg daily.

CALCIUM ANTAGONISTS

Only slow-release verapamil is licensed currently for treatment of hypertension in the United States. The calcium antagonists lower BP by blunting the basal arteriolar tone and the renal and aldosterone response to angiotensin. They are mildly salt depleting.

Advantages

They are especially effective in the elderly or in those with severe hypertension. They may not require salt restriction. These agents are especially useful in patients with angina and those with severe, low-renin hypertension (e.g., black patients).

Disadvantages

Verapamil often causes constipation and nifedipine occasionally causes diarrhea. Nifedipine causes edema in about 10% of patients. Verapamil and diltiazem blunt AV node conduction.

Drug Interactions

Verapamil and diltiazem depress atrioventricular conduction and must be used with caution with beta-blockers.

Verapamil and diltiazem increase plasma digoxin levels by decreasing digoxin clearance. Dosage adjustments are required.

Drugs and Doses

Verapamil slow release (Calan SR), 120-240 mg daily.

Diltiazem (Cardizem), 30-90 mg three times daily.

Nifedipine (Procardia), 10-60 mg three times daily.

INTRAVENOUS AGENTS

These drugs are considered in detail in Chapter 20.

OTHER

Reserpine and adrenergic neuron antagonists (e.g., guanadrel, guanethidine, bretylium) are used only occasionally because of frequent adverse effects.

RESULTS OF CLINICAL TRIALS IN HYPERTENSION

Treatment of malignant or severe hypertension undoubtedly prolongs life. Results from placebo-controlled trials of treatment (for an average of 5 years) of mild hypertension (average diastolic blood pressure, 100 mmHg) have shown that death from stroke is reduced by 50%, but myocardial infarction is reduced by less than 10%. These trials used diuretics as the primary treatment except the Medical Research Council trial, which compared a diuretic with propranolol; there was no overall benefit with the diuretic (see references in the Report of the Joint National Committee on Detection, Evaluation, and Treatment of High Blood Pressure for further information). Clearly, successful lowering of BP with a diuretic does not necessarily eliminate the excess risk of myocardial infarction.

Five trials have shown that beta-blockers significantly reduce the risk of reinfarction in normotensive patients after a primary myocardial infarction. Therefore, beta-blockers are strongly indicated in patients with a previous myocardial infarction.

Large placebo-controlled clinical trials have not yet reported on mortality or morbidity in mild hypertensives treated with drugs other than diuretics or beta-blockers. However, ACE inhibitors reduce mortality in patients with severe cardiac failure. Therefore, ACE inhibitors should be used when possible to manage hypertension in such patients.

SUGGESTED READING

Genest J, Kuchel O, Hamet P, Cantin M. Hypertension: physiopathology and treatment. New York: McGraw-Hill Book Company, 1983.

Glassock RJ. Current therapy in nephrology and hypertension. Philadelphia: BC Decker Inc, 1987.

McMahon FG. Management of essential hypertension: the new low dose era. New York: Futura Publishing Co, 1984.

The 1988 Report of the Joint National Committee on Detection, Evaluation, and Treatment of High Blood Pressure. Arch Intern Med 1988;148:1023-1038.

Chapter 20

Hypertensive Emergencies

Edward D. Frederickson

DEFINITION

Hypertension becomes an emergency when there is rapidly progressive end-organ damage or an imminent risk of death. This chapter describes the etiology, pathophysiology, and management of six important categories of emergency hypertension.

MALIGNANT HYPERTENSION

Despite its decreasing frequency, malignant hypertension remains a critical problem since prompt and appropriate management can save a patient's life. The clinical features include a diastolic blood pressure (BP) above 120 mmHg, papilledema with retinal hemorrhages and exudates, albuminuria, microscopic hematuria, and renal failure. Papilledema signifies cerebral edema. Occasionally, malignant nephrosclerosis occurs without papilledema.

Malignant hypertension is unstable since the severe hypertension induces further vascular and renal damage, which accelerates the process. These patients often have pre-existing essential hypertension which has frequently been poorly treated. Laboratory findings are inconsistent but often include a hyperkalemic metabolic alkalosis, a raised erythrocyte sedimentation rate, and a microangiopathic hemolytic anemia. Renal failure develops rapidly if malignant hypertension is not controlled. Proteinuria is common. There may be an active urinary sediment with red cells, white cells, and granular casts. Occasionally there is gross hematuria. The plasma renin activity and aldosterone levels are usually markedly elevated.

The life expectancy of patients with untreated malignant hypertension is only 2-6 months. However, effective control of hypertension before irreversible end-organ damage has occurred carries a good prognosis. These patients require urgent therapy, usually with intravenous drugs. Therefore, they should be managed in an intensive care unit. Initially, sublingual nifedipine or intravenous labetolol may be used in the emergency room before the patient is transferred to the intensive care unit. These drugs have a rapid onset of action and a short half-life. Dangerous hypotension is an occasional problem. Thereafter, an arterial line is placed and intensive treatment initiated, usually with intravenous sodium nitroprusside. Loop diuretics are used in patients who are volume expanded. However, some patients with malignant hypertension have severe vasoconstriction without volume expansion; diuretics should be avoided in these cases.

It is important not to reduce the blood pressure to normal levels too rapidly. Initially, the severe intimal proliferation and edema of small blood vessels limits organ perfusion; blood flow is therefore pressure dependent. Thus, an abrupt fall in BP can compromise perfusion of critical organs such as the brain and kidney and precipitate a stroke or renal failure. The initial aim should be to lower the diastolic BP to 100-110 mmHg within the first hour. This level can usually be maintained for 12-24 hr. It is wise to allow 36-48 hr before attempting to reduce BP to normal. Such gradual lowering of hypertension allows cerebral and renal vessels to accommodate and resume some autoregulatory function.

NEUROLOGICALLY UNSTABLE PATIENTS WITH HYPERTENSION

This includes patients with transient ischemic attacks, thrombotic or embolic cerebrovascular accidents (CVAs), intracranial or subarachnoid hemorrhages, and hypertensive encephalopathy. The Cushing reflex, which is initiated by increased intracranial pressure, is characterized by severe hypertension, bradycardia, and hyperventilation. Its reversal requires relief of the increased cerebral pressure. It is sometimes difficult to determine whether the primary event is a CVA complicating hypertension or the Cushing reflex complicating increased intracranial pressure. Therefore, computed axial tomography (CAT) is useful in the assessment of patients with hypertension and neurologic deterioration to determine whether hypertension is secondary to an intracerebral hemorrhage. A study of patients with a subarachnoid hemorrhage has demonstrated that a calcium-channel antagonist, nimodipine, reduces the associated vasospasm and decreases mortality. It is unclear whether other calcium antagonists have a similar beneficial effect.

Hypertensive encephalopathy is caused by patchy cerebral ischemia and generalized edema. Normally, the blood brain barrier is protected from the effects of hypertension by cerebral vasoconstriction. However, at a diastolic BP above approximately 120 mmHg, cerebral hyperperfusion occurs. Hypertensive encephalopathy is most likely to complicate sudden or severe increases in BP since patients with prolonged hypertension are protected by hypertrophy of the resistant vessels.

Patients with an unstable neurological examination require a very cautious approach to treatment of hypertension. Increased intracranial pressure, which can occur with powerful vasodilators such as hydralazine or minoxidil, may increase cerebral blood flow and, thereby, raise intracranial pressure further. Moreover, a sudden reduction in BP in the absence of effective cerebral autoregulation may induce cerebral ischemia or even infarction. Thus, the guidelines outlined above for the management of patients with malignant hypertension should be used in those with an unstable neurological examination. Nitroprusside is the drug of choice; its action can be titrated precisely and quickly and its actions include venodilation as well as arterial dilatation.

HYPERTENSION AND CARDIAC INSTABILITY

The direct effects of hypertension exacerbate angina by increasing cardiac work and oxygen demand and decreasing subendocardial perfusion, while the effects of prolonged hypertension add a further strain by inducing left ventricular hypertrophy. However, hypertension may be caused or exacerbated by coronary insufficiency which activates the sympathetic nervous system. Therefore, hypertension and coronary insufficiency require aggressive management. In the absence of congestive heart failure or bronchospasm, a beta-1 antagonist such as metoprolol, which can be given intravenously, is effective. Calcium-channel antagonists are alternatives. Nifedipine has the advantage of not decreasing cardiac contractility or depressing the conduction system.

Hypertension may precipitate acute left ventricular failure. Clearly, reversal of systemic hypertension is important to diminish the left ventricular afterload. Initial therapy with morphine sulfate, diuretics, and vasodilators is appropriate. Nifedipine is useful since it lowers BP and dilates the coronary arteries. Intravenous nitroglycerine also dilates the coronary arteries and lowers left ventricular preload by venodilatation. Sodium nitroprusside is both an arterial- and a venodilator. However, this drug is a powerful dilator of normal coronary vessels and may steal blood flow from ischemic regions of the myocardium. Diuretics should be used cautiously in patients with acute congestive heart failure (CHF) secondary to ischemia or myocardial infarction since the blood volume is not necessarily expanded and the ischemic left ventricle, which is often stiff and noncompliant, may depend upon preload to maintain cardiac output. Also, there is an abrupt rise in peripheral vascular resistance following intravenous loop diuretics given to patients with cardiac failure. This is probably due to further stimulation of the renin-angiotensin system and activation of sympathetic nerves. Thus, placement of a Swan-Ganz catheter is often very useful prior to diuresis to monitor the response to therapy.

Patients who have had recent coronary artery bypass grafts placed, or other arterial or major surgery, require aggressive control of any hypertension to avoid rupturing suture lines. The agents of choice include calcium-channel antagonists such as nifedipine and sympatholytic agents. After cardiac or coronary surgery, increased sympathetic stimulation leads to tachycardia and increased cardiac work which may promote ischemia. Therefore, vasodilators should be used sparingly or with appropriate beta-blockade to moderate the cardiac reflex responses.

ACUTE DISSECTING AORTIC ANEURYSM

Acute aortic dissection is an emergency which requires an integrated medical and surgical approach. Patients require initial medical therapy to decrease the shearing force on the aorta. The aortic wall shear is determined both by the mean arterial pressure and by its rate of rise which is set by cardiac contractility. Beta-blockers are a critical part of management since they reduce both blood pressure and cardiac contractility. Other useful drugs include verapamil, which has a negative inotropic action, and clonidine, which inhibits sympathetic activity. Sodium nitroprusside is used often but only after effective beta-blockade. Vasodilators such as hydralazine and minoxidil, which lead to increased sympathetic activity, can increase the shearing stress; however, they can be considered if fully effective and sustained beta-blockade is ensured. Ganglionic blockade with trimethaphan is logical since the antihypertensive response can be regulated by the degree of tilt and reflex responses are prevented. However, this drug causes many severe and adverse effects including paralytic ileus and urinary retention and is reserved for occasional emergency use.

SYMPATHETIC HYPERTENSION

Exaggerated sympathetic activity or sympathomimetic drug action can cause hypertension in several settings: pheochromocytoma, the clonidine withdrawal syndrome, administration of a sympathomimetic, or ingestion of tyramine by a patient taking a monoaminoxidase inhibitor, and drug abuse with cocaine, amphetamine, or phencyclidine. In each of these settings there is evidence of sympathomimetic overactivity with paroxysmal or unstable hypertension, usually accompanied by tachycardia and often by fever. The extremities may be mottled, cold, and cyanotic despite sweating. Patients complain of palpitations and headaches and they can experience panic and be deluded, or even psychotic. There may be nausea, vomiting, diarrhea, or abdominal cramps. Physical findings include pupillary dilation and piloerection. Orthostatic hypertension is frequently due to a reduced plasma volume and impaired cardiovascular reflexes. The marked increase in cardiac work, which is caused by hypertension and increased contractility, can precipitate angina or even a myocardial infarction.

The treatment of sympathetic hypertension should be directed at reducing the extreme peripheral vasoconstriction. Alpha-1 blockade with prazosin or phentolamine is a logical initial choice. More prolonged blockade can be achieved with phenoxybenzamine, which is a noncompetitive alpha-antagonist used in patients with pheochromocytoma. Such patients require complete alpha-blockade and plasma volume expansion prior to surgery (see Chapter 19). Beta-blockade is contraindicated initially, as unopposed alpha activity increases the vasoconstriction induced by a high concentration of catecholamines. However, following complete alpha-blockade, a small dose of a beta-blocker can be used to control tachycardia.

The treatment of choice for clonidine withdrawal is to reinstitute the drug. Subsequently, most patients should be weaned off clonidine over the next 2-3 weeks to prevent recurrences.

PREGNANCY-INDUCED HYPERTENSION

Hypertension occurs in 5% of all pregnancies and accounts for 25,000 infant deaths in the United States each year. Blood pressure normally falls during the first two trimesters but returns toward normal during the last trimester. The definition of pregnancy-induced hypertension is a rise in blood pressure of 30/15 mmHg or an absolute level above 140/90 mmHg. Fetal mortality increases sharply above these levels of blood pressure (see Figure 20-1).

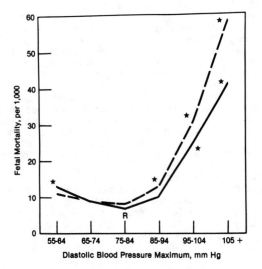

Figure 20-1. Fetal mortality in relation to the maximal diastolic blood pressure recorded during 38,636 pregnancies by the Collaborative Perinatal Project. Total series (solid line) is contrasted with patients manifesting comcomitant proteinuria of any degree (broken line). Asterisks designate mortality rates significantly different (P<.01) from rate of those patients with normal maximal diastolic values (R). (From Friedman EA, Neff RK. JAMA 1978;239:2249. Copyright 1978, American Medical Association.)

Preeclampsia is defined as hypertension with proteinuria, edema, or both, usually developing after the 20th week of gestation. It occurs most frequently in young nulliparous females but recurs during 25% of subsequent pregnancies. Eclampsia, which develops from pre-eclampsia, includes seizures and coma. Encephalopathy may develop at blood pressures of only 150/90 mmHg, suggesting that the upper limit of cerebral blood flow autoregulation is lowered in pregnancy.

Hypertension presenting during the first or second trimester of pregnancy is usually due to essential or secondary hypertension. However, the decrease in BP and increase in glomerular filtration rate which normally occurs during the first two trimesters may mask chronic hypertension or underlying mild renal parenchymal disease. These may become overt only during the last trimester.

The initial treatment for pregnancy-induced hypertension is to admit the patient to the hospital for rest. This controls hypertension in approximately 85% of patients. For those whose diastolic BP persists above 95 mmHg, antihypertensive drug therapy is appropriate. The use of drugs during pregnancy is always of concern. However, alpha-methyldopa and hydralazine have been used extensively. Labetolol, which is an alpha- and beta-blocker, is currently being evaluated. Many drugs are contraindicated (Table 20-2).

Magnesium sulfate ($MgSO_4$) is used frequently to prevent convulsions and control blood pressure. A bolus intravenous dose is followed by a continuous infusion adjusted to suppress the patellar reflexes without causing somnolence or depressed respirations. $MgSO_4$ should be used sparingly in patients with renal failure. It should be continued for 12-24 hours after delivery to prevent postpartum seizures.

Patients with chronic severe hypertension or significant renal insufficiency should be advised against pregnancy or counseled concerning a therapeutic abortion. Patients with mild or moderate hypertension, which is controlled by drugs, should usually be maintained on these medications unless they are contraindicated (Table 20-1). They require care in a high risk obstetrical clinic.

Table 20-1 Recommended Drugs in Hypertensive Emergencies

Parenteral Agents	Initial Dose	Comments
Sodium nitroprusside	0.5 µg/kg/min titrated upward every 3 to 5 min	Advantage-precise BP control. Disadvantage-metabolized to cyanide and thiocyanate; accumulation occurs after 3-5 days of therapy (more rapidly in renal failure); thiocyanate levels should be maintained below 10 mg/dl.
Labetolol	20 mg IV bolus followed by repeated doses or an infusion starting at 2 mg/min	Advantage-large dose range; increased alpha-antagonism at high doses. Disadvantage-may induce CHF or bronchospasm.
Hydralazine	5-10 mg IM or IV	Advantage-reasonably safe with monitoring. Disadvantage-reflex sympathetic activation may cause cardiac ischemia.
Trimethaphan	3-4 mg/min as an IV drip	Advantage-used to decrease shear in patients with dissecting aortic aneurysms. Disadvantage-paralytic ileus, urinary retention, and tachyphylaxis.
Phentolamine	5-10 mg IV	Advantage-used for short-term control of increased circulatory catecholamine actions. Disadvantage-tachycardia, abdominal pain, cramps, diarrhea, and vomiting.
Diazoxide	50-100 mg boluses each 10 min up to 300 mg	Advantage-prolonged action of 1-12 hr. Disadvantage-can cause profound hypotension; largely replaced by sodium nitroprusside.

Table 20-1 Recommended Drugs in Hypertensive Emergencies (cont'd)

Oral agents	Dose	Comments
Clonidine	0.2 mg p.o. followed by 0.1 mg every hr	Advantage-very effective, no cardiac stimulation, depression, or bronchospasm. Disadvantage-induces somnolence and mental depression; can cause a withdrawal syndrome.
Nifedipine	10 mg bite and swallow	Advantage-rapid onset, very effective. Disadvantage-short half-life requiring frequent dosing; causes flushing, tachycardia, and occasional severe hypotension.
Labetolol	200-400 mg orally	Advantage-combined with IV dosing. Disadvantage-may induce CHF or bronchospasm.
Metoprolol	50 mg q6h	Advantage-may be started intravenously during cardiac ischemia. Disadvantage-may induce CHF or bronchospasm.
Hydralazine	25 to 50 mg	Advantage-effective with beta-blockade. Disadvantage-sympathetic activation promotes cardiac ischemia; lupus syndrome.

Table 20-2 Antihypertensive Drugs in Pregnancy

α_2-Receptor agonists	Alpha-methyldopa (0.5 to 3 g per day) is used extensively; its safety and efficacy have been supported in trials. Neonatal tremors have been reported; other side effects are the same as in the nongravid population. Clonidine can cause embryopathy in animals and is not currently recommended.
β-Receptor antagonists	These agents currently are undergoing extensive testing; they appear to be safe and effective, e.g., atenolol (50 to 100 mg per day), metoprolol (50 to 225 mg per day), and propranolol (40 to 240 mg per day). They may cause fetal and neonatal bradycardia and hypoglycemia, and animal data suggest they may decrease the ability of the fetus to tolerate hypoxic stress.
α- and β-Receptor antagonists	Labetolol may be as effective as alpha-methyldopa but has not been fully studied. There is a possible association with retroplacental hemorrhage.
Arteriolar vasodilators	Hydralazine (50 to 200 mg per day) is used frequently as adjunctive therapy with methyldopa and β-receptor antagonists. There has only been fragmentary experience with minoxidil which is, thus, not recommended at present.
Converting-enzyme inhibitors	Captopril is associated with fetal death in animals and, therefore, is not used in pregnancy.
Diuretics	Most authorities discourage their use, although some continue them if they were effective in controlling hypertension before gestation. Some use diuretics when blood pressure control is poor despite other agents, the fetus is immature, and pregnancy termination is the only alternative.
Miscellaneous	Calcium-channel antagonists and serotonin antagonists (e.g., ketanserin) are currently under investigation. Ganglion-blocking agents and nitroprusside are contraindicated.

Reprinted with permission from Lindheimer MD, Katz AI. Hypertension in pregnancy. N Engl J Med 1985;131:675-680.

SUGGESTED READING

MALIGNANT HYPERTENSION

Glasscock RJ. Hypertensive emergencies. In: Current therapy in nephrology and hypertension-2. Toronto: BC Decker Inc, 1987;296-300.

Kaplan NM. Hypertension crises. 4th ed. Clinical hypertension. Baltimore: Williams & Wilkins, 1986;7:273-281.

Smith MC, Dunn M. Renovascular and renal parenchymal hypertension. In: Brenner BM, Rector FC, eds. 3rd ed. The kidney. WB Saunders, 1986;27:1221-1257.

NEUROLOGICALLY UNSTABLE PATIENTS

Allen GS, Ahiv, HS, Preziosi TJ, et al. Cerebral arterial spasm - a controlled trial of nimodipine in patients with subarachnoid hemorrhage. N Engl J Med 1983;308:619-624.

CARDIAC INSTABILITY

Given BD, Lee TH, Stone PH, Dzau VT. Nifedipine in severely hypertensive patients with congestive heart failure and preserved ventricular function. Arch Intern Med 1985;145;281-285.

Mann T, Cohn PF, Homan L, Green LH, Markis JE, Phillips DA. Effect of nitroprusside on regional myocardial blood flow in coronary artery disease. Circulation 1978;57:732-737.

AORTIC DISSECTION

Slater EE, DeSanctis RW. Dissection of the aorta. Med Clin North Am 1979;63:141-154.

SYMPATHETIC HYPERTENSION

Bravo EL, Gifford RW, Jr. Pheochromocytoma: diagnosis, localization, and management. N Engl J Med 1984;311:1298-1303.

Houston MC. Abrupt cessation of treatment in hypertension. Consideration of clinical features, mechanisms, prevention, and management of the discontinuation syndrome. Am Heart J 1981;102:415-430.

HYPERTENSION IN PREGNANCY

Friedman EA, Neff RK. Hypertension-hypotension in pregnancy: correlation with fetal outcome. JAMA 1978;239:2249-2251.

Kaplan NM. Hypertension in pregnancy and the pill. In: Clinical hypertension. 4th ed. Baltimore: Williams & Wilkins, 1986;10:345-374.

Lindheimer MD, Katz AI. Hypertension in pregnancy. N Engl J Med 1985;131:675-680.

Chapter 21

Acute Renal Failure

Nicolas J. Guzman
John C. Peterson

DEFINITION

Acute renal failure is defined as the abrupt deterioration of the ability of the kidney to excrete nitrogenous wastes. This leads to acute retention of nitrogen products, a condition known as azotemia.

CLASSIFICATION

Acute renal failure can be divided into three categories.

PRERENAL AZOTEMIA

Rapidly reversible decrease in glomerular filtration rate (GFR) due to renal hypoperfusion.

ACUTE (PARENCHYMAL) RENAL FAILURE

Decrease in GFR due to a) tubular cell damage from hypoperfusion or nephrotoxic injury (also known as acute tubular necrosis or ATN); b) glomerular, tubulointerstitial, or vascular inflammation; c) thrombotic or embolic renovascular occlusion.

OBSTRUCTIVE UROPATHY (POSTRENAL AZOTEMIA)

Decrease in GFR due to obstruction of the genitourinary tract.

This chapter will concentrate on prerenal azotemia and ATN.

PRERENAL AZOTEMIA

Prerenal azotemia is responsible for 50% of the cases of acute renal failure seen in hospitalized patients.

PATHOPHYSIOLOGY

Renal autoregulation ensures that glomerular blood flow and capillary hydrostatic pressure are maintained over a wide range of perfusion pressures (mean arterial pressure of 60-120 mmHg). However, systemic hypotension also triggers hormonal and neural responses such as stimulation of the renin-angiotensin-aldosterone axis, antidiuretic hormone release, and the sympathetic nervous system which redistributes blood flow away from the renal cortex and leads to avid tubular reabsorption of sodium, water, and urea. As a result, urine volume and sodium output decline and the osmolality increases. The blood urea nitrogen (BUN) increases before changes in serum creatinine become apparent. Further reductions in renal blood flow decrease GFR, and if renal hypoperfusion is sustained or severe, acute renal failure will ensue. Nonsteroidal anti-inflammatory drugs (NSAIDs) and angiotensin-converting enzyme (ACE) inhibitors interfere with some of these compensatory mechanisms and reduce GFR in prerenal patients (see Chapter 27).

ETIOLOGY

Common Causes of Prerenal Azotemia

- Intravascular volume depletion
  Hemorrhage
  Gastrointestinal losses (e.g., diarrhea, vomiting, nasogastric suction)
  Renal losses (e.g., osmotic diuresis, diuretics, adrenal insufficiency)
  Skin losses (e.g., burns, excessive sweating)
  Sequestration in third spaces (e.g., pancreatitis, peritonitis, massive trauma with crush injury)

- Reduced cardiac output
  Cardiogenic shock
  Congestive heart failure
  Pericardial tamponade
  Massive pulmonary embolism

- Systemic vasodilatation
  Anaphylaxis
  Antihypertensive drugs
  Sepsis
  Drug overdose

- Systemic or renal vasoconstriction
  Anesthesia
  Surgery
  Alpha adrenergic agonists or high dose dopamine
  Hepatorenal syndrome

- Impaired renal autoregulation
  Nonsteroidal anti-inflammatory drugs
  Angiotensin-converting enzyme inhibitors

- Hyperviscosity syndromes
  Multiple myeloma or macroglobulinemia
  Polycythemia

CLINICAL PRESENTATION

Findings Suggestive of Prerenal Azotemia

- Symptoms
  History of fluid losses (vomiting, diarrhea, polyuria, burns, etc.)
  Use of NSAID or ACE inhibitors
  Thirst
- Signs
  Fluid deficit by intake/output balance (output >intake)
  Weight loss (catabolic patients may lose >1 lb/day)
  Oliguria
  Orthostatic hypotension (decrease in systolic blood pressure >10 mmHg) and pulse rise (>10/min)
  Tachycardia
  Flat neck veins in the supine position
  Lack of sweat
  Dry skin and mucosae with loss of skin turgor
- Laboratory tests
  Hemoconcentration (increased albumin and hematocrit)
  Serum BUN/creatinine >20*
  Urine osmolality >500 mOsm/kg H_2O
  Urinary sodium <20 mEq/l
  FE_{Na} <1 %
- Special monitoring
  Low central venous pressure, pulmonary capillary wedge pressure, and cardiac output
  Evidence of congestive heart failure, tamponade, sepsis, cardiogenic shock

*Can also occur with increased protein catabolism such as steroid therapy, sepsis, burns, surgery, high fever, and gastrointestinal bleeding

Prerenal azotemia often results from failure to fully replace fluid and electrolyte losses. Body weight is a useful indicator of volume status.

INVESTIGATIONS

Examination of the urine is very helpful. Typical findings in oliguric patients who have not had recent diuretic therapy include:

- Urine specific gravity >1.030
- Urine osmolality >500 mOsm/kg H_2O
- Urine sodium concentration <20 mEq/l
- Fractional excretion of sodium (FE_{Na}) <1%

$$FE_{Na} = \frac{U_{Na} \times P_{Cr}}{P_{Na} \times U_{Cr}} \times 100$$

The FE_{Na} also can be low in some nonoliguric forms of acute renal failure (see section on acute renal failure).

MANAGEMENT

In patients with prerenal azotemia, rapid and aggressive volume replacement is essential to prevent renal failure. A useful protocol consists of administering a fluid challenge of 300-500 ml of isotonic saline intravenously (IV) over 30-60 min; a more gradual infusion of 100-150 ml/hr is required in the elderly or when the cardiovascular status is fragile. The fluid challenge may be repeated once or twice at hourly intervals while the urine output and cardiovascular status are monitored closely. Thereafter, maintenance fluid replacement should be continued to maintain the urine output between 1-2 ml/min. If there are doubts regarding the patient's cardiovascular status, a Swan-Ganz catheter should be inserted to monitor central venous pressure, pulmonary capillary wedge pressure, and cardiac output. In patients with prerenal azotemia from causes other than volume depletion (e.g., congestive heart failure, pericardial tamponade, drug overdose), the underlying disorder should be corrected.

ACUTE TUBULAR NECROSIS

DEFINITION

The term acute tubular necrosis (ATN) describes an abrupt decrease in GFR due to tubular cell damage as a consequence of renal hypoperfusion or nephrotoxic injury. While ATN is usually accompanied by oliguria (urine output less than 500 ml/24 hr), some patients will continue to excrete 1-2 l of urine per day. The hallmark of ATN is the acute onset or worsening of azotemia which is not immediately reversible after withdrawal of the causative agent.

INCIDENCE

In the hospital population the incidence of ATN varies from 1% of all admissions to a general medical or surgical ward to as high as 50% in patients undergoing emergency abdominal aortic aneurysm resection, 20% in those undergoing open heart surgery or sustaining severe trauma, and 10% in patients undergoing elective abdominal aortic surgery. The mean incidence of ATN in a general hospital is approximately 5%.

ETIOLOGY

Renal hypoperfusion leading to ischemia with inadequate restoration of renal perfusion accounts for 50% of cases. Ischemic damage may occur also in the absence of systemic hypotension, as is the case in more than 50% of patients with postsurgical ATN.

The other major cause of ATN is nephrotoxic injury from either exogenous (25%) or endogenous (20%) toxins. Approximately 70% of patients with ATN will have more than one possible cause for their renal failure. The accompanying display lists a variety of agents that can induce nephrotoxic injury.

Some Toxic Causes of ATN

- Exogenous toxins
    - Antibiotics (e.g., aminoglycosides, cephalosporins, tetracyclines, amphotericin B, pentamidine)
    - Radiographic contrast media
    - Heavy metals (e.g., mercury, lead, arsenic, bismuth)
    - Chemotherapeutic agents (e.g., cisplatin, methotrexate, mitomycin)
    - Immunosuppressive agents (e.g., cyclosporine)
    - Organic solvents (e.g., ethylene glycol, carbon tetrachloride)
    - Pesticides
    - Fungicides

- Endogenous toxins
    - Myoglobin
    - Hemoglobin
    - Calcium
    - Uric acid
    - Oxalate

PATHOPHYSIOLOGY

- **Back-leak of filtered tubular fluid due to damaged tubular epithelium.** Filtered fluid leaks back from the tubular lumen into the peritubular vasculature across a disrupted tubular epithelial barrier. This mechanism is important in nephrotoxic ATN.
- **Deposition of tubular debris with tubular obstruction.** This is important in early ischemic ATN.
- **Alterations in renal hemodynamics leading to reduction in total renal blood flow and redistribution of renal blood flow away from the outer cortex.** This may play a role in both types of ATN.
- **Alterations in the permeability barrier for glomerular filtration.** The importance of this mechanism is unclear.

Regardless of the pathogenetic mechanism, the final result of ATN is always impaired renal function with progressive azotemia and, in most cases, impaired water and electrolyte handling.

CLINICAL PRESENTATION AND LABORATORY FINDINGS

Most patients with ATN present with an acute rise in serum creatinine and oliguria. Some patients, particularly those with nephrotoxic injury, are nonoliguric initially. Complete anuria rarely occurs in ATN and its presence should suggest obstructive uropathy, bilateral cortical necrosis, vascular occlusion, or rapidly progressive glomerulonephritis. A smaller number of patients will present at a later stage with complications such as volume overload leading to congestive heart failure and pulmonary edema, peripheral edema, hypertension, or hyperventilation and dyspnea from metabolic acidosis. Occasionally uremia, characterized by lethargy, anorexia, nausea, vomiting, and abdominal pain, is the presenting feature. Frequently the patients will have marked electrolyte disturbances consisting of severe azotemia, hyperkalemia, high anion gap metabolic acidosis, and hyponatremia due to volume expansion. The daily rate of rise in serum creatinine with total renal failure ranges between 0.5 and 1.0 mg/dl. A more rapid increase should suggest the presence of a hypercatabolic state or massive muscle destruction. Other metabolic abnormalities include hyperphosphatemia, hypermagnesemia, hypocalcemia, and hyperuricemia.

Careful examination of the urine reveals an active urine sediment with renal tubular epithelial cells, cellular debris, cellular and coarse granular ("muddy" brown or "ugly-looking") casts. Hematuria and red blood cell casts are rare. White blood cells or white blood cell casts suggest acute interstitial nephritis or pyelonephritis. Significant pigmenturia or crystalluria usually points to the etiology of ATN. Eosinophiluria may be seen in interstitial nephritis.

In the setting of oliguria and acute azotemia, and in the absence of recent diuretic therapy, a high FE_{Na} (>1%), a urine osmolality less than 350 mOsm/kg H_2O, and a urine sodium concentration >40 mEq/l are characteristic of ATN. These urinary diagnostic indices are helpful in trying to differentiate between ATN and prerenal azotemia; however, a low FE_{Na} (<1%) can occur in ATN, particularly the non-oliguric types, when associated with radiocontrast media, sepsis, burns, liver failure, edematous states, and interstitial nephritis.

CLINICAL COURSE

The clinical course of ATN can be divided into three phases.

Initiating Phase

This is defined as the period between the onset of decreased renal function and the occurrence of established renal failure when renal failure can still be reversed by treating the underlying disorder or removing the offending agent.

Maintenance Phase

Renal failure is not immediately reversible. Duration may vary from a few hours to 6 or more weeks. Renal function usually improves spontaneously after 10 to 16 days in oliguric patients and 5 to 8 days in nonoliguric patients. Most complications occur during this phase.

Recovery Phase

Renal function begins to improve and BUN and serum creatinine return toward normal. Oliguric patients increase their urine output and may sometimes enter a polyuric phase, which can result in serious fluid and electrolyte imbalance. Recovery of renal function usually occurs within 4 weeks but occasionally takes up to 12 months. In a few patients, particularly those with previous underlying renal disease, renal function may never return to baseline.

SELECTED CLINICAL ASPECTS OF ATN

EXOGENOUS NEPHROTOXINS

Antibiotics

Aminoglycosides. ATN occurs in 10-26% of patients receiving gentamicin, tobramycin, or amikacin even when plasma levels are maintained within the therapeutic range. Nephrotoxicity correlates better with total cumulative aminoglycoside dose than plasma levels. ATN, which is usually nonoliguric, becomes clinically apparent after 5-10 days of therapy. The following predispose to ATN during aminoglycoside therapy: advanced age, pre-existing renal disease, volume depletion, and recent exposure to other nephrotoxins. Early findings include isosthenuria due to nephrogenic diabetes insipidus, tubular proteinuria, and Fanconi's syndrome with proximal renal tubular acidosis, glycosuria, and aminoaciduria. Tubular magnesium and potassium wasting may lead to hypomagnesemia and hypokalemia. With more severe nephrotoxicity, azotemia ensues. Recovery may be slow (months) or incomplete. Tobramycin appears to be as nephrotoxic as gentamicin.

Amphotericin B. Nephrotoxicity occurs in most patients after a cumulative dose of 2 to 3 g; it is rare below 600 mg. Distal nephron damage is manifested as polyuria with isosthenuria (nephrogenic diabetes insipidus), hypokalemia, and distal renal tubular acidosis. Renal vasoconstriction contributes to ATN. Salt repletion and mannitol may be protective.

Radiographic Contrast Media

The reported incidence of ATN following administration of classic contrast media ranges from 1 to 50%. Renal failure usually occurs 1 or 2 days after exposure; it is characterized by a persistent nephrogram, a low FE_{Na}, and a high urine specific gravity. ATN can be prevented by adequate hydration with saline and/or mannitol given immediately prior to the contrast load. New nonionic radiographic contrast agents may have less nephrotoxicity. The following are associated with an increased risk for ATN from contrast media:

- Advanced age
- Pre-existing renal disease
- Volume depletion or any other prerenal state
- Diabetes mellitus, especially with vascular complications
- Multiple myeloma
- Large or repeated doses of contrast
- Recent exposure to other nephrotoxic agents

Cyclosporine

Cyclosporine nephrotoxicity is usually dose dependent; blood levels help to predict the renal failure (see Chapter 25).

Cisplatin

Cisplatin nephrotoxicity, which occurs in 50-75% of patients that receive it, usually causes severe tubular magnesium wasting; however, ATN and chronic renal insufficiency have also been described. Toxicity can be reduced by hydration, mannitol, and a slow infusion of cisplatin in chloride-containing solutions.

Organic Compounds

Ethylene glycol is an occasional cause of poisoning and ATN. Renal failure is associated with deposition of calcium oxalate crystals inside the tubules and the diagnosis can be made by identifying these crystals in the urine. Patients with ethylene glycol poisoning almost always require hemodialysis in addition to ethanol treatment.

ENDOGENOUS NEPHROTOXINS

Pigments

Rhabdomyolysis can be caused by:

- Direct damage to muscles (e.g., trauma, crush injury, burns).
- Ischemia and/or increased muscle metabolism (e.g., seizures, strenuous exercise, heat stroke, hyperthermia, prolonged compression, shock, vascular occlusion).
- Metabolic disorders (e.g., ketoacidosis, hypokalemia, hypophosphatemia).
- Muscle diseases (e.g., dermatomyositis, polymyositis).
- Toxins (e.g., alcohol, heroin, CO poisoning, snake bite, brown recluse spider bite).
- Severe infections.

A common clinical presentation is that of the alcoholic patient who, after a prolonged binge during which starvation and volume depletion have occurred, develops ketoacidosis, hypokalemia, and hypophosphatemia. The release of large amounts of myoglobin from necrotic muscle, particularly in the presence of volume depletion and acidosis, precipitates ATN. One-third of patients with rhabdomyolysis will develop ATN.

The clinical features of rhabdomyolytic ATN include: muscle pain, dark brown urine, a positive orthotoluidine test for blood in the urine ("dipstix," usually with uniform staining), hyperkalemia, hyperphosphatemia, hyperuricemia, early hypocalcemia, and late hypercalcemia. Elevated serum creatine phosphokinase and myoglobin levels indicate ongoing rhabdomyolysis.

ATN can be prevented by vigorous volume replacement with isotonic saline (200-300 ml/hr), mannitol (12.5-25 g IV in 30 min) or furosemide (40-300 mg IV every 4-6 hr) to maintain a urine output between 100 and 200 ml/hr, and urine alkalinization to a pH above 7 with intravenous sodium bicarbonate (1 mEq/kg/dose). However, this last goal is often difficult to achieve and the use of large amounts of alkali may induce tetany in hypocalcemic patients. When ATN develops, the patient is usually so severely hypercatabolic that early and frequent hemodialysis is almost always required. The prognosis for recovery of renal function is good. Mortality, however, varies from 5 to 10%.

Massive intravascular hemolysis, as seen in severe transfusion reactions and snake bites, may cause significant hemoglobinuria and ATN. Strategies for prevention and treatment of hemoglobinuric ATN are the same as those for myoglobinuric ATN.

Crystals

Hyperuricemic ATN can be precipitated by chemotherapy for leukemia and lymphoma or by tumors with high cell turnover (e.g., lymphoproliferative and germ cell neoplasms). Preventive measures include vigorous hydration, alkaline diuresis, and allopurinol. These should be initiated several days before chemotherapy and maintained during the induction period. Hyperkalemia and hyperphosphatemia commonly complicate hyperuricemic ATN. The plasma uric acid level is frequently above 20 mg/dl. Renal failure results from intratubular deposition of uric acid crystals. Hemodialysis is the treatment of choice.

Multiple Myeloma

ATN may occur in patients with multiple myeloma from tubular damage by light chains, intratubular casts, or from complications such as hypercalcemia, hyperviscosity, volume depletion, and infections. These patients are also very susceptible to contrast-induced ATN.

Pregnancy

ATN precipitated by septic abortion remains a frequent problem in certain areas. ATN in late pregnancy is usually associated with eclampsia, abruptio placentae, peripartum hemorrhage, amniotic fluid embolism, or prolonged intrauterine fetal death. The pathogenetic mechanisms appear to be a combination of renal hypoperfusion from vasospasm and formation of fibrin thrombi inside the glomerular capillaries. Disseminated intravascular coagulation is a frequent complication. Most patients develop ATN although partial or complete cortical necrosis leading to end-stage renal disease can occur.

Rare forms of pregnancy-associated acute renal failure include acute fatty liver with ATN and postpartum acute renal failure. In the former, acute renal failure is associated with liver disease of multiple etiologies; the only effective treatment is termination of the pregnancy. Postpartum acute renal failure is a form of thrombotic microangiopathy with histologic findings suggestive of malignant hypertension. There is no effective therapy.

Hepatorenal Syndrome

This is a progressive decline in renal function in patients with advanced liver disease (usually cirrhosis), in the absence of other identifiable causes. There is marked renal vasoconstriction; the urine sodium concentration is usually below 10 mEq/l and the FE_{Na} is <1%. The syndrome usually develops in the hospital after aggressive diuretic therapy, paracentesis, infection, surgery, or gastrointestinal bleeding. The mortality is very high (>95%) and is usually due to liver failure, infection, or hemorrhage. There is no effective therapy. Colloid infusions can occasionally improve renal perfusion and increase diuresis but the effect is very short-lived; repeated infusions cause volume expansion which increases the risk of bleeding from esophageal varices. In some patients, the insertion of a peritoneo-venous (LeVeen) shunt has reversed the syndrome.

DIAGNOSTIC APPROACH TO THE PATIENT WITH ACUTE AZOTEMIA

After excluding a spurious elevation in serum creatinine concentration (see Chapter 1), the next step is to determine whether the azotemia is acute or chronic. In the absence of recent renal function tests, the presence of one or more of the following features is suggestive of chronic renal disease:

- History
   Family history of renal disease, e.g., polycystic kidney
   disease
   Chronic disease causing renal insufficiency, e.g.,
   diabetes mellitus

- Symptoms
   Polyuria, nocturia, edema, or hematuria
   Anorexia, nausea, vomiting, abdominal pain, lethargy, or
   pruritis
   Symptoms of chronic urinary obstruction or infections

- Signs
   Uremic fetor and frost
   Hypertension
   Peripheral neuropathy

- Routine tests
   Normocytic, normochromic anemia
   Radiologic evidence of renal osteodystrophy
   Bilateral small or scarred kidneys on ultrasound

Once chronic renal failure has been excluded, the next step is
to identify patients with prerenal azotemia (see pages 197 and 198) or
urinary tract obstruction. All patients should have a single bladder
catheterization, a complete urinalysis, and a renal ultrasound to
search for obstruction. Renal ultrasound may be nondiagnostic early
in its course. Whenever the index of suspicion is high, ultrasound
should be repeated and further diagnostic tests (e.g., hippuran
renogram, retrograde pyelogram, computed tomography) undertaken.

Findings Suggestive of Obstructive Uropathy

- History of previous urinary tract obstruction or infections.
- Findings suggestive of bladder outflow obstruction (e.g.,
   dysuria, nocturia, frequency, hesitation, weakening of stream,
   enlarged prostate, distended bladder, flank mass, or
   tenderness).
- History of diseases known to predispose to papillary necrosis
   (e.g., diabetes mellitus, sickle cell, or analgesic abuse).
- Pelvic or retroperitoneal disease or surgery.
- Complete anuria or wide variations in urine output.
- Normal urinalysis in the setting of progressive renal failure.

ACUTE RENOVASCULAR DISEASE

Etiology

   Aortic aneurysm (dissection, thrombosis)
   Renal artery dissection or thrombosis (trauma, postangioplasty)
   Embolism (thrombus, cholesterol)
   Thrombotic microangiopathy
   Renal vein thrombosis

Findings Suggestive of Acute Renovascular Disease

- Hypertension (new onset or accelerated)
- Evidence of aortic or renal arterial disease (aortic aneurysm, abdominal bruits, reduced or absent femoral pulses)
- Vascular disease elsewhere (peripheral, cerebral)
- Source for arterial embolization (infective endocarditis, atrial fibrillation, recent myocardial infarction)
- Evidence of cholesterol embolization (recent aortic catheterization, livedo reticularis, elevated erythrocyte sedimentation rate (ESR), peripheral eosinophilia, low complement levels, thrombocytopenia)
- Evidence of thrombotic microangiopathy (thrombocytopenia, microangiopathic anemia, fever, neurologic abnormalities)
- Nephrotic syndrome associated with proximal tubular dysfunction (suggests renal vein thrombosis)

ACUTE INTERSTITIAL NEPHRITIS (see Chapter 14)

Findings Suggestive of Acute Interstitial Nephritis

- History
  Previous allergic reaction
  Exposure to relevant drugs (e.g., penicillins, NSAID, sulfonamides)

- Signs
  Fever
  Skin rash
  Arthralgias
  Lymphadenopathy

- Laboratory tests
  Peripheral blood: thrombocytopenia, eosinophilia
  Urinalysis: pyuria, white blood cells casts, eosinophiluria (Pyuria and bacteriuria suggest acute pyelonephritis.)

ACUTE GLOMERULONEPHRITIS AND VASCULITIS (see Chapter 4)

Findings Suggestive of Glomerulonephritis or Vasculitis

- Signs
  Fever
  Skin rash
  Arthralgias
  Evidence of systemic disease or pulmonary involvement

- Laboratory tests
  Elevated ESR, low complement levels
  Positive serology for collagen vascular disease
  Urinalysis: hematuria and red blood cell casts

ACUTE TUBULAR NECROSIS (ATN)

The diagnosis of ATN is made only after exclusion of all of the other conditions mentioned. The following findings suggest ATN:

- History of renal hypoperfusion or exposure to nephrotoxins, particularly in patients with risk factors for ATN.
- Urinalysis with coarse granular casts and renal tubular epithelial cells.
- Pigmenturia or crystalluria.
- Oliguria associated with:
    urine osmolality <350 mOsm/kg H_2O
    urinary sodium >40 mEq/l
    FE_{Na} >1%
- Normal-sized kidneys on ultrasound

Most patients with acute renal failure will be diagnosed on clinical grounds alone. A group of patients remain, however, in whom the diagnosis is unclear and a kidney biopsy is needed. Kidney biopsy should normally be performed in patients in whom acute renal failure persists beyond 4-6 weeks in the absence of a known etiology.

COMPLICATIONS OF ACUTE RENAL FAILURE

These result from accumulation of nitrogenous wastes, disordered handling of water and electrolytes, and inability to excrete acid metabolites. They develop more rapidly and are more severe in oliguric and catabolic patients. Life-threatening complications include:

- **Hypervolemia** causing hypertension and congestive heart failure
- **Hyperkalemia** causing severe arrhythmias
- High anion gap **metabolic acidosis**
- **Hyponatremia** leading to central nervous system dysfunction
- **Uremia** leading to neurological dysfunction, gastrointestinal bleeding, platelet dysfunction, and, rarely, pericarditis
- **Infections**, particularly sepsis, pneumonia, and urinary tract are common (30-70% incidence) and are the leading cause of mortality

Less serious complications include hyperphosphatemia, hyperuricemia, hypocalcemia, hypercalcemia, hypermagnesemia, anemia, and thrombocytopenia.

MANAGEMENT

First, all reversible factors must be rapidly and exhaustively sought and treated. Conversion of oliguric to nonoliguric ATN may facilitate management but does not clearly reduce morbidity or mortality. This may be initiated by administering mannitol (12.5-25 g IV) or a loop diuretic such as furosemide (80-400 mg IV) and repeated once if no response is seen after 1 hour. However, mannitol may precipitate congestive heart failure and high doses of loop diuretics may impair hearing. Complications can be prevented by close monitoring of fluid and electrolyte balance, and by serial assessment of clinical and biochemical parameters as indicated below.

Fluid Intake

Restrict fluids to match measurable plus insensible losses (usually <1 l/day in oliguric patients).

Diet

Electrolytes. Restrict to match measured losses. For Na this is usually <2 g or 86 mEq/day and for K is usually <1.5 g or 40 mEq/day.

Protein. Restrict to 0.6 g/kg/day (high biologic value).

Carbohydrates. Provide at least 100 g/day.

Weight. Allow for loss of 0.5 lb/day due to catabolism.

Hyperalimentation. Consider this especially in catabolic patients.

Biochemical Monitoring

Serum Na. Avoid hyponatremia by restricting free water.

Serum K. Treat hyperkalemia with sodium bicarbonate, glucose plus insulin, Kayexalate, or dialysis. Use calcium gluconate to antagonize the cardiac effects of potassium (see Chapter 7).

Serum Bicarbonate. Maintain above 15 mEq/l.

Serum PO_4. Control hyperphosphatemia with phosphate binders such as aluminum hydroxide, 30-60 ml 4 to 6 times a day.

Serum Ca. Hypocalcemia rarely requires therapy; treat only if symptomatic or IV sodium bicarbonate is used.

Drugs

Avoid magnesium-containing medications.

Adjust drug dosages for level of renal function (see Chapter 27).

Dialysis

Early dialysis simplifies management and nutritional support. Hemodialysis, continuous arteriovenous hemofiltration, and peritoneal dialysis are all effective (see Chapters 23 and 24).

Indications for Dialysis in Oliguric Patients

- Severe hyperkalemia, particularly in catabolic patients.
- Volume overload resulting in congestive heart failure or severe hypertension.
- Severe metabolic acidosis (pH <7.20).
- Symptomatic uremia, e.g., encephalopathy, hemorrhagic gastritis.
- BUN >100 mg/dl.
- Uremic pericarditis.

The predialysis BUN and creatinine should be maintained below 100 mg/dl and 8 mg/dl, respectively.

PROGNOSIS

The mortality from acute renal failure is 20-50% in a medical setting and 60-70% when surgically related. This high mortality is mainly due to the nature of the underlying disorders. Factors associated with an increased mortality include: advanced age, severe underlying disease, and multiple organ failure. The leading causes of death are infections, progression of the underlying disease, gastrointestinal hemorrhage, and fluid and electrolyte disturbances. Patients who survive usually regain enough renal function to avoid chronic dialysis. Despite current technological advances in critical care, mortality has not changed significantly during the past 20 years. Therefore, the importance of prevention of acute renal failure cannot be overemphasized.

SUGGESTED READING

Hou SH, Bushinsky DA, Wish JB, Cohen JJ, Harrington JT. Hospital-acquired renal insufficiency: a prospective study. Am J Med 1983; 74:243-248.

Pru C, Kjellstrand C. Urinary indices and chemistries in the differential diagnosis of prerenal failure and acute tubular necrosis. Semin Nephrol 1985;5(3):224-233.

Rasmussen HH, Ibels LS. Acute renal failure. Am J Med 1982;73:211-218.

Schrier RW. Acute renal failure: pathogenesis, diagnosis and management. Hosp Prac 1981:93-112.

Chapter 22

Chronic Renal Failure

John C. Peterson

DEFINITION

Chronic renal failure (CRF) exists when renal function has been diminished by pathologic renal damage. This includes a broad spectrum of functional impairment extending from a creatinine clearance of 70 ml/min (mild impairment) to as low as 5 ml/min. In contrast, end-stage renal disease (ESRD) is present when there is so little remaining function that patients require replacement therapy in the form of dialysis or transplantation (see Chapters 23-25).

INCIDENCE

In 1986, over 90,000 patients were being treated for ESRD. Similar data are not available for patients with chronic renal failure.

ETIOLOGY

Major Causes of CRF in Adults

- Glomerulonephritis
- Hypertension (nephrosclerosis)
- Diabetic nephropathy
- Hereditary renal disease
    Polycystic kidney disease
    Alport's syndrome
- Obstructive uropathy
- Interstitial nephritis

PATHOPHYSIOLOGY

PROGRESSION OF CRF TO ESRD

Although the initial damage to the kidneys may be due to any one of a variety of conditions, when the plasma creatinine exceeds 2.0 mg/dl (177 mmol), progression to ESRD is common. The reason for this progression is unknown. Suggested causes include hypertension, hyperfiltration, secondary hyperparathyroidism, and unknown "toxic factors" related to the uremic state. Infection, when present, can also contribute.

One factor which may play a significant role in the progressive loss of renal function is secondary hyperparathyroidism, presumably due to phosphorus retention with elevation of the calcium x phosphorus product and deposition of calcium phosphate in soft tissue including the renal parenchyma. Since therapy with vitamin D and calcium can induce a similar loss of renal function after parathyroidectomy, this effect can occur in the absence of parathyroid hormone (PTH). Conversely, human studies have shown a decline in the rate of progression of renal failure with restriction of phosphorus intake. Thus, an early and vigorous attempt to control serum calcium and phosphorus levels may be helpful in slowing progression of renal failure.

The concept of hyperfiltration injury in remnant nephrons has been proposed as a major factor in the progression of chronic renal disease to end-stage. According to this theory, diffuse renal injury leads to heterogeneity of single nephron glomerular filtration rate (GFR) in "remnant nephrons." The end result is glomerulosclerosis. Animal studies have shown increased blood flow and hydraulic pressure across glomerular capillary walls. In various models, these changes can be attributed to mediators of the immune response or to vasoactive hormones. Human studies suggest a delayed progression of the hyperfiltration injury by the use of angiotensin-converting enzyme inhibitors to control systemic hypertension and "normalize" the transcapillary hydraulic pressure.

UREMIA

Although initial injury to the kidney may arise from a wide spectrum of diseases, the ensuing renal failure produces abnormalities which are similar in all such patients, the so-called "uremic syndrome." Uremia is defined as the retention of excessive waste products of protein metabolism, but this syndrome is also marked by abnormalities of fluid and electrolyte homeostasis as well as endocrine and metabolic derangements.

Fluid and Electrolyte Changes

As GFR decreases, the fractional excretion of electrolytes and water increases. This homeostatic mechanism can prevent severe abnormalities of fluid and electrolytes until the GFR is less than 5 ml/min.

Because the ability to concentrate or dilute the urine is impaired, restriction of water intake may result in hypernatremia and volume contraction, whereas, if water or salt intake is excessive, edema and/or hyponatremia may result (see "Treatment" section for therapeutic guidelines).

In general, serum potassium is also well regulated by increased aldosterone levels and increased fecal excretion until the GFR is less than 5 ml/min. Thus, hyperkalemia with CRF implies excessive intake, competitive inhibitors of aldosterone, use of potassium-sparing diuretics, or type IV hyperkalemic distal tubular acidosis in which aldosterone levels are inadequate for the prevailing serum potassium level or the tubule may be unresponsive to an adequate level of aldosterone (see Chapter 9). Finally, if metabolic acidosis develops acutely the transcellular shift of potassium may also overwhelm the impaired defense mechanism with resultant hyperkalemia.

The fractional excretion of calcium, magnesium, and phosphorus is also increased as GFR declines. Although serum magnesium and phosphorus values are rarely elevated until the GFR is less than 5 ml/min, the serum levels of PTH are increased when the GFR is 70-80% of normal and dihydroxy vitamin D_3 (1,25 D_3) levels are depressed when the GFR reaches 40-50% of normal. Hypocalcemia is very common in CRF due to decreased gastrointestinal absorption (low 1,25 D_3 levels) as well as bone resistance to the action of PTH. The interpretation of these findings led to the "trade-off hypothesis" which states that maintenance of normal serum phosphorus and calcium levels is obtained through elevation of PTH levels and resultant bone dissolution (uremic osteodystrophy). In this process, the accumulation of net acid is buffered by bone salts to defend the blood pH. Because of this "bone buffering" and the maintenance of tubular proton secretion until extremely low levels of GFR are reached, the acidosis of renal failure is rarely severe (pH usually above 7.32).

Endocrine (Hormonal) Changes in Uremia

Abnormal hormonal levels are common in the uremic state.

- The diseased kidney is unable to produce appropriate levels of some hormones - e.g., erythropoietin and 1,25 D_3.
- The normal kidney is involved in degradation of certain hormones. The diseased kidney cannot perform these actions and, therefore, elevated levels of prolactin, luteinizing hormone, gastrin, insulin, glucagon, and PTH are common.
- If ischemic, the kidney may produce elevated levels of renin with resultant elevation of angiotensin II and aldosterone.
- Certain hormones may be elevated as part of the adaptive response to regulate fluid or electrolyte balance - e.g., PTH elevation in response to low serum calcium.

Retained Waste Products

Though many aspects of altered metabolic pathways in uremia have been studied, the specific toxin(s) remains unknown. Because blood urea nitrogen (BUN) reflects protein metabolism and represents the largest quantity of retained nitrogen in CRF, its role as a toxin has also been studied. Patients in whom urea was added to the dialysate during hemodialysis became symptomatic (fatigue, nausea, vomiting) only when the BUN was greater than 150 mg/dl for longer than 1 week. In CRF an increase in BUN is invariably associated with elevations of other nitrogenous waste products (ammonia, guanidine, guanidine succinic acid, methyl-guanidine), but definitive demonstration that any can account for uremic symptomatology is lacking.

The strongest evidence that nitrogenous waste products play a toxic role in uremia is indirect. Walser, Mitch, and coworkers demonstrated a marked improvement in well-being of uremic patients after supplementing their diets with the ketoanalogues of essential amino acids. This substitution lowered the catabolism of tissue protein while simultaneously reducing nitrogen intake, thereby stimulating nitrogen reutilization.

CLINICAL FEATURES

The initial symptoms of CRF are subtle and often ignored. A generalized symptom complex of lethargy, malaise, and weakness is common. The major symptoms listed below are organized by organ systems:

- General: fatigue, weakness
- Skin: pruritis, easy bruisability, edema
- Cardiovascular: dyspnea on exertion, retrosternal pain on inspiration (pericarditis)
- Gastrointestinal: anorexia, nausea, vomiting, singultus
- Genitourinary: nocturia, impotence
- Neuromuscular: restless legs, numbness and cramps in legs
- Neurologic: generalized irritability and inability to concentrate, decreased libido

Physical examination of patients with CRF generally reveals only nonspecific findings.

- General: sallow-appearing with debilitated appearance
- Skin: pallor, ecchymoses, excoriations, edema, xerosis
- HEENT: uriniferous breath
- Pulmonary: rales, pleural effusion
- Cardiovascular: hypertension, flow murmur or pericardial friction rub, cardiomegaly
- Neurologic: stupor, asterixis, myoclonus, peripheral neuropathy

EVALUATION OF THE PATIENT WITH CRF

Initially it is important to document not only the degree of renal impairment (and its cause, if possible), but also to determine whether there exist any potentially reversible factors contributing to the severity of renal dysfunction.

Laboratory evaluation is required to establish the level of renal function as well as to exclude any reversible component.

The urine culture and ultrasound yield valuable information. Infection rarely causes CRF in the absence of obstruction. Ultrasonography will reveal the kidney size (usually <10 cm in CRF, although diabetes, myeloma, and amyloid may all produce normal to large kidneys in the presence of CRF) and contour (polycystic kidney disease). These evaluations can be undertaken simultaneously with a 24-hr urine collection for creatinine clearance and total protein excretion. If lean body mass is not changing, the daily urinary creatinine excretion is relatively constant. However, once the creatinine clearance is below 25 ml/min, this measurement may exceed the true GFR (as measured by inulin clearance) by as much as 20-30% due to secretion of creatinine. Once the creatinine clearance falls below 5 ml/min, the values again approximate the inulin clearance.

Reversible Factor	Test Required
• Infection	Urinalysis, culture, and sensitivity
• Obstruction	Bladder catheterization, then ultrasonography
• Nephrotoxic agents	Drug history (nonsteroidal anti-inflammatory agents, analgesics, antibiotics, radiocontrast agents)
• ECF volume depletion	Diuretic use or severe Na restriction; supine and upright BP
• Hypertension	Measure BP, chest X-ray
• Congestive heart failure	Physical examination, chest X-ray
• Pericarditis	Echocardiography

• Electrolyte abnormalities
    Hypokalemia
    Hypercalcemia
    Hyperuricemia (usually >15 mg/dl)
	Serum electrolytes, Ca, PO_4, uric acid

DIFFERENTIAL DIAGNOSIS

The specific findings in various disease states are discussed in Chapters 4, 5, and 14. Once renal failure is substantial, the cause of the underlying renal disease is less important than attention to monitoring the decline of renal function with constant vigilance against reversible factors tending to hasten that decline.

MONITORING THE PATIENT WITH CRF

After the initial evaluation of renal function has been performed and reversible factors have been excluded, the physician must focus on serial measurement of parameters reflecting the patient's clinical course. Creatinine clearance is the best means of monitoring renal function, although serum creatinine may be used. A linear decline in renal function can be established by plotting the reciprocal of the serum creatinine ($1/S_{Cr}$) versus time. If changes in the slope of this curve occur, reversible factors should be sought.

Once the patient is known to have CRF, a set of bone X-rays, particularly of the hands and feet, should be obtained to seek evidence of secondary hyperparathyroidism (subperiosteal reabsorption along radial sides of digital bones of the hand or vascular calcification).

The parameters listed below are suggested at routine follow-up visits (usually monthly) until a definite pattern of decline of function is established:

- History: uremic symptoms (check for worsening)
- Physical examination: weight, supine and upright BP and pulse, skin turgor, pericardial friction rub, edema, reflexes and sensation in extremities
- Laboratory tests: BUN, creatinine, electrolytes, calcium, phosphorus, albumin, complete blood count, ferritin (6-month intervals), PTH (6-month intervals)
- X-ray tests: chest X-ray and bone films (every 6 months)

TREATMENT

The goals of therapy in the patient with CRF are:

- Correction of reversible factors hastening the loss of renal function
- Correction of fluid and electrolyte abnormalities
- Prevention of further loss of renal function
- Reduction of uremic symptoms by lowering the quantity of retained nitrogenous waste products while maintaining adequate protein nutrition

CORRECTION OF REVERSIBLE FACTORS

As previously discussed (see "Evaluation of the Patient With CRF"), reversible factors such as urinary tract infections, obstruction, extracellular fluid (ECF) volume contraction, or congestive heart failure should be assiduously sought and treated.

Drugs

The use of drugs in patients with CRF is a two-edged sword in that the effectiveness of an agent may be outweighed by toxicity since many agents depend upon renal degradation or excretion for elimination. A detailed analysis of the use of drugs in CRF is provided in Chapter 27. Certain drugs should not be used in the presence of CRF due to specific toxicities.

- Nitrofurantoin: causes peripheral neuropathy
- Amiloride ⎤
- Triamterene ⎬ may cause severe hyperkalemia
- Spironolactone ⎦
- Sulfonylureas: cause prolonged hypoglycemia
- Nonsteroidal anti-inflammatory agents may acutely decrease renal function by depressing renal blood flow; additionally they may cause nephrotic syndrome and/or an interstitial nephritis (Drug-induced interstitial nephritides are discussed in Chapter 14.)
- Tetracyclines: increase protein catabolism

Avoid the use of intravenous contrast media - in the presence of renal dysfunction it may cause irreversible renal failure (especially in patients with multiple myeloma or diabetic nephropathy). If a dye procedure is necessary, acute hemodialysis can be employed to remove the contrast immediately following the procedure.

Avoid pregnancy which may accelerate progression of CRF; risks are greatest in patients with hypertension, serum creatinine >1.5 mg/dl, and those with active renal disease.

CORRECTION OF FLUID AND ELECTROLYTE ABNORMALITIES

Sodium and Water

The limits of salt excretion are narrowed in CRF. An obligatory daily salt excretion predisposes patients to volume contraction during severe salt restriction. The 24-hr urinary sodium excretion can be measured during a period of stable weight and the dietary sodium intake adjusted to allow a trace of ankle edema in the early evening. In general, a 6-g NaCl diet ("no added salt") is a good starting point. The patient should be encouraged to keep a record of daily weights and notify his physician of any change in excess of 5 pounds over a 48-hr period. At the time of routine clinic visits the weight chart, as well as supine and upright BP measurement, will allow assessment of volume status.

Because dietary sodium intake will frequently be an amalgam of sodium chloride and sodium bicarbonate, the following equivalent measures are useful:

1 g $NaHCO_3$ contains 12 mEq Na
1 g NaCl contains 17 mEq Na
1 g of sodium equals 43 mEq Na

Note: In patients who require salt restriction, a warning should be given to prevent the use of "salt substitutes" as these compounds contain up to 45 mEq KCl per teaspoonful and are potentially lethal.

Water

Since osmolality is well regulated until the creatinine clearance is less than 5 ml/min, hyponatremia in the CRF patient requires water restriction only with evidence of total body salt and water overload (edema); in the euvolemic or hypovolemic CRF patient with hyponatremia, the most common etiology is diuretic therapy. Water restriction would only worsen ECF contraction. These patients frequently have an increased BUN to creatinine ratio and are best managed by withdrawal of diuretics or judicious replacement of salt.

Diuretics

Thiazide diuretics, when given alone, become less effective when the GFR is below 30 ml/min. Loop diuretics (furosemide, ethacrynic acid, or bumetanide; see Chapter 28) are preferred. Because retained organic anions compete for tubular secretion, the patient with CRF requires higher doses of these diuretics. It is reasonable to start with 40 mg of furosemide or 1 mg of bumetanide and double the dose until the desired effect is achieved. If diuresis is not achieved with 240-300 mg of furosemide as a single daily· dose, addition of metolazone (2.5 or 5 mg every day) is a useful adjunct. The effectiveness of metolazone in this setting is due to its more distal tubular site of action which prevents compensation to the effects of furosemide.

Acidosis

Patients with CRF are acidotic because their kidneys cannot excrete the approximate 1 mEq/kg/day of acid generated by metabolism of dietary protein. In general, maintenance of serum total CO_2 levels above 18-20 mEq/l will provide symptomatic relief as well as preventing catabolism of skeletal muscle. $NaHCO_3$ can be given as 650 mg tablets three times a day and titrated to obtain a total CO_2 of 20 mEq/l. Alternatively, $CaCO_3$ has been suggested since it alleviates the hypocalcemia of CRF. Unfortunately, it is not as effective as $NaHCO_3$ in the treatment of acidosis.

Potassium

Potassium homeostasis is generally intact until GFR is severely depressed (less than 5 ml/min). When hyperkalemia does occur it is due to either a) decreased urine output (diminished distal tubular sodium delivery or b) deficient aldosterone synthesis or effectiveness.

Treatment of acute hyperkalemia involves the use of $CaCl_2$ and/or $NaHCO_3$ and is addressed in Chapter 7. Chronic hyperkalemia is best treated by dietary potassium restriction and, failing that, by use of a negatively charged resin equilibrated with sodium - sodium polystyrene sulfonate (Kayexalate). The usual dose is 15-30 g in either juice or sorbitol (acts as a cathartic) once per day. Potassium losses are estimated at 1 mEq/kg/1 g of polystyrene excreted in the stool.

Calcium and Phosphorus

The maintenance of normal serum phosphorus levels can prevent renal osteodystrophy and progression of renal failure. The serum phosphorus should be maintained between 3.5 and 4.0 mg/dl (1.1-1.3 mmol/l). Dietary sources very rich in phosphorus should be restricted - e.g., eggs, dairy products (cream, cheese, milk), and meat. Most patients also require "phosphate-binding" compounds. Because of the long-term risks of aluminum-induced bone disease (see Chapter 23) the standard regimen is now a combination of $CaCO_3$ (can use "Tums") and $Al(OH)_3$ in a ratio of 2 $CaCO_3$ tabs: 30 cc $Al(OH)_3$ interspersed during each meal.

Until serum phosphorus is controlled, vitamin D should not be given. Balance studies have shown that patients with CRF require 1000-1500 mg Ca/day to maintain balance. If supplements of $CaCO_3$

and/or Ca gluconate do not normalize serum calcium (and if serum phosphorus remains controlled), therapy with 1,25 D_3 may be initiated with 0.25 μg/day, which can be increased at 2- to 4-week intervals to normalize serum calcium.

PREVENTION OF FURTHER LOSS OF RENAL FUNCTION

As discussed under pathophysiology, the hyperfiltration injury is ameliorated by reduction of transcapillary hydraulic pressure by use of converting enzyme inhibitors and a low protein diet.

Hypertension

Treatment with angiotensin-converting enzyme inhibitors is preferable, but serial checks of serum creatinine are important to detect an abrupt worsening of GFR, which can occur in cases of bilateral renal artery stenosis (GFR is angiotensin dependent), nephrotic syndrome, and volume depletion due to diuretics. Details are discussed in Chapters 17 and 18.

Dietary Protein Restriction

Dietary protein increases renal plasma flow and GFR in humans and animals. Over long periods of time this has been proposed to cause progressive injury resulting in glomerulosclerosis. The recent literature regarding the protective effect of low protein diets in patients with CRF suggests that protein restriction (with appropriate attention to increasing the biologic value of remaining dietary protein) may also be appropriate in patients with CRF. The recommendation is for 0.6 g/kg/day of protein of high biologic value supplemented by an amount equal to urinary protein loss. Such therapy is investigational at present. If attempted, it requires collaboration with a trained dietitian and regular assessments of dietary compliance with measures of urea excretion (see Chapter 26).

THERAPY OF SPECIFIC UREMIC SYMPTOMS

Pruritis

If unresponsive to dietary protein restriction and/or normalization of serum phosphorus, use of diphenhydramine at bedtime is frequently effective.

Gastrointestinal Symptoms

Anorexia, musty or metallic tastes, and early morning nausea and vomiting usually respond well to dietary protein restriction, but they may resurface as the patient approaches end-stage. At this time, the abnormal taste may be treated with half-strength hydrogen peroxide gargles (decreases oral bacteria which contain urease, converting urea to ammonia).

Anemia

If the anemia is not normocytic and normochromic, a search should be instituted for iron deficiency (serum ferritin) or folic acid/B_{12} deficiencies. Reversal of anemia by recombinant human erythropoietin is effective in relieving much of the symptom complex previously ascribed to uremia. When it is available, most authorities anticipate current use of androgens and/or the risks of repetitive transfusions will be abrogated.

When conservative management fails to control uremic symptoms and signs, dialysis (see Chapters 23 and 24) or transplantation (Chapter 25) should be undertaken. Indications for initiation of dialysis or transplantation include:

- Volume overload unresponsive to diuretic therapy (usually manifest as CHF or hypertension)
- Pericarditis
- Progressive renal osteodystrophy
- Progressive neuropathy (usually motor worse than sensory)
- Diabetic complications including gastroparesis, peripheral vascular disease, or early, progressive retinopathy
- Bleeding diathesis
- Noncompliant or irresponsible patient with hyperkalemia

SUGGESTED READING

Alfrey AC. Chronic renal failure. In: Schrier RW, ed. Renal and electrolyte disorders. 3rd ed. Boston: Little, Brown, and Company Inc, 1986:461-494.

Johnson WJ, Hagge WH, Waggner RD, et al. Effects of urea loading in patients with far-advanced renal failure. Mayo Clin Proc 1972;47:21-29.

Miller RW. The patient with chronic azotemia, with emphasis on chronic renal failure. In: Schrier RW, ed. Manual of nephrology. 2nd ed. Minneapolis: McGraw-Hill, Inc, 1987:149-183.

Rose BD, Brenner BM. Mechanisms of progression of renal disease. In: Rose BD, ed. Pathophysiology of renal disease. 2nd ed. Minneapolis: McGraw-Hill, Inc, 1987:119-138.

Chapter 23

Hemodialysis

Gerald B. Stephanz, Jr.
C. Michael Bucci

INTRODUCTION

Hemodialysis (HD) is now the predominant method of treatment of uremia. The technique, pioneered by Wilhelm Kolff in the 1940s, was first applied to patients with chronic renal failure by Belding Scribner at the University of Washington in 1960. As the problems of vascular access, anticoagulation, and production of reliable and convenient dialyzers were solved, hemodialysis became accepted as practical therapy for acute and chronic renal failure.

The Medicare End-Stage Renal Disease (ESRD) Program, established in 1972, led to availability of dialysis to virtually all nationwide. Currently there are approximately 80,000 patients receiving HD in the United States. This number continues to rise despite the increased success of continuous ambulatory peritoneal dialysis (CAPD) and renal transplantation (see Chapters 24 and 25). The average yearly cost is approximately $25,000 per patient.

DEFINITIONS

DIALYSIS

Dialysis is defined as the movement of solute and water through a semipermeable membrane (the dialyzer) which separates the patient's blood from the dialysate. Three processes occur simultaneously during dialysis in the extracorporeal dialysis circuit: diffusion, ultrafiltration, and osmosis.

DIFFUSION

Diffusion is the movement of solutes across the dialyzer and is dependent on the concentration gradient between plasma water and dialysate.

ULTRAFILTRATION

Ultrafiltration is the bulk flow of solute and water through the dialyzer in the direction of the hydrostatic pressure difference. It is the principle method of fluid removal.

OSMOSIS

Osmosis is the passage of solvent (water) through the dialyzer in the direction of the osmotic concentration gradient.

HIGH-FLUX DIALYSIS

High-flux dialysis (HFD) or high efficiency dialysis uses a highly permeable dialyzer and high blood and dialysate flow rate to shorten treatment time (2 1/2 hr compared to 4 hr for conventional HD). Hemofiltration and hemoperfusion will be discussed later in this chapter.

INDICATIONS FOR HEMODIALYSIS

Most hospitalized patients with acute renal failure are successfully managed without dialysis (see Chapter 21). A list of indications and contraindications for acute HD is shown below.

Indications/Contraindications for Hemodialysis in Renal Failure

Indications
- Relative
  - Hyperkalemia (see Chapter 7)
  - Diuretic unresponsive volume overload
  - Intractable acidosis
  - Symptomatic azotemia
  - Toxin exposure (drugs/radiocontrast agents)

- Absolute
  - Uremic pericarditis

Contraindications
- Relative
  - Hypotension unresponsive to pressors
  - Terminal illness
  - Organic brain syndrome

Factors to be considered before initiating HD in patients with **chronic renal failure** should include age, renal diagnosis, comorbid conditions, patient preference, and logistics. The timing of therapy is dictated by serum chemistries and symptoms. At present, most patients who are not preterminal from another progressive illness, or so mentally incompetent to present a danger to themselves or others, are offered dialysis therapy.

Patient survival has not improved significantly despite advances in dialysis knowledge and technology, perhaps because of the inclusion of patients with multisystem disease in the ESRD program. Increased age, poor left ventricular function, and diabetes mellitus greatly increase the risk of death on HD.

VASCULAR ACCESS

Provision of dialysis requires reliable repeated access to the patient's circulation which is capable of providing blood flow of 150-400 ml/min. Ideally, the access should be created well before the need for chronic dialysis.

ACUTE VASCULAR ACCESS

Subclavian (or internal jugular) venous catheters have become the preferred temporary/acute vascular access in many centers. Modern catheters provide dual lumens for bidirectional blood flow. They are relatively safe, easy to insert, and may be left in place for extended periods. Possible complications include bleeding, infection, thrombosis of the vessel, pneumothorax, and air embolus.

Temporary dialysis catheters should not be used as routine intravenous lines since breaks in sterile technique greatly increase the risk of infection and catheter thrombosis. Catheters are filled with a concentrated heparin solution between dialysis treatments; both catheter ports should be aspirated prior to use in an emergency. Catheters obstructed by clot have been successfully cleared using thrombolytic agents (streptokinase, urokinase).

Femoral vein catheterization is widely used for temporary access but is not suitable for ambulatory patients.

In the presence of systemic bacteremia or local infection, temporary dialysis catheters should be removed, the appropriate cultures taken (including through the infected line prior to removal and culture of the catheter tip), and systemic antibiotics administered (empiric therapy aimed at Gram-positive organisms).

External arteriovenous Scribner shunts are now largely limited to acute care situations.

CHRONIC VASCULAR ACCESS

Arteriovenous Fistula

The arteriovenous fistula (AVF) is the preferred vascular access for chronic hemodialysis. Fistulae are created by the surgical anastomosis of artery and vein, most commonly the radial artery to the cephalic vein in the nondominant arm. When progression to ESRD is imminent, an effort should be made to spare the nondominant arm from venipuncture and arterial puncture. The AVF provides an autologous access capable of the required blood flow while having the highest patency and lowest complication rates of all forms of access. The complications of chronic vascular access are listed below.

An AVF may last for years; therefore, it is important to protect the access when the patient is hospitalized. Admission orders should include the admonition of "no blood pressure or needle sticks" in the access arm. Examination of the functioning AVF reveals a palpable pulsation (thrill) and bruit by auscultation. When an established AVF is acutely thrombosed, early surgical intervention (within 24-48 hr) is required.

Arteriovenous Grafts

When the patient's own vessels are inadequate to create an AVF, materials such as an autologous saphenous vein, a modified human umbilical vein, a bovine heterograft or a polytetrafluoroethylene graft (PTFE, Gortex-TM) can be used to form a conduit from artery to vein. Most graft complications relate to thrombosis and infection. Graft removal is usually required to resolve an infection. As in patients with prosthetic heart valves, antibiotic prophylaxis should precede procedures for which bacteremia is anticipated.

Complications of Chronic Vascular Access

- Thrombosis
- Infection*
- Failure to develop adequate venous outflow
- Ischemic limb
- Venous hypertension syndrome
- Skin erosion*
- High output cardiac failure

*More common in vascular grafts

HEMODIALYSIS--THE PROCEDURE

The equipment used for hemodialysis prepares the dialysate, regulates dialysate and blood flow past a semipermeable membrane ("artificial kidney" or dialyzer), and monitors functions on various aspects of the dialysate and extracorporeal blood circuit. Heparin administration provides systemic anticoagulation.

For a detailed discussion of water preparation, dialysate proportioning systems, and machine monitoring functions, readers are referred to dialysis texts listed at the end of the chapter.

Blood and dialysate are perfused on opposite sides of a semipermeable membrane in a countercurrent direction for maximal efficiency of solute removal. Dialysate composition, the characteristics and size of the membrane in the dialyzer, and blood and solute flow rates all affect solute removal.

DIALYSATE COMPOSITION

The electrolyte composition of dialysate is similar to plasma except for substances varied to compensate for the metabolic abnormalities of ESRD or the particular clinical situation for which dialysis is employed. Standard glucose concentration of dialysate is 200 mg/dl; sodium, potassium, and calcium concentrations are prescribed as the clinical situation dictates. High sodium baths (140-148 mEq/l) are used to prevent intradialytic hypotension, severe muscle cramping, and prophylactically in acute dialysis to avoid the dialysis disequilibrium syndrome. Low calcium baths may be used in the acute and chronic therapy of hypercalcemia.

The dialysate buffer base may be either acetate or bicarbonate. In the absence of liver dysfunction, acetate is converted mole per mole into bicarbonate. Acetate may cause hypotension, nausea and vomiting, hypoxia, and headache. Bicarbonate dialysis, although more costly, usually ameliorates these symptoms. It is the therapy of choice in patients with respiratory compromise, hemodynamic instability, liver disease, severe metabolic acidosis, and in high flux dialysis.

DIALYZERS

Hollow fiber and parallel plate dialyzers are used in the vast majority of dialysis treatments. Hollow fiber dialyzers are composed of approximately 10,000 small diameter fibers through which blood circulates. Parallel plate dialyzers consist of a parallel arrangement of membrane sheets that form compartments through which blood flows. Commonly used membranes include cuprophane (a cellulose-based copper-containing membrane), cellulose acetate, and several high porosity synthetic copolymer membranes (polyacrylonitrile, polymethyl-methacrylate, and polysulfone). Cuprophane membranes more commonly produce allergic and "first use" reactions. Allergic reactions are marked by pruritis and respiratory embarrassment upon initiation of dialysis. They may be prevented by rinsing the dialyzer, but once they occur, cessation of dialysis, treatment with antihistamines, and expectant management of respiratory difficulty are required. A clinical complex of chest and back discomfort, pruritis, nausea, and malaise occurring within the first 30 minutes of dialysis is termed "first use syndrome"; the syndrome is associated with dialyzer membrane-induced leukopenia and complement activation. The symptoms are lessened if the dialyzer is reprocessed for continued use. Symptomatic treatment is suggested if the syndrome is not severe; otherwise discontinuation of dialysis and a change of dialyzer membranes is indicated.

In comparison with cuprophane membranes, the synthetic copolymer membranes exhibit better biocompatibility (less allergic and first use reaction), improved ultrafiltration characteristics (greater volume removal), and increased solute clearance, especially in the "middle molecule" (molecular weight 300-2000) region. These membranes are used in high flux dialysis and hemofiltration; a disadvantage of the synthetic membranes is their high cost. Reprocessing or "reuse" of these dialyzers is commonly performed.

Increasing the size of the membrane increases the solute and volume removal but may cause hypotension, muscle cramping, and the dialysis disequilibrium syndrome.

AIMS OF DIALYTIC THERAPY

Incomplete understanding of the pathogenesis of uremia and failure to identify "the" uremic toxin make it difficult to define an adequate dialysis prescription. Although a predialysis blood urea nitrogen (BUN) concentration of less than 80 mg/dl is one guide to therapy, correlation of toxic manifestations of uremia to plasma BUN is often poor. The National Cooperative Dialysis Study (NCDS) has shown less morbidity in chronic stable dialysis patients maintained at time-averaged concentration urea (TAC-urea, calculated from pre- and postdialysis BUN, dialysis time, and intradialytic time) levels of 50 mg/dl than at higher levels.

The prescription for dialysis therapy is increasingly guided by urea kinetic modeling as high flux dialysis assumes greater prominence in chronic dialytic therapy. Key concepts in this model include the protein catabolic rate (a measure of the dietary protein intake), residual renal function, and the dimensionless parameter Kt/V UREA, where K is a dialyzer urea clearance, t is dialysis treatment time, and V is the body urea distribution volume. This ratio determines the magnitude of decline of BUN during a dialysis and it serves as a measure of the dose of dialysis related to urea removal. This ratio should be at least 1.0 to minimize uremic symptoms.

A beneficial effect is seen on survival in post-traumatic **acute renal failure** if serum BUN concentration is maintained at 70 mg/dl or less.

COMPLICATIONS OF HEMODIALYSIS

Complications Related to Hemodialysis

- Acute
    Hypotension
    Muscle cramps
    Dialyzer reactions
    Hypoxemia
    Disequilibrium syndrome
    Bleeding
    Arrhythmias

- Chronic
    Anemia
    Bleeding
    Transfusion-related diseases [hepatitis B, human
      immunodeficiency virus (HIV)]
    Metabolic bone disease
    Acquired renal cystic disease
    Pericarditis

HYPOTENSION

Hypotension, which occurs during 30-50% of dialysis treatments, has been related to acetate dialysis, "low" sodium dialysate (130-135 mEq/L), atherosclerotic heart disease, autonomic neuropathy, and bio-incompatibility of dialyzer membranes. Prevention of symptomatic hypotension can be achieved by accurate determinations of "dry weight" (the weight below which the chronic HD patient has orthostatic hypotension) and holding or reducing antihypertensive medications immediately prior to dialysis.

MUSCLE CRAMPS

Muscle cramps are common especially during rapid ultrafiltration. Preventative measures include maintenance of interdialytic fluid restriction, in order to gain no more than 1-2 kg between treatments (to lessen the need for prolonged ultrafiltration), stretching exercises, and, if clinically disabling, quinine sulfate administration (260-325 mg nightly and prior to dialysis).

DIALYSIS DISEQUILIBRIUM SYNDROME

The dialysis disequilibrium syndrome is believed to result from osmotic shifts causing intracellular brain edema. The syndrome is rare; it is seen most commonly in the first dialytic treatments in acute renal failure.

Symptoms can occur during or after the procedure and include headache, lethargy, nausea, muscular twitching, and malaise, with progression to mental status changes and seizures, and even cardiorespiratory arrest. Recognition of high risk patients and the use of "high" sodium dialysates, smaller surface area dialyzers, and lower blood flow rates will lessen osmotic shifts. Predialysis mannitol infusion (25-50 g) may lessen the frequency and severity of symptoms but carries a risk of pulmonary edema and increasing thirst (with increased interdialytic weight gain).

HYPOXEMIA

Hypoxemia during dialysis is important in patients with compromised cardiopulmonary function. Research to date implicates membrane bioincompatibility and acid-base changes induced by acetate metabolism. Predisposed patients should be given supplemental oxygen and dialyzed with synthetic copolymer membranes against bicarbonate baths.

ARRHYTHMIAS

Acidosis, hypoxemia, hypotension, removal of antiarrhythmic agents during dialysis, and hypokalemia and hypomagnesemia (especially in patients taking digoxin) all contribute to arrhythmias in predisposed patients (those with arteriosclerotic heart disease).

BLEEDING

Uremia causes platelet dysfunction which is best assessed by measuring the bleeding time. The action of heparin may be reversed by protamine sulfate, but if protamine sulfate is administered in excess, it has an anticoagulant effect. Dialysis may be attempted without heparin if indicated. Cryoprecipitate (risks of transfusion-related diseases) and 1-deamino-8-arginine vasopressin (DDAVP) can be used when uremic bleeding has been unresponsive to adequate dialysis therapy.

ANEMIA

The causes of anemia in ESRD include decreased red blood cell production and survival and loss in blood lines and dialyzers. In initial clinical trials, recombinant human erythropoietin has been effective in reversal of the anemia; complications of therapy include hypertension and vascular access thrombosis.

TRANSFUSION-RELATED DISEASES

The incidence of hepatitis B has decreased dramatically since the screening of donor blood and implementation of isolation techniques. Hepatitis B vaccine induces a response in 40-70% of hemodialysis patients. Current recommendations of the Centers for Disease Control state that HIV-positive patients should be treated similarly to chronic hepatitis B surface antigen carriers. False-positive screening tests for HIV infection occur in 5% of dialysis patients.

METABOLIC BONE DISEASE

The causes of metabolic bone disease include secondary hyperparathyroidism, iron (blood transfusions or iron supplements) or aluminum bone deposition (from aluminum-containing antacids used as phosphate binders), and a unique form of amyloid deposition (beta-2 microglobulin) related to poor clearance of beta-2 microglobulin by cuprophane dialysis membranes. Clinical features common to dialysis bone disease include muscle weakness, carpal-tunnel syndrome, bone pain, arthralgias, and fractures or bone cysts.

Treatment of bone disease begins with limitation of serum phosphate to less than 5.5 mg/dl with dietary phosphate restriction and phosphate-binders (see Chapter 22); parathyroid hormone levels should be followed routinely. Serum aluminum levels and bone biopsies delineate bone histology and guide management.

ACQUIRED RENAL CYSTIC DISEASE

Multiple renal cysts develop in the kidneys of approximately 40-50% of patients and increase to 80% in those dialyzed for more than 3 years. An increasing hematocrit in an HD patient suggests a renal adenoma; these tumors have malignant potential. HD patients should be screened by ultrasonography or computed tomography after 3 years on dialysis.

PERICARDITIS

Two distinct patterns of pericarditis are encountered in patients with renal failure: uremic and dialysis-associated. **Uremic pericarditis** (see Chapter 22) is a presenting feature of renal failure and generally responds to the initiation of dialysis therapy.

Dialysis-associated pericarditis appears during seemingly adequate maintenance HD and has a worse prognosis. A hemorrhagic pericardial effusion is usually present; tamponade is frequent.

Treatment of dialysis-associated pericarditis is controversial because of lack of prospective clinical studies. Echocardiograms should be followed serially during treatment to gauge success or failure of therapy. Nonsteroidal anti-inflammatory medications (e.g., indomethacin, 50 mg three times a day) may relieve symptoms (chest pain, fever). Conventional wisdom dictates a trial of intensive dialysis (7-10 days of consecutive dialysis). If this fails or tamponade ensues, percutaneous pericardiocentesis with steroid instillation, placement of a pericardial window, or pericardiectomy may be necessary.

HEMOFILTRATION

Hemofiltration (HF; also called hemodiafiltration and diafiltration) relies on ultrafiltration rather than diffusion to move solutes across a high porosity semipermeable membrane. In HF, blood pressure alone provides the driving force for the ultrafiltrate. Large volumes of ultrafiltrate (500 ml/hr) with a composition similar to plasma water can be generated and are replaced by a balanced electrolyte solution (modified by the clinical situation; see Table 23-1) in amounts determined by desired fluid losses or gains. The solutions are separated by a four-pronged manifold until infused. The quantity of solute removed is a function of the amount of ultrafiltrate generated.

Table 23-1 **CAVH Replacement Solutions**

Solution	Contains (mEq/l)	
One liter 0.9% NS + 7.5 ml 10% $CaCl_2$	Na	147
One liter 0.9% NS + 1.6 ml 50% $MgSO_4$	K	0.0
One liter 0.9% NS	Cl	115
One liter D_5W + 1530 mEq	$NaHCO_3$	37.5
	Ca	2.4
	Mg	1.4
	Glu	125 mg/dl

HF can be used in acute and chronic renal failure; chronic HF is rarely used in the United States because of the cost of preparing the large amount of replacement fluid. Continuous arteriovenous hemofiltration (CAVH) is employed to treat acute renal failure. Adequate ultrafiltration can be achieved with mean arterial blood pressures as low as 70 mmHg.

Indications for CAVH

- ARF (with hemodynamic instability)
- Postoperative ARF
- Need for parenteral nutrition in ARF
- Cardiogenic shock with pulmonary edema
- Diuretic-unresponsive CHF

Arteriovenous access is obtained with large bore catheters, most commonly in the femoral vessels. Systemic heparinization is required.

Replacement fluid is usually given pre-dilution (before the inlet portion of the hemofilter).

Advantages/Disadvantages of CAVH

- Advantages
    Ease of initiation
    Gradual correction of uremia and electrolyte/acid-base abnormalities
    Precise fluid control
    Rare hypotension
    Large volumes of parenteral nutrition may be administered
    Less technically demanding

- Disadvantages
    Intensive care unit setting only
    Poor emergent treatment for hyperkalemia/acidosis
    Systemic heparinization
    Possible inability to control nitrogen balance (intermittent HD needed)
    Requires adequate vascular (arterial) access
    Access site infection
    Requires strict fluid monitoring

A frequent problem in CAVH is a sudden decrease in ultrafiltrate caused by kinked blood lines, hypotension, blood leaks, or plasma hemoconcentration. A 50- to 100-ml bolus of normal saline (with the arterial line momentarily clamped) can be used to check for a clotted hemofilter.

Variations of CAVH exist using external pumps to augment blood flow and modified peritoneal dialysis solution as a continuous dialysate.

DIALYTIC TECHNIQUES IN DRUG OVERDOSE

HD and a related technique, hemoperfusion, are occasionally helpful in the management of overdose of medications or toxins. Charcoal hemoperfusion utilizes coated or uncoated charcoal particles to absorb toxins; it is limited by the production of hemolysis and thrombocytopenia.

Drugs and Toxins Removed by Hemodialysis

- Alcohols (methanol)
- Aspirin
- Ethylene glycol
- Lithium
- Mannitol
- Radiocontrast dye
- Theophylline*

*Hemodialysis or hemoperfusion is effective.

In acute poisonings HD has the advantage of correcting any acid-base and electrolyte disturbances. The previous display gives a listing of medications removed by HD/hemoperfusion. Antidepressants and benzodiazapines are poorly removed by dialytic techniques. In any poisoning dialysis should be considered only when supportive measures are ineffective or there is impending irreversible organ toxicity.

OTHER CONSIDERATIONS IN THE CARE OF DIALYSIS PATIENTS

DIET/FLUIDS

Please refer to Chapter 26 on dietary therapy. In general, anuric patients should have their total fluid intake limited to 1-1.5 liters per day (including intravenous and oral maintenance fluids), unless extrarenal losses are excessive.

DISCHARGE PLANNING

The referring dialysis unit and physician should be told of any changes in therapy and notified well in advance of anticipated discharge to plan outpatient dialysis for patients with chronic renal failure.

DRUGS

Please refer to Chapter 27. Many drugs are removed by HD, including antibiotics and antiarrhythmics. Therefore, supplemental doses or alteration of the dosing schedule may be required.

PSYCHOSOCIAL

Patient and family adjustment to renal replacement therapy may be difficult. Consultation with psychiatry, psychology, or social work can help with changes in patient self-image, financial arrangements, and logistical support.

SUGGESTED READING

Blagg CR. The end-stage renal disease program: here are some of the data. JAMA (ed) 1987;257:662-663.

Fraser CL, Arieff AI. Nervous system complications in uremia. Ann Intern Med 1988;109:143-153.

Golper, TA. Continuous arteriovenous hemofiltration in acute renal failure. Am J Kidney Dis 1985;6:373-386.

Hakim RM, Lazarus JM. Medical aspects of hemodialysis. In: Brenner BM, Rector FJ, eds. The kidney. 3rd ed. 1986:1791-1846.

Henderson LW, Mion C, Man NK, eds. Contemporary management of renal failure. Kidney Int 1988;33(Suppl 24):S1-S197.

Manis T, Friedman EA. Dialytic therapy for irreversible uremia (two part). N Engl J Med 1987;301:1260-1265, 1321-1328.

Chapter 24

Peritoneal Dialysis

Gerald B. Stephanz, Jr.

With the advent of improved peritoneal access and dialysate devices in the mid-1970s, peritoneal dialysis (PD) has provided an acceptable alternative to hemodialysis for many uremic patients who cannot tolerate or accept hemodialysis.

DEFINITION

PD uses the peritoneal membrane to exchange solutes and fluid with the bloodstream. Peritoneal instillation of dialysate provides both a chemical gradient for movement of solute and an osmotic gradient for removal of fluid.

INCIDENCE

Approximately 17% of all patients undergoing chronic dialysis in the United States are on PD. Continuous ambulatory peritoneal dialysis (CAPD) accounts for 13% of the chronic dialysis population in the United States and about 30% in Europe.

PERITONEAL DIALYSIS TECHNIQUES

Dialysate (commonly 2 liters) is instilled into the peritoneal cavity by gravity and allowed to equilibrate (or dwell) for a set time while retained metabolites diffuse into the dialysate. Thereafter the solution is drained into plastic bags and the cycle repeated. Reliable access to the peritoneum and the appropriate choice of dialysate solutions are critical for successful PD.

Catheters

Traditionally, acute access to the peritoneum was achieved with stiff plastic catheters, 25-30 cm long, with a removable metal trocar extending through the catheter to facilitate insertion. Hazards of insertion include perforation of bowel (producing diarrhea with a strong positive reaction for glucose after dialysate instillation) and bladder (producing a miraculous increase in urine output with dialysate instillation).

The Tenckhoff catheter is now generally preferred for acute and chronic PD. It is approximately 30 cm in length, flexible, and has intra-abdominal, subcutaneous, and external portions. The intra-abdominal portion may be either straight or coiled (to prevent omental wrapping and obstruction) and contains a number of outflow ports. The subcutaneous portion has one or two cuffs at the skin surface and in the deep subcutaneous tissue, to provide anchorage and a barrier to bacterial invasion. The external portion is attached to a connecting tube which attaches ("spikes") to dialysate bags.

Dialysate

Effective PD requires effective diffusion gradients between the blood and dialysate to correct the accumulation of uremic solutes. Table 24-1 provides representative values for composition.

Table 24-1 Composition of Blood and Commercial Dialysate

Solute	Blood (mEq/l)	Dialysate (1.5%) (mEq/l)
Na	140	132-141
K	4.0	0
Cl	100	101-107
HCO₃	26	0
Lactate	0.3-1.3	45
Ca(ionized)	3.0	3.5
Mg	1.5	0.5-1.5
PO₄	2.5	0
Glucose	100 mg%	1500 mg%
pH	7.35-7.45	5.0-5.8
Osmolality	280-300	340

Several points concerning dialysate content are worth noting.

Potassium is omitted from the dialysate. Occasionally PD patients who develop hypokalemia require that K be added to the dialysate.

Phosphate is poorly dialyzed. Thus, nearly all PD patients will require phosphate-binding medications.

Metabolic acidosis complicating chronic renal failure can be moderated by providing a buffer base in the dialysate. Sodium bicarbonate is not used routinely because it forms insoluble salts with calcium and magnesium; lactate is used as the buffer base, and if liver function is normal, lactate will be metabolized mole per mole to bicarbonate.

Hypertonic glucose in the dialysate provides the osmotic gradient for fluid removal (ultrafiltration). It is available in concentrations of 1.5, 2.5, and 4.25%. If not drained from the peritoneal cavity, glucose will ultimately be absorbed. Table 24-2 illustrates the expected ultrafiltrate volume per dialysate glucose concentration and dwell time with a normal peritoneal membrane.

Peritonitis has variable effects in the volume of ultrafiltrate, which may be reflected clinically by dehydration or volume overload.

Table 24-2 **Net Peritoneal Ultrafiltration**

Solution*	Dwell Time	Ultrafiltrate
1.5%	1-2 hr	+400 cc
1.5%	3-4 hr	+200 cc
4.25%	4-6 hr	+900 cc
4.25%	14 hr	-500 cc

* Two liter exchanges

Continuous Ambulatory Peritoneal Dialysis (CAPD)

This method is usually performed by the patient. It is a closed system consisting of the peritoneum, the catheter, connecting tubing, and a plastic container of dialysate. Fluid (2 liters commonly in adults) is instilled into the peritoneal cavity for 4-8 hr per cycle; four daily exchanges are the norm. Empty bags remain connected to the catheter via a connecting tube and are carried under the patient's clothing until they are lowered for gravity drainage at the end of the dwell time. Advantages of CAPD include patient independence and freedom from a machine. The most important disadvantage is infection.

Continuous Cyclic Peritoneal Dialysis (CCPD)

This method uses an automated cycler to perform 3 or more exchanges overnight after which there is a single all-day ambulatory exchange. Advantages of CCPD include fewer breaks in the sterile system and the convenience.

Intermittent Peritoneal Dialysis (IPD)

This method is now reserved for acute renal failure or PD-associated peritonitis. The operator can vary the dialysate glucose concentration, peritoneal volume, and cycling time. A typical protocol is 2-liter exchanges, inflow periods of 10-15 minutes, and total cycle times (inflow, dwell, and outflow) of 1 hr. The dialysate can be exchanged by automated cycling. Disadvantages of IPD include a higher risk of infection, confinement of the patient to bed during dialysis, and a large commitment of nursing time.

FACTORS AFFECTING THE EFFICIENCY OF PERITONEAL DIALYSIS

PD requires an adequate area of contact between the bloodstream and dialysate solution. The three barriers to solute transfer are the capillary endothelium, the capillary basement membrane, and the peritoneal lining.

Alteration of the architecture or function of the peritoneum can lead to ineffective dialysis. Peritonitis, diabetes mellitus, vasculitis, systemic lupus erythematosus (SLE), scleroderma, and malignant hypertension can all limit peritoneal diffusion. Alternatively, acute peritonitis (described later in this chapter) can increase membrane permeability, leading to protein losses and decreased ultrafiltration; with antibiotic treatment transport properties return in approximately 1 week.

DIALYSATE-RELATED FACTORS

Improved solute clearance (K, urea, etc.) can be achieved by decreasing the cycling time, or increasing the dwell volumes, or both. However, both can be uncomfortable and higher dwell volumes are associated with atelectasis.

Although warming PD solutions will theoretically enhance solute clearance, in practice, the effect is negligible. Warming of dialysate is primarily for patient comfort; dry heat (warming ovens, microwave ovens) is recommended.

INDICATIONS FOR PERITONEAL DIALYSIS

The indications for dialysis have been discussed in the chapters on acute (Chapter 21) and chronic renal failure (Chapter 22). Indications and contraindications for PD are listed below.

Peritoneal Dialysis: Indications and Contraindications

- Indications
  Cardiovascular instability (hypotension, arrhythmias)
  Inadequate/unreliable vascular access
  Contraindication to systemic heparinization
  Patient preference
  Logistics (poor access to hemodialysis)

- Major Contraindications
  Peritoneal fibrosis/resection/adhesions
  Pleuroperitoneal communication (hydrothorax)
  Recent abdominal surgery
  Severe catabolic states
  Recent aortic prosthesis (infection)
  Colostomy or nephrostomy (infection)
  Respiratory compromise

- Minor Contraindications
  Peripheral vascular disease
  Hernias or diverticular disease
  Hyperlipidemia
  Obesity

- Contraindications For Self-Care
  Physical or mental handicaps (including blindness)

PD is a logical alternative to continuous arteriovenous hemofiltration (see Chapter 23) in which vascular access is a problem or systemic heparinization is contraindicated.   PD may be inadequate to remove nitrogenous wastes in severely catabolic cases of acute renal failure, especially in those receiving hyperalimentation.

PD has been favored over hemodialysis for diabetics with renal failure who often have cardiovascular instability and poor peripheral circulation, which interferes with the formation and maintenance of a vascular access. The continuous slow ultrafiltration provided by PD avoids rapid shifts of fluid that may precipitate angina or vascular collapse. Regular insulin may be administered in the dialysate as the sole form of insulin replacement; because of the long daytime dwell in CCPD, subcutaneous insulin must also be used.   The dialysis texts listed at the end of this chapter provide details on the use of intraperitoneal insulin.

The relative advantages and disadvantages of PD are listed below.

Advantages and Disadvantages of PD Compared to Hemodialysis

- Advantages of PD
  Minimal risk of disequilibrium syndrome (Chapter 23)
  Less hemodynamic stress per treatment
  Improved clearance of "middle molecules" (Chapter 23)
  No systemic anticoagulation
  Transfusion requirements minimized
  Technically more simple
  Patient independence (chronic therapy)
  Less dietary restriction (chronic therapy)

- Disadvantages of PD
  Less effective in treatment of hypercatabolic acute renal
   failure
  Less efficient solute/fluid removal
  Infection
  Catheter malfunction
  High protein/amino acid loss in dialysate
  Worsening hypertriglyceridemia

CLINICAL PROBLEMS IN PERITONEAL DIALYSIS

Approximately 50% of patients using CAPD will be hospitalized for complications during the first year of therapy.   Some common problems are listed in the accompanying display.

INFECTIONS

A major cause of morbidity in the PD patient is infection involving the peritoneal cavity (peritonitis) or the dialysis catheter (exit site, cuff or tunnel abscess).

Peritonitis

Approximately 60% of patients undergoing CAPD develop peritonitis during the first year of dialysis; an incidence of 1.6 to 2 episodes of peritonitis per patient per year has been recorded. Recurrent peritonitis, occurring in up to 20% of patients, is a leading cause of CAPD failure and transfer to hemodialysis. Lack of compliance with aseptic technique, low socioeconomic status, and concurrent exit site or tunnel infections have been shown to be important risk factors in the development of peritonitis. Age, sex, and presence of diabetes mellitus do not appear to be associated with an increased incidence of peritonitis.

Clinical Complications of Peritoneal Dialysis

- Inflammatory
  - Peritonitis
  - Exit site infections
  - Tunnel abscess
  - Eosinophilic peritonitis

- Mechanical
  - Catheter inflow/outflow blockage
  - Bleeding
  - Leakage
  - Hernias
  - Perforated viscus

- Metabolic
  - Hyperglycemia
  - Protein depletion
  - Hyperlipidemia
  - Obesity

- Pulmonary
  - Hydrothorax
  - Pleural effusion
  - Atelectasis

Patients with peritonitis note a turbid dialysate and symptoms of outflow obstruction (abdominal pain, fever, nausea, and vomiting). The dialysate white blood count (WBC) exceeds 100 cells/mm^3; greater than 50% are neutrophils. The PD fluid should be Gram stained and sent for bacterial culture and sensitivity and WBC with differential. Blood cultures are rarely positive unless severe systemic signs and symptoms are present.

Approximately 70% of these peritonitis episodes are caused by Gram-positive organisms from the skin (coagulase-negative staphylococci, *Staphylococcus aureus*, *Streptococcus viridans* and enterococci), while 20% are caused by Gram-negative coliform organisms. Peritoneal cultures positive for several organisms or for anaerobic organisms suggest a perforated viscus. Infections due to fungi and mycobacteria should be considered in "culture negative" cases. Candida species, responsible for the majority of fungal peritonitis episodes, are easily and quickly recovered without special culture media.

Intraperitoneal or intravenous antibiotics should be used without delay to treat bacterial peritonitis. Three rapid exchanges can be followed by an exchange with a loading dose of antibiotics. The maintenance dose is added to successive exchanges. Patients receiving intraperitoneal antibiotics can be managed as outpatients.

Patients should be admitted to the hospital if they are severely ill or have not improved within 24-48 hr.

A first generation cephalosporin and an aminoglycoside are used empirically until culture and sensitivity results are available. For uncomplicated cases of Gram-positive peritonitis, 7-10 days of therapy is indicated. Gram-negative peritonitis may require 2 weeks or more of therapy. Table 24-3 lists the peritoneal dosage of antibiotics commonly employed. Semisynthetic penicillin doses should not be combined with aminoglycosides since complexes may form.

Table 24-3 **Intraperitoneal Antibiotic Dosage* in the Treatment of Peritonitis**

Antibiotic	Loading Dose	Maintenance Dose
Cephalosporin (cefazolin, cephapirin, cephalothin)	10 mg/kg	250 mg
Amikacin	10 mg/kg	30 mg
Gentamicin	1.7 mg/kg	10 mg
Tobramycin	1.7 mg/kg	10 mg
Ampicillin	1 g	100 mg
Azlocillin	2 g	200 mg
Cefotaxime	1 g	250 mg
Clindamycin	600 mg	100 mg
Metronidazole	15 mg/kg IV	20 mg
Nafcillin	2 g	200 mg
Penicillin	2,000,000 U	100,000 U
Piperacillin	2 g	200 mg
Ticarcillin	2 g	200 mg
SMZ/TMP	800/160 mg	50/10 mg
Vancomycin	1 g	30 mg

*Per 2 liter exchange

Patients in the hospital are best managed by IPD with cycling. Protein losses increase with peritonitis and may require increased dietary protein intake. Heparin (500-1000 units/l, not systemically absorbed) should be added to the dialysate if fibrin is noted in the dialysate.

In general, WBC counts should decrease to less than 100 cells/mm^3 after 3 days of therapy. Failure of WBC counts to decrease may signify polymicrobial infections, inappropriate antibiotic selection, or the need to remove the catheter. Recurrent (three or more) episodes of peritonitis with the same organism, perforated viscus, or fungal and mycobacterial peritonitis generally require removal of the peritoneal catheter.

Exit Site Infection/Tunnel Abscess

The exit site is the skin surrounding the PD catheter; the "tunnel" is the pathway of the catheter from the skin to the peritoneum. Routine care of the exit site includes daily cleaning with soap or povidone-iodine solution; a dressing is not necessary.

Exit site infections cause erythema, pain, drainage, and induration; responsible organisms are similar to those described for PD peritonitis. Oral (first generation cephalosporin) or intraperitoneal antibiotics may be employed for a minimum of 2 weeks. Persistent or recurrent infection, tunnel abscess, or peritonitis usually requires removal of the catheter.

Tunnel abscess is diagnosed by pain, erythema, induration, and warmth over the tunnel. Proper therapy includes surgical drainage (if a dual-cuffed catheter is present, removal of the superficial cuff will allow drainage of the tunnel), oral or intraperitoneal antibiotics, and usually catheter removal.

"Sterile" Peritonitis

Causes other than infections may cause cloudy dialysate. Peritoneal reactions related to particulate matter in the dialysate may cause inflammatory reactions. Endotoxin contamination of the dialysate has been associated with sterile peritonitis.

Eosinophilic peritonitis is a condition usually occurring within the first 2 weeks of initiation of PD and is most often asymptomatic. Dialysate will have increased protein as well as eosinophils, with greater than 20% eosinophils. Eosinophilic peritonitis clears without treatment; the etiology is unknown but may relate to unspecified particulate matter or to low dialysate pH.

Catheter Obstruction

Inflow obstruction occurs after catheter insertion. It is caused by kinking of the catheter or intraluminal obstruction from blood clots or fibrin. The catheter will have to be replaced in most instances of inflow obstruction; thrombolytic agents have been used to clear catheters obstructed by fibrin or coagulated blood. Addition of heparin, 500-1000 units per liter of dialysate, will help prevent fibrin and blood clot deposition.

Outflow obstruction commonly causes increased retention of dialysate (respiratory insufficiency, volume overload, metabolic complications). It is usually caused by catheter tip displacement from the pelvic cavity (seen on a plain roentgenogram of the abdomen) or omental "wrapping" of the catheter (creating a ball-valve effect). Frequently, the catheter will have to be replaced. Unexplained poor outflow drainage can be caused by constipation; enemas or suppositories will then re-establish flow.

Dialysate Leaks

An exit-site leak is detected by a positive reaction for glucose; up to one third of patients on CAPD will experience a leak sometime during therapy. Approximately 50% of leaks become infected. Leakage may also occur into the subcutaneous tissue (pitting edema of the abdomen, scrotal or labial swelling). Leaks may be treated by a purse-string suture around the catheter exit site, bed rest (to avoid increased intra-abdominal pressure), smaller dwell volumes, or discontinuation of dialysis for 2 weeks.

Pain

Pain at the catheter insertion site suggests local bleeding. Diffuse abdominal pain implies either peritonitis, intra-abdominal bleeding, or visceral perforation (complicating acute catheter insertion or due to erosion from chronic placement). Pain in the rectum, lower abdomen, or back suggests the tip of the catheter is deep in the pelvis; pain in the bladder suggests the catheter is in or on the bladder; Shoulder pain suggests referred pain from diaphragmatic irritation. In these instances pain is often relieved with changes in patient position or withdrawal of the catheter by several centimeters.

SUGGESTED READING

Diaz-Buxo JA. Intermittent, continuous ambulatory and continuous cycling peritoneal dialysis. In: Nissenson AR, Fine RN, Gentile DE, eds. Clinical dialysis. 1st ed. New York: Appleton-Century-Crofts, 1984:263-396.

Golper TA, Bennett WM, McCarron DA, eds. Pharmacotherapy of renal disease and hypertension. In: Brenner BM, Stein JH, eds. Contemporary issues in nephrology. New York: Churchill Livingstone 1987;17:21-48.

Levey AS, Harrington JT. Continuous peritoneal dialysis for chronic renal failure. Medicine 1982;61:330-339.

Nissenson AR, Fine RN, eds. Dialysis therapy. 1st ed. Philadelphia: Hanley and Belfus, Inc, 1986.

Nolph KD, Linblad AS, Novak JW. Current concepts: continuous ambulatory peritoneal dialysis. N Engl J Med 1988;318:1595-1600.

Nolph KD. Peritoneal dialysis. In: Brenner BM, Rector FC, eds. The kidney. 3rd ed. Philadelphia: WB Saunders Company, 1986:1847-1906.

Peterson PK, Matzke G, Keane WF. Current concepts in the management of peritonitis in patients undergoing continuous ambulatory peritoneal dialysis. Rev Inf Dis 1987;9:604-612.

Chapter 25

The Renal Transplant Patient

Daniel R. Salomon

DEFINITION

Kidney transplantation is a surgical procedure which involves the removal of a kidney from the donor and the implantation of this organ into the recipient patient. If the organ has been harvested from a patient who has been declared legally dead, it is called a cadaveric renal transplant. When the kidney has been donated by a parent or sibling, it is called a living related donor transplant.

DEMOGRAPHICS

Of the 90,000 patients with end-stage renal disease on chronic dialysis in the United States, approximately 12,000 are awaiting a cadaveric kidney transplant. Approximately 10,000 kidney transplants are performed each year in the United States (2,000 living related donor and 8,000 cadaveric). This is an increase from 6,000 in 1983. Donor organ availability has become a major limitation to the expansion of transplantation.

PATIENT SELECTION FOR TRANSPLANTATION

The last decade has seen several major changes in the selection of patients for transplantation. Recently, a number of institutions have demonstrated that diabetic patients can be successfully transplanted using lower steroid doses and better medical management of hypertension and opportunistic infections. The age limits for kidney transplantation have been relaxed and patients in their 60s and early 70s are often considered. Transplanting patients before they require dialysis therapy avoids some of the long-term complications of renal failure and dialysis such as aluminum-related and uremic bone disease, transfusion-related hepatitis and iron overload, and the cardiac dysfunction associated with anemia and uremia. Finally, there has been an increase in transplantation in patients with more unusual causes of renal failure such as amyloidosis and sickle cell disease and in patients with malignancies that are in full remission.

ACUTE KIDNEY TRANSPLANT DYSFUNCTION

ETIOLOGY

Transplant Surgery Procedures and Acute Postoperative Complications

The kidney transplant is placed retroperitoneally below the pelvic brim. Usually, the vascular anastomoses are made to the external iliac vessels, but sometimes the internal or common iliac vessels are chosen. The donor's ureter is tunneled through the bladder muscle and the kidney is placed at an angle such that the vessels and ureter face downward and medially into the pelvis. It is important to recognize and treat surgical complications before considering the diagnosis of acute transplant rejection.

Acute Postoperative Complications

- Arterial
    Rupture with hemorrhage
    Thrombosis
    Stenosis

- Lymphatic
    Lymphocele
    Ureteral obstruction
    Ascites

- Urologic
    Urine leak
    Ureteral stenosis
    Bladder dysfunction

- Perirenal infection/abscess

Technical problems with the anastomoses are common causes of early transplant dysfunction (1-4 weeks). The renal artery anastomosis may be too tight resulting in acute renal ischemia or infarction. The ureteral anastomosis may break down resulting in a urinary leak. The blood supply of the transplanted ureter is tenuous and depends on a very small set of vessels originating in the renal pelvis. Thus, there is a real possibility of infarction at the distal or anastomotic end of the ureter leading to a urinary leak or eventually to fibrosis and obstruction.

Any pre-existing problems with the patient's urine outflow such as a neurogenic bladder (typical of diabetes mellitus, congenital uropathy, or after trauma), uretheral strictures, or prostatic hypertrophy may cause acute obstruction and renal transplant dysfunction.

Pelvic dissection can disrupt lymphatics and lead to accumulation of large amounts of lymphatic fluid around the kidney transplant. The resulting lymphocele may cause ureteral obstruction or, if it drains into the peritoneum, it may cause ascites.

The renal artery, vein, and ureter are potential targets for transplant rejection resulting in fibrosis and stenosis. These problems typically occur 3 to 12 months after transplantation. Renal artery stenosis leads to renal vascular hypertension and renal ischemia, while ureteric stenosis results in urinary tract obstruction and hydronephrosis.

The kidney transplant is placed in a limited space in the retroperitoneum. Thus, any perirenal collection of blood, urine, pus, or lymph will increase the pressure on the kidney and obstruct the relatively low pressure ureter and renal pelvis.

Acute Tubular Necrosis and Primary Graft Dysfunction

Acute tubular necrosis (ATN) occurs in 20-50% of patients receiving cadaveric donor transplants. The cadaveric organ is often harvested at another institution. It is preserved in an iced saline solution called Uro-Collins for transport. This period of cold ischemia usually lasts 24-36 hr during which time the potential recipient is tissue matched, the organ is shipped to the transplanting institution, and the selected patient is prepared for surgery. Clearly this period of ischemia will result in a variable degree of renal tubular damage that may be superimposed on that sustained prior to harvesting the kidney. ATN causes delayed graft function after surgery. It requires postoperative dialysis and lasts about 7-14 days before spontaneous resolution. The key issue in a patient with a poor urine output is to distinguish ATN from a surgical complication or acute rejection. This will be discussed at the end of this section.

Acute Rejection

Acute rejection can be divided into acute vascular or acute cellular rejection, although both types may occur together.

Acute vascular rejection. This is defined by injury to the vascular endothelium (endovasculitis) to the tunica media and muscularis of the arteries (transmural vasculitis) or to the glomerular capillaries (transplant glomerulitis). This vascular tissue injury may be mediated by antibodies directed at the human leukocyte antigen (HLA) antigens of the donor expressed on the endothelial cell surfaces of the transplanted kidney. Antibody binding activates the complement and clotting cascades, recruits polymorphonuclear leukocytes and macrophages, and may promote invasion by activated T cells. The end result is endothelial cell swelling, fibrin and platelet thrombi, reduced blood flow, and relative ischemia of dependent tissue.

Acute cellular rejection. Acute cellular rejection is defined by the tubulointerstitial accumulation of activated, killer-type T lymphocytes and invasion of tubular epithelial cells called emperipolesis. In addition, other cells including macrophages, polymorphonuclear leukocytes, and plasma cells can be found in the interstitial cell infiltrates. Antibodies do not play any identifiable role.

The immunologically specific phase of tissue damage is succeeded by a nonspecific acute inflammatory response. This includes the activation of the complement and clotting cascades, the recruitment of macrophages and polymorphonuclear leukocytes, and the release of such soluble mediators as platelet aggregating factor and prostaglandins.

INVESTIGATION AND MANAGEMENT OF ACUTE KIDNEY TRANSPLANT DYSFUNCTION

Acute Surgical Complication

If the patient develops acute kidney transplant dysfunction within the first month, the first step is to exclude a surgical complication. The next step is to examine the patient for a tender or swollen graft, fever, an increase in tube drainage, or bleeding. Sometimes a urinary leak can be diagnosed by measuring the creatinine concentration of the tube drainage; it will be 30-100 mg/dl as compared to a serum concentration of 1-15 mg/dl. A falling hematocrit suggests a perirenal hemorrhage, while fever and a swollen kidney suggest acute infection or rejection. The most helpful noninvasive diagnostic tests are ultrasound and renal scan. The ultrasound permits rapid exclusion of urinary tract obstruction and perirenal fluid collections. The hippuran scan measures renal blood flow and, thus, may exclude graft thrombosis.

Acute Rejection

The next step is to diagnose rejection as the cause of acute kidney dysfunction. There is no single laboratory test that will identify rejection. It can be diagnosed with certainty only with a transplant biopsy. However, clinical judgment is essential. For example, a sudden increase in serum creatinine concentration 2 weeks after transplantation is very suggestive of rejection; most clinicians would initiate therapy without a biopsy. On the other hand, fever, malaise, a falling WBC, and mild liver function abnormalities suggest acute cytomegalovirus (CMV) infection. The patient should be biopsied before consideration of antirejection therapy. Patients that are treated initially for acute rejection and fail the first course of therapy should be biopsied. Finally, patients with delayed graft function suggestive of ATN should be biopsied after the first week to exclude acute rejection. There are two ways of managing acute rejection.

Steroid pulse. Traditionally, 1 g of methylprednisolone (Solu-Medrol^R) is given intravenously for three consecutive days. Alternatively, lower doses of Solu-Medrol^R or high doses of oral prednisone can be used.

Antibody therapy. Antithymocyte globulin (ATG) or anti-lymphocyte serum (ALS) is used to destroy the T cells that invade the rejecting kidney. Recently, monoclonal antibodies (e.g., OKT3 or Orthoclone T3) have been used to target the T cell antigen receptor complex and destroy lymphocytes involved in acute rejection. Therapy with muromonab-CD3 (Orthoclone OKT^{R}3) requires 5 mg intravenously daily for 14 consecutive days.

The choice of therapy is still controversial. While monoclonal antibodies are new, expensive, and require a course of longer therapy, they avoid many steroid side effects and are probably somewhat more effective.

Successful therapy is reflected, after a lag period of several days, by an increased urine output, decreased fever and graft tenderness, and a falling creatinine. The major complication of any anti-rejection therapy is infection. Pulse steroids can also cause hyperglycemia, mental status alterations (even psychosis), muscle weakness, or arthralgias and acute gastritis. Monoclonal antibody infusion can cause acute serum sickness with fever, chills, pulmonary edema, and, occasionally, seizures.

ATN. This is usually a consequence of donor organ preservation prior to transplantation and warm ischemia during the surgical procedure. Thus, ATN will present as oliguria almost immediately after surgery, although the urine output may fall sometimes in the second 24 hr after surgery. ATN usually resolves within 7-14 days. Since ATN does not preclude the development of acute rejection, it is our practice to biopsy any patient with primary graft dysfunction after 7-10 days. Up to 60% of these patients have an unexpected acute rejection superimposed on the ATN.

ATN results from any form of ischemia or tissue injury to the transplanted kidney. For example, both acute vascular and tubulo-interstitial cellular rejection cause concomitant ATN that is pathologically indistinguishable from that complicating organ preservation. Therefore, the history must be evaluated carefully before deciding the significance of ATN on a biopsy. It may take 5-7 days for the ATN to resolve and renal function to improve after successful therapy for acute rejection.

CHRONIC KIDNEY TRANSPLANT DYSFUNCTION

ETIOLOGY

The most common causes of chronic transplant dysfunction are chronic rejection and recurrent or *de novo* kidney disease.

Chronic Rejection

Drugs suppress, but do not abolish, the immune response. Therefore, prolonged survival of the kidney transplant depends on continued effective use of immunosuppressive drugs. Thus, noncompliance is a common cause of late rejection episodes. However, even with excellent compliance a low grade immune response may persist and gradually destroy the kidney over several years. The transplant biopsy demonstrates extensive vascular damage including intimal proliferation, luminal obliteration, and interstitial atrophy and fibrosis. The glomeruli will demonstrate so-called transplant glomerulopathy.

Recurrent or De Novo Kidney Disease

Many kidney diseases can recur in the transplanted kidney. Diabetes mellitus or uncontrolled hypertension will often result in long-term transplant damage. Several types of glomerulonephritis may recur after transplantation: focal glomerular sclerosis, IgA nephropathy, membranoproliferative glomerulonephritis, membranous glomerulonephritis, and anti-glomerular basement membrane glomerulonephritis. Fortunately, the majority of patients do not lose their graft function. Systemic lupus erythematosus rarely recurs in transplanted patients for reasons that are unknown. Also, the kidney transplant is not protected from the development of a *de novo* kidney disease, the most common of which is membranous glomerulonephritis.

INVESTIGATION AND MANAGEMENT

The clinical picture of chronic rejection is slowly progressive renal dysfunction over many months or years. The patients are typically asymptomatic until progressive anemia, hypertension, fluid excess, and other features of chronic renal failure develop. An ultrasound is required to exclude urinary tract obstruction. The urinalysis is helpful to differentiate recurrent or *de novo* glomerulonephritis which is often associated with an active urinary sediment (see Chapter 4). However, a renal transplant biopsy is often required to distinguish chronic rejection from recurrent or *de novo* disease. Acute rejection can occur even years after surgery and appropriate therapy may quickly improve kidney function.

Unfortunately, there is no specific therapy for chronic rejection. Aggressive control of systemic hypertension is critical in prolonging graft function. The potential benefit of dietary protein restriction has not been established in renal transplant patients.

OTHER COMPLICATIONS OF KIDNEY TRANSPLANTATION

HYPERTENSION

At least 70% of patients with a successful renal transplant will have hypertension that is often evident within the first week after surgery. In the immediate postoperative period hypertension may cause seizures in cyclosporine-treated patients, particularly in children and those receiving the drug intravenously. The long-term clinical consequences of hypertension are described in Chapter 17. Transplant patients may be at increased risk for hypertension-related complications because of their previous renal failure and lipoprotein abnormalities which often persist following transplantation.

The etiology of hypertension in transplant patients is multifactorial. Volume overload is caused by steroids. Cyclosporine can increase vascular tone and renin-angiotensin levels. The transplant, or the patient's own native kidneys, may generate excess renin.

Transplant renal artery stenosis can complicate the surgical procedure or the effects of rejection on the vessel. The hypertension is difficult to control and progressive renal insufficiency is common. Angiotensin-converting enzyme inhibitors can cause a dramatic increase in the serum creatinine, which fortunately reverses when the drug is discontinued. Such a rise should prompt further evaluation including renal angiography. The decrement in glomerular filtration rate (GFR) is ascribed to an abrupt reduction of angiotensin-induced efferent arteriolar tone, leading to a fall in glomerular capillary pressure and, hence, in the GFR.

Post-transplant hypertension often requires a loop diuretic. The use of central acting drugs, vasodilators, and beta-blockers is similar to that described for any hypertensive patient. Calcium-channel antagonists like verapamil and diltiazem inhibit hepatic clearance of cyclosporine and can cause a 3- to 5-fold increase in the drug levels within days. Nifedipine does not have this interaction.

When hypertension is attributed to renal artery stenosis, per-cutaneous balloon angioplasty is often successful and carries a low morbidity. Where the hypertension is uncontrollable but there is no evidence of renal artery stenosis, bilateral native nephrectomies or ablation of the native kidneys with alcohol administered directly into the renal arteries can be considered.

INFECTION

Infection is a major cause of both morbidity and mortality. Immunosuppressive drugs inhibit the patient's immune response to infectious agents. Any infection, however mild initially, may develop rapidly into a life-threatening situation. For example, a simple cystitis can develop into Gram-negative sepsis and shock within 24 hr.

Viral infections, especially herpes simplex and cytomegalovirus (CMV), are also major problems. The former is usually limited to a few oral lesions but may progress to severe stomatitis and esophagitis, or even to disseminated acute hepatic failure and encephalitis. Acyclovir, either oral or intravenous, is effective. CMV infection typically presents from 3-18 weeks after transplantation with unex-plained fever, malaise, falling WBC, mild liver function abnormali-ties, nausea, and often mild renal dysfunction suggesting rejection. It is critical to diagnose CMV infection by demonstration of a rising IgM titer or viral isolation in urine or blood since antirejection therapy can cause CMV infection to progress rapidly to life-threaten-ing interstitial pneumonia and acute hemorrhagic gastroenteritis. In patients with severe CMV infection, an investigational drug called Ganciclovir (manufactured by Syntex) has been used successfully.

Finally, opportunistic infections caused by *Pneumocystitis carinii*, nocardia, aspergillus, legionella, and candida species can cause pneumonitis. Transplant patients presenting with interstitial pneumonia must be evaluated very aggressively and a tissue diagnosis established quickly. There is a "window of opportunity" early before the patient becomes too ill to permit invasive diagnosis. This opportunity can be lost very rapidly!

OTHER

Transplant patients have an increased risk of malignancy from immunosuppressive drugs. Since the most common are squamous and basal cell skin cancers, sunscreens are strongly recommended and suspicious skin lesions should be evaluated promptly by biopsy. Lymphoma is the next most common malignancy. Cancers of the gastrointestinal (GI) tract are also common, particularly colon and stomach, and there is an increased risk of genitourinary malignancy.

Bone disease reflects the deranged calcium and bone homeostasis of the preceding end-stage renal disease and the osteoporosis caused by chronic steroid administration. Acute hip pain after transplantation suggests aseptic necrosis of the hip. This can also occur in the shoulder and ankles. The use of magnetic resonance imaging (MRI) permits the diagnosis of aseptic necrosis well before the classic X-ray changes.

IMMUNE RESPONSE AND IMMUNOSUPPRESSIVE DRUGS

The immune response is the basis for understanding how rejection occurs and how the different immunosuppressive drugs work. The immune response is depicted in Figure 25-1. The response is divided into three phases - HLA antigen recognition, induction, and amplification.

The induction phase involves a series of signals delivered by soluble mediators called cytokines or lymphokines to the T cells activated during recognition of the HLA antigens and expressing specific cell surface receptors for these soluble mediators. If the correct sequence of signals is received by the killer T cells, they will enter the proliferative phase of the immune response. The recognition and inductive phases of the immune response provide the precise information on the nature and location of the donor cells to permit the killer T cells of the proliferative phase to successfully target and destroy the transplant.

The antibody-forming machinery of the B cell system is also activated by the immune response in a complex interaction with T cell activation. These anti-HLA antibodies are important mediators of acute vascular rejection. Finally, the immune response also generates suppressor T cells that deliver negative signals to the helper and killer cells. These suppressor cells may play a key role in successful transplantation and the mechanisms of the immunosuppressive drugs.

In this context the mechanisms of the three basic immunosuppressive drugs can be discussed. Note that the immunosuppressive drugs are also effective in combinations because of their multiple sites of action.

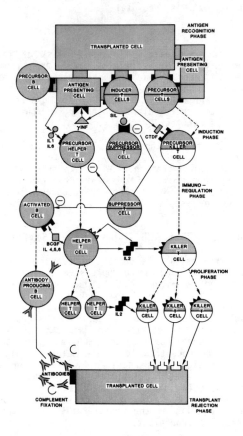

Figure 25-1 A schematic diagram of the immune response in transplantation.

STEROIDS

Steroids inhibit the activation of the macrophages and, thus, block the release of interleukin 1 (IL1). They also inhibit macrophage release of inflammatory cytokines such as leukotrienes and prostaglandins. Finally, steroids inhibit T cell activation by other mechanisms that are not IL1 dependent.

AZATHIOPRINE (IMURAN)

Azathioprine inhibits proliferation of the activated T cells and, thus, blocks the development of the proliferative phase of the immune response.

CYCLOSPORINE

Cyclosporine inhibits the activation of helper T cells and the release of several critical T cell-derived lymphokines including gamma interferon and interleukins 2, 3, 4, and 5. This inhibits the induction phase of the immune response at several sites and explains why cyclosporine is such a powerful immunosuppressive drug.

SPECIAL CONSIDERATIONS IN THE USE OF CYCLOSPORINE

The introduction of cyclosporine in 1978 enhanced the success of kidney, heart, liver, and pancreas transplantation. However, this drug is not without major problems that affect its application to kidney transplantation.

Because cyclosporine is such a potent immunosuppressive drug, the intensity of the immune response in acute rejection is often attenuated enough to modify the classic clinical presentation such that fever and a swollen or tender graft are rarely seen. Similarly, the incidence of rejection has been reduced significantly, particularly when all three drugs are used in combination. Therefore, a higher index of suspicion must be attached to even mild but unexplained increases in serum creatinine. Since cyclosporine is also nephrotoxic, it is often difficult to decide whether a rising creatinine is due to rejection or cyclosporine toxicity. Measurement of the whole blood drug level is very useful although there is no precise drug level which proves toxicity. Levels above 500 ng/ml suggest toxicity, whereas levels under 250 ng/ml might suggest acute rejection. (There are multiple assays for cyclosporine; these correlations are for the whole blood methods which are generally considered the best.) In many cases a transplant biopsy is necessary since cyclosporine toxicity may coincide with acute rejection.

Cyclosporine is very hydrophobic and its GI absorption is highly dependent on bile acids. Therefore, the patient should take the drug at approximately the same time each morning with breakfast. Alterations in biliary tract function secondary to surgery, liver disease, or bowel motility disorders such as those associated with diabetes mellitus or acute viral gastroenteritis can reduce cyclosporine levels by 30-50%. The poor correlation between dose and blood levels mandates frequent dose adjustments in the first 6 months. Blood levels must be followed very carefully as they can change quickly. A large number of drugs can alter cyclosporine absorption or metabolism.

Drugs That Increase and Decrease Cyclosporine Levels

Increase	Decrease
• Ketoconazole	• Phenytoin
• Cimetidine	• Phenobarbital
• Ranitidine	• Ethambutol
• Verapamil	• Sulfamethoxazole
• Diltiazem	• Ethanol
• Erythromycin	• Cholestyramine

Cyclosporine toxicity can also involve the nervous system with fine intention tremor, altered mental clarity and judgment, anxiety, paresthesias, and an increased seizure risk. Gingival hyperplasia, hirsutism, dry eyes, and mild hepatotoxicity are common. Cyclosporine causes the same increased risk of infection and malignancy as steroids and azathioprine.

SUGGESTED READING

Amend WC, Hess AD, Humes HD, Vincenti F, eds. Cyclosporine in clinical use. New York: World Medical Press, 1987.

Croker BC, Salomon DR. Pathology of the renal allograft. In: Tisher CC, Brenner BM, eds. Renal pathology with clinical and functional correlations. Philadelphia: JB Lippincott, 1989;1518-1554.

Morris PJ, ed. Kidney transplantation, principles and practice. 3rd ed. London: Greene and Stratton, 1987.

Salomon DR, Strom TB. Diagnosis and therapy of renal transplant rejection. In: Garavoy M, Guttmann R, eds. Renal Transplantation. Edinburgh: Churchill Livingstone, 1986;125-157.

Chapter 26

Nutrition in Renal Failure

Edward D. Frederickson
Patti Dean

INTRODUCTION

The purpose of this discussion is to outline general nutritional concepts and provide specific recommendations for the most common situations encountered in renal patients. In renal failure, increased levels of nitrogen-containing metabolites, urea, and larger peptides and amino acids, collectively termed the "middle molecules," produce the uremic syndrome. Other substances also accumulate to produce toxic syndromes. These include phosphorus, which induces secondary hyperparathyroidism, and aluminum, which causes osteomalacia, encephalopathy, and microcytic anemia.

In patients with renal insufficiency [glomerular filtration rate (GFR) <70 but >5 ml/min], carefully controlled low protein diets not only control the uremic syndrome but may also reduce the progressive course of the disease.

GENERAL NUTRITIONAL CONCEPTS

CALORIC REQUIREMENT

Patients with renal failure have normal energy requirements in the absence of a systemic illness. Renal patients on hemodialysis frequently consume fewer calories than needed, which accounts for some degree of protein malnutrition. Continuous ambulatory peritoneal dialysis (CAPD) patients are more likely to meet their caloric needs because of the glucose absorbed from the dialysate. Patients on low protein diets and patients losing protein either through peritoneal dialysis or the nephrotic syndrome require additional caloric intake as carbohydrate to "spare" the essential amino acids for protein synthesis rather than for metabolism to provide basal energy requirements.

The basal energy expenditure (BEE) in kilocalories is given by the Harris Benedict equation.

BEE (males) = 66.5 + [13.7 x weight (kg)] + [5.0 x height (cm)] - [6.8 x age]

BEE (females) = 655.1 + [9.6 x weight (kg)] + [1.7 x height (cm)] - [4.7 x age]

The caloric requirement (Kcal) equals the BEE times a factor of 1.3 for maintenance or 1.7 for catabolic patients.

Renal patients are frequently catabolic. Therefore, they should be monitored closely for calorie-protein malnutrition with measurements of body weight, triceps skin-fold thickness, midarm muscle circumference, serum albumin, serum transferrin, and the total lymphocyte count.

MACRONUTRIENTS

PROTEIN

The typical American diet contains 1.4-1.6 g/kg of protein/day. The minimal protein requirements for renal patients are the same as normal people (0.6-0.8 g/kg/day) but are lower (0.45-0.6 g/kg/day) if only high biologic value protein is consumed. Biologic value of a protein source is determined by the efficiency with which it is utilized for protein synthesis. Eggs, milk, and fish have the highest biologic value, followed by poultry and beef. Protein derived from grains is used less efficiently. Very low protein diets can be used if they contain supplements of essential amino acids (EAA) or a combination of EAA and ketoacids (KA). KA, which are currently experimental, are the alpha ketoanalogues of EAA. Therefore, they provide the carbon skeleton without the nitrogen; the liver transaminates these compounds back to the corresponding amino acid.

The compliance of a patient on a protein-restricted diet can be checked by measuring the urine urea nitrogen ($U_{UN}V$):

$$I_N \text{ (nitrogen intake)} = U_{UN}V + NUN \text{ (nonurea nitrogen)}$$

The nonurea nitrogen (NUN) is estimated as follows:

$$NUN \text{ (g)} = 0.031 \times \text{body weight (kg)}$$

The I_N can be converted to daily protein intake using the formula:

$$\text{Protein intake} = \frac{6.25 \cdot I_N}{\text{g nitrogen}}$$

Example: A 70-kg patient without edema with a stable blood urea nitrogen and weight excretes 5 g urea N/day.

$$I_N = 5 \text{ g urea N/day} + 0.031 \text{ g/kg} \times 70 \text{ kg nonurea}$$

$$I_N = 5 + 2.17 = 7.17 \text{ g N/day}$$

Protein intake = 6.25 x 7.17 = 48.8 g/day

FATS

Fifty to 70% of patients with chronic renal failure have abnormal serum lipids. A reduction of lipoprotein lipase causes hypercholesterolemia and hypertriglyceridemia. Triglycerides are further elevated in patients on peritoneal dialysis by dextrose absorption from their dialysate. Dialysis does not restore normal lipoprotein lipase activity.

Current clinical guidelines recommend a total blood cholesterol level of 200 mg/dl or lower; above 240 mg/dl is considered high risk. Individuals with higher cholesterol levels should have a lipoprotein analysis performed to determine the level of low-density lipoprotein (LDL) cholesterol which should be below 140 mg/dl after a 12- to 24-hr fast. Dietary recommendations for reducing LDL cholesterol and total cholesterol include:

• Attain and maintain ideal body weight.
• Reduce fat intake to 25-30% of calories consumed.
• Decrease saturated fats to 10%, substituting mono- and polyunsaturated fat.
• Reduce the total cholesterol intake to 150-250 mg/day.

In order to reduce triglyceride levels it is recommended to reduce dietary fat intake as well as simple sugars and ethanol.

To provide adequate calories for a patient on protein restriction, it is frequently necessary to add large amounts of fruits (also limited by potassium restrictions), sugars, syrups, and fats. However, it is often impossible to restrict protein, simple sugars, and fats to ideal levels and meet caloric needs.

CARBOHYDRATES

The chief sources of carbohydrates are grains, vegetables, fruits, sugars, and syrups. Complex carbohydrates are polysaccharides and are less likely to cause hypertriglyceridemia. Carbohydrates are of primary importance in the renal diet for the following reasons:

• They are a major energy source.
• They can spare protein, especially when given with amino acids.
• They minimize the formation of ketones from fat by allowing complete oxidation of fatty acids.
• They provide dietary fiber.

Dietary carbohydrate control is recommended in patients with poorly controlled diabetes and/or hypertriglyceridemia. Simple sugars are to be avoided. Carbohydrate intake for CAPD patients must also take into consideration the dextrose absorbed from the dialysate.

MICRONUTRIENTS

SODIUM AND CHLORIDE

Chronic renal failure leads to a variable degree of salt retention or, less commonly, salt wastage. Acute renal failure frequently causes oliguria with salt retention, but a polyuric phase may occur with marked wasting of sodium, chloride, and volume. The nephrotic syndrome and other edematous states can cause severe salt retention. Most hypertension associated with chronic renal disease is a consequence of volume overload, and the salt restriction is a main focus of therapy. A diet with 100 mEq of sodium chloride contains 2.3 g of sodium and 3.5 g of chloride.

POTASSIUM

The degree of potassium restriction necessary in the renal diet is dependent upon the plasma potassium concentration, body size, urinary potassium excretion, and the amount of potassium removed by dialysis. Dietary K restriction involves limiting fruits, vegetables, legumes, dairy products, and meat. The protein content of a diet may dictate the degree of potassium restriction that is feasible. For example, 40 g of protein contain about 26 mEq or 1 g of potassium. In general, 1 mEq of potassium per kg body weight represents a moderate potassium restriction which will avoid hyperkalemia in most situations.

PHOSPHORUS

As the GFR falls, phosphorus is retained. To avoid hyperphosphatemia, dietary phosphorus must be restricted and phosphate binding resins should be given. Dietary phosphorus intake can be limited by restriction of dairy products, dried legumes, meat, fish, poultry, and eggs. Aluminum-containing antacids have routinely been used to bind dietary phosphorus. It is now recognized that significant amounts of aluminum can be absorbed leading to osteomalacia, microcytic anemia, and encephalopathy. Calcium carbonate is also a phosphate binder but is not as effective. It is recommended to lower very high phosphorus levels (>6 mg/dl) initially with aluminum hydroxide and to substitute calcium carbonate for maintenance. Phosphate binders must be taken with food. Calcium carbonate is also used as a calcium supplement and in this situation it should not be taken with food.

VITAMINS AND MINERALS

Water-soluble vitamin deficiencies can develop in the uremic patient due to anorexia, dietary restrictions, altered metabolism, or dialysate losses. Currently it is recommended to supplement folic acid, vitamin C, and pyridoxine. Some recommend supplementation of thiamine, riboflavin, and pantothenic acid. Precise recommendations have not been established for vitamin B_{12}, thiamine, and riboflavin.

Fat-soluble vitamins A, E, and K do not require supplementation. Indeed, vitamin A supplements can be toxic in renal failure.

Many renal patients have low zinc levels due to low intake and decreased intestinal absorption. Symptoms such as hypogeusia, hair loss, and impotence may be improved with zinc supplementation.

Iron deficiency in renal patients often contributes to anemia. Deficiency is likely to occur due to blood loss during hemodialysis or gastrointestinal bleeding. These patients also may have poor dietary intake of FeSO$_4$.

Both aluminum and magnesium excretion are impaired in renal failure. Aluminum toxicity may develop due to excessive aluminum in the water supply, dialysate, or with use of aluminum phosphate binding agents. Magnesium overload may occur with the use of magnesium-containing antacids.

SPECIFIC RECOMMENDATIONS

ACUTE RENAL FAILURE (PREDIALYSIS)

Protein

Approximately 0.5-0.8 g protein/day is required to reduce nitrogen metabolism and retention of which 75-80% should be of high biologic value.

Calories

The stress of acute renal failure (ARF) typically requires 45-50 Kcal/kg for weight maintenance and protein sparing. High calorie, low protein nutritional supplements are often necessary to provide adequate calories without excessive protein.

Fat

Maintaining high caloric intake requires liberal use of fats.

Carbohydrates

Caloric needs necessitate liberal use of carbohydrates. Only with hyperglycemia should simple carbohydrates be restricted.

Sodium

During the oliguric phase, the daily sodium intake should be restricted to 1-1.5 g (43-65 mEq). This must be liberalized during the diuretic phase.

Potassium

Hyperkalemia is frequent in the oliguric phase due to diminished excretion and cellular K release. It may be necessary to restrict dietary potassium to 35-50 mEq/day. During the diuretic phase of ARF, excretion may become excessive requiring supplemental potassium.

Phosphorus

Restrict intake to 0.5-1 g and prescribe phosphate-binding resins.

Magnesium

Magnesium-containing antacids (Maalox, MOM, Riopan) are contraindicated.

CHRONIC RENAL FAILURE (PREDIALYSIS)

Calories

Caloric requirements are determined by BEE and the activity level. Low protein diets require assurance of adequate caloric intake to "spare" protein.

Protein

GFR	Recommendation
>70 ml/min	No specific limitation
25-70 ml/min	0.55 to 0.6 g/kg/day (70% of high biologic value)
5-24 ml/min	0.55 to 0.6 g/kg/day (70% of high biologic value) or 0.28 g/kg/day + 10-20 g/kg/day of EAA or KA supplements
<5 ml/min	Progress to dialysis and increase protein intake to avoid protein malnutrition

Fat

Cholesterol and triglycerides are frequently elevated. Therefore, if possible, only 30% of the total calories should be in the form of fat with a limit of 10% from saturated fat.

Carbohydrates

Complex carbohydrates are used if hypertriglyceridemia is present.

Sodium Chloride

Restrict sodium chloride to control hypertension or edema in the range of 1-3 g sodium or 3-6 g sodium chloride (50-100 mEq) daily.

Potassium

Hyperkalemia may be a problem at low GFR or if the patient has a hyperkalemic renal tubular acidosis. If so, restrict K to 50-70 mEq/day.

Phosphorus

Dietary phosphorus should be limited to 0.5 to 1.0 g/day and phosphate-binding resins should be used if the GFR is <40 ml/min to prevent secondary hyperparathyroidism.

HEMODIALYSIS

Calories

Determined by BEE and activity level. Adjustments should be made for desired weight reduction or weight gain.

Protein

For greater catabolic requirements, provide 1-1.2 g/kg/day.

Fat

If the caloric level is adequate, fat should be limited to approximately 30% of the total calories with only 10% from saturated fat.

Carbohydrates

The remainder of caloric needs should be provided by carbohydrate sources.

Sodium

Restriction is based on blood pressure, fluid balance, and weight gain. Include approximately 1-3 g of sodium or 2-6 g of sodium chloride (34-100 mEq) daily.

Potassium

Provide 50-70 mEq/day or 1 mEq/kg/day.

Phosphorus

Restrict phosphorus to 0.8-1.2 g/day and use phosphate binders.

Vitamins and Minerals

Established recommended daily supplements include:

Folic acid	1 mg
Vitamin C	100 mg
Vitamin B$_6$	10 mg
Pantothenic acid	5-20 mg
Riboflavin	1.6-2.0 mg

Calcium supplementation, frequently in combination with vitamin D$_3$, is recommended to maintain normal serum calcium levels. The need for **iron** supplementation should be identified by serum ferritin levels.

CAPD

Calories

Needs are assessed by BEE times the activity factor with adjustments for desired weight gain or loss. Calories absorbed from dialysate must be considered as part of the caloric intake. The absorption rate has been estimated as approximately 70%.

1.5% Dextrose = 102 Kcal/2 l (.70) = 71 Kcal
2.5% Dextrose = 170 Kcal/2 l (.70 = 119 Kcal
4.25% Dextrose = 306 Kcal/2 l (.70) = 214 Kcal

Protein

Some protein loss into the dialysate is common. An intake of 1.2-1.3 g protein/kg/day is recommended. If hypoalbuminemia is present, 1.5 g/kg/day is recommended.

Fat

Serum cholesterol and triglycerides are frequently elevated in CAPD patients. Ideally, 30% of dietary calories should be derived from fat sources with a limit of 10% from saturated fat.

Carbohydrates

The remainder of calories should be provided from carbohydrates. Emphasis should be placed on use of complex carbohydrates to reduce hypertriglyceridemia.

Sodium

Restrict sodium if necessary to control fluid balance or hypertension.

Potassium

If hyperkalemia is present, restrict to 50-70 mEq/day. Otherwise, limit intake to 80 mEq/day.

Phosphorus

Moderate phosphorus restriction of 0.8 g/day is recommended.

Vitamins

Follow recommendations for the hemodialysis patient.

RENAL TRANSPLANT

Immunosuppressive medications have nutritional implications that require dietary modification. The medications are initiated in relatively high doses compared to maintenance levels and have a more pronounced effect on nutritional status. With maintenance doses, a regular diet may be resumed, unless hypertension or other complicating factors require dietary modification.

NEPHROTIC SYNDROME

Protein

In some patients proteinuria and protein catabolism can be reduced with a low protein diet while maintaining a neutral or even a positive nitrogen balance and serum albumin (S_{Alb}) level. Protein restriction should be prescribed cautiously. The current recommendation for adults is 0.8 g/kg/day plus urinary losses. It is important that the protein be of high biologic value. Failure to reduce proteinuria and to obtain an increased S_{Alb} should prompt discontinuation of protein restriction to avoid severe malnutrition.

Fat

Hyperlipidemia is included in the definition of the nephrotic syndrome. These patients have a greater cardiovascular risk with the marked elevations in cholesterol and triglycerides. High-density lipoprotein fractions are decreased because this smaller protective lipoprotein is easily filtered in the urine. Specific recommendations are to reduce the calories derived from fat sources to 30%, to reduce daily cholesterol intake to 300 mg, and to reduce the percentage of saturated fats, obtaining a polyunsaturated:saturated ratio between 3 and 10.

Carbohydrates

Complex carbohydrates decrease hypertriglyceridemia.

Sodium

Salt reduction is required to decrease edema. The specific recommendation is 1-3 g sodium or 3-6 g sodium chloride (50-100 mEq) daily.

Potassium

Losses induced by diuretics may need to be replaced.

Calcium

Hypocalcemia parallels hypoalbuminemia but is complicated by poor intestinal absorption secondary to decreased vitamin D binding protein. Recommended dietary calcium is at least 800 mg/day.

Vitamin D$_3$

Vitamin D deficiency may result from urinary losses of vitamin D-binding protein and the bound vitamin, therefore, cholecalciferol (Vitamin D$_3$ - 400 IU/day) should be supplemented. The liver and kidney usually continue to hydroxylate vitamin D appropriately so 1,25-OH-D$_3$ is unneccessary unless renal insufficiency ensues.

SUGGESTED READING

Mitch WE, Klahr S. Nutrition and the kidney. Boston: Little, Brown, and Company, 1988.

CHRONIC RENAL DISEASE

Mitch WE. The influence of the diet on the progression of renal insufficiency. Ann Rev Med 1984;35:249-264.

PHOSPHORUS IN CHRONIC RENAL FAILURE

Slatopolsky E, Weerts C, Stokes T, et al. Alternative phosphate binders in dialysis patients: calcium carbonate. Semin Nephrol 1986;6(4 Suppl 1):35-41.

NEPHROTIC SYNDROME

Kaysen GA. Effect of dietary protein intake on albumin homeostasis in nephrotic patients. Kidney Int 1986;29:572-577.

PERITONEAL DIALYSIS

Kopple JO, Blumenkrantz MJ. Nutritional requirements for patient undergoing continuous ambulatory peritoneal dialysis. Kidney Int 1983;24:(S16)295-302.

RENAL TRANSPLANTATION

Hoy WE, Sargent JA, Freeman RB, et al. The influence of glucocorticoid dose on protein catabolism after renal transplantation. Am J Med Sci 1986;291:241-247.

Chapter 27

Use of Drugs in Renal Failure

Edward D. Frederickson

INTRODUCTION

This discussion will outline pharmacokinetic principles and provide specific information about the prescribing of commonly used drugs in renal failure (see Tables 27-1 - 27-4). The activity of any drug is related to the concentration of free drug in the tissue compartment where the effect occurs (Fig. 1). The kidney is a major route of drug elimination both through excretion and metabolism. Patients with renal disease and also elderly patients who have relative renal insufficiency secondary to normal aging are more likely to develop dose-related drug toxicity. Drug interactions are also more common in renal patients as they are frequently receiving many drugs. Uremia alters gastrointestinal absorption, hepatic metabolism, and protein affinity of many compounds. Protein binding of drugs is also diminished by hypoalbuminemia. Active metabolites, which in a normal state are eliminated, may accumulate in renal insufficiency and may produce an increased desired primary effect or perhaps an undesired secondary action.

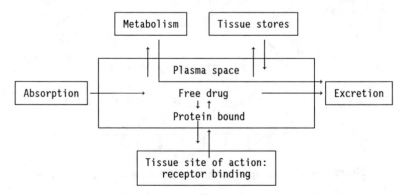

Fig. 27-1. Relationship of absorption, distribution, protein binding, and excretion of a drug and its concentration at the locus of action.

The elimination of almost all drugs is by first order kinetics. Notable exceptions include ethanol, salicylates, and phenytoin at high plasma concentrations. First-order elimination means that the rate at which a drug is removed (dx/dt) is directly proportional to the amount of drug in the body at that time and an elimination rate constant (k). The amount of drug removed over a period of time is directly proportional to the total amount of drug in the body at time (t), X_t, and the elimination rate constant (k). Therefore:

(eq 1) $dx/dt = -kX_t$

where X_t is the total amount of drug in the body at time (t). Equation 1 can be rearranged and integrated from time 1 (t_1) to time 2 (t_2) yielding equation 2, which defines the elimination rate constant k.

(eq 2) $\ln X_2/X_1 = -k\Delta t$ or $\ln X_1/X_2 = k\Delta t$

X_1, X_2 can be expressed as the ratio of the total amount of drug in the body or as the actual plasma concentrations.

Defining the **elimination rate constant** for a drug is very helpful, as one can then project the time at which a patient will have a specific drug concentration.

The half-life ($T_{\frac{1}{2}}$) of a drug is given by the time at which the drug concentration at t_2 is one half of the drug concentration at t_1. Since $(X_1)/(X_2) = 2$, equation 3 simplifies to:

(eq 3) $\ln 2 = kT_{\frac{1}{2}}$ or $T_{\frac{1}{2}} = 0.693/k$

The **apparent volume of distribution**, V_D, is the second key pharmakokinetic parameter to be considered. V_D is the sum of all of the relative volumes of each tissue compartment in which the drug is distributed. A very large V_D implies avid tissue binding with the concentration of the drug in some compartments being larger than the plasma or central compartment. A small V_D reflects confinement of the drug in the central compartment by plasma protein binding. Calculation of V_D requires back extrapolation of the linear elimination phase of the natural logarithm of the concentration versus time curve (Figure 27-2).

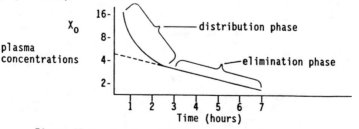

Figure 27-2. Semilogarithmic concentration versus time curve.

The dose of a drug at t_0 approximates the total amount of drug in the body assuming complete absorption or intravenous administration.

(eq 5) (X_0) = dose/V_D

This equation can be generalized such that:

(eq 6) $V_D = X_t/(x_t)$ where X_t equals the total amount of drug in the body and (x_t) is the plasma concentration at time t.

The third concept is **plasma clearance** (Cl), which is the volume of plasma cleared of a drug per unit of time. The clearance multiplied by the plasma concentration (X_t) is equal to the product of the elimination rate constant (k) and the total amount of drug in all tissue compartments(X_t) at any given time (t).

(eq 7) kX_t = Cl (x_t) or k $X_t/(x_t)$ = Cl

eq 6 can be substituted such that

(eq 8) $k = Cl/V_D$

substituting eq 4; (eq 9). $T_{\frac{1}{2}} = 0.693\ V_D/Cl$

Thus, the half-life of a drug is dependent upon its apparent volume of distribution and its plasma clearance.

Example: A 75-kg man has acute oliguric renal failure and Gram-negative sepsis. A loading dose of 150 mg of gentamicin is given intravenously. When should the next dose be given and how much? The peak gentamicin level is 7.5 mg/l and the level at 24 hr is 40 mg/l.

Step 1: Calculate an approximate V_D (assuming rapid distribution). The peak level measured at 30 min equals 7.5 mg/l. Thus, V_D = dose/(X_0) = 150 mg/7.5 mg/l = 20 liters.

Step 2: Obtain a 24-hr plasma level and calculate an elimination rate constant; if (X_{24}) = 4.0 then

ln X_1/X_2 = ln 7.5/4.0 = k (24 hr)

Therefore k = 0.03 hours^{-1}. This elimination rate constant can be used to calculate the time a desired plasma trough level will be reached. If the desired trough is 1.5 mg/l, then the next dose should be given in:

$$\frac{\ln\ (X_1)/(X_2)}{k} = \frac{\ln\ 4.0/1.5}{0.03} = 32.7\ hr$$

Step 3: The size of the next dose should be equal to the product of the desired increment and volume of distribution. If the desired peak level is 6.0 mg/l, then:

$[(X_2)-(X_1)]\ V_D$ = (6.0 mg/l - 1.5 mg/l) 20l = 90 mg

CLEARANCE

The total plasma clearance of a drug (Cl_T) is equal to the sum of renal elimination (Cl_R), hepatic metabolism and conjugation (Cl_H), and other metabolic and excretory pathways in other tissues (Cl_O).

(eq 10) $Cl_T = Cl_R + Cl_H + Cl_O$

Renal elimination of drugs is determined by glomerular filtration, active secretion primarily in the proximal tubule, and reabsorption. Protein bound drugs are poorly filtered, but they may be efficiently cleared by proximal secretion. Unbound drugs are usually freely filtered at the glomerulus; their renal elimination depends upon volume of distribution, glomerular filtration rate (GFR) and drug reabsorption. Drugs with large volumes of distribution and large tissue reservoirs are not available for glomerular filtration. The GFR can be estimated using an empiric relationship developed by Cockcroft and Gault:

$$GFR \ (ml/min) \approx \frac{(140-age) \times lean \ body \ weight \ (kg)}{Cr(mg\%) \times 72}$$

(multiply by 0.85 for females)

The proximal tubule is normally very active metabolically. Following luminal endocytosis, peptides and other compounds are degraded by lysosomes. Neutral uncharged compounds are highly reabsorbed, whereas, charged molecules will become trapped in the lumen based on the pH of the urine and the pK_A of the compound.

Hepatic metabolism gains importance in patients with renal insufficiency. Whenever possible, drugs with significant hepatic elimination should be used. Uremia can impair hepatic metabolic pathways, e.g., the reduction of drugs such as hydrocortisone and the acetylation of drugs like isoniazid. Conjugation to glycine may also be impaired. In renal failure, previously minor hepatic metabolic pathways may become the major mechanism for elimination of a drug; therefore, concomitant hepatic failure can result in severe overdosage and toxicity.

PROTEIN BINDING

Alterations in protein binding are common in renal failure. Protein affinity for drugs is decreased by competitive binding from small peptides and other metabolites and by acidosis. Patients with the nephrotic syndrome or hypoalbuminemia secondary to peritoneal dialysis or protein malnutrition will also have decreased plasma protein binding of drugs. This leads to an increase in the apparent V_D. Therefore, at a given dose, the total plasma concentration will be diminished. An offsetting factor is that the percentage of free drug in the plasma will increase such that the effective activity of a particular dose may remain unchanged or increase slightly. It is important to remember to adjust the therapeutic range downward such that a low plasma level is not misinterpreted as subtherapeutic.

Alternatively, the free drug concentration can be measured. The normal therapeutic range of phenytoin is 10-20 μg/ml; this decreases progressively with uremia or hypoalbuminemia.

BIOAVAILABILITY

Gastrointestinal absorption of drugs is largely unchanged by mild or moderate renal insufficiency. However, many patients with renal disease have gastrointestinal motility disorders, the most common being diarrhea and/or gastroparesis in the diabetic patient. Aluminum-based antacids used as phosphate binders may cause profound constipation. Contact time for intestinal absorption is the most important factor in drug absorption. Therefore, constipation may increase bioavailability and diarrhea decrease it. The peak level obtained following the oral intake of a drug is also a function of drug absorption. Most drugs are absorbed in the proximal small intestine. The peak height of the plasma concentration versus time curve will be increased and occur earlier with more rapid gastric emptying. Delayed gastric emptying will delay and diminish the peak concentration and total drug absorption.

HEMODIALYSIS OF DRUGS

The degree to which a drug is removed by hemodialysis is directly proportional to the plasma concentration of free drug (not bound to plasma proteins) and to the clearance characteristics of the dialysis membrane. Hemodialysis clearance is inversely proportional to the amount of tissue binding or V_D. Many drugs, particularly antibiotics, are removed by hemodialysis and it is important to supplement the dose after a treatment. Occasionally symptoms will occur because of an inadequate drug level toward the end of a treatment. Arrhythmias may break through because N-acetyl procainamide, the acetylated active metabolite of procainamide, is dialysable. Opiates and ethanol are dialysable and their removal can precipitate withdrawal or inadequate analgesia. Drug intoxications are occasionally treated by hemodialysis. The most important are methanol and ethylene glycol, which are water soluble and readily removed with hemodialysis. There also is a role for dialysis in severe salicylate intoxication, but usually this can be managed by a brisk alkaline diuresis.

PERITONEAL DIALYSIS OF DRUGS

Drugs are poorly removed by peritoneal dialysis. Drug administration in the dialysate fluid is similarly a difficult way to obtain a systemic drug level. Antibiotics are frequently used intraperitoneally to treat dialysis-related peritonitis, and removal of systemic antibiotics can be avoided by placing therapeutic drug levels into the dialysate. Insulin can be given intraperitoneally, which avoids injections and provides an improved physiologic delivery as it is absorbed directly into the portal vein. Erythropoietin is also effective intraperitoneally. Intraperitoneal heparin is useful to prevent fibrin clot formation without causing systemic effects.

TABLES

The following tables provide specific information about the most commonly used drugs in renal patients. The information is a guideline and should be used to start therapy with the understanding that individual adjustments will be the rule rather than the exception. Included is information on the major route of elimination, the normal volume of distribution, the percentage of protein binding, the normal $T_{\frac{1}{2}}$ and the $T_{\frac{1}{2}}$ in end-stage renal failure (ESRD), the degree to which the drug is dialyzed, and a dosage adjustment factor. The adjustment factors have been borrowed from William Bennett, M.D., and are based on virtual complete loss of renal function; they should be extrapolated downward by multiplying by the percentage of decline in GFR from normal. For example, if the remaining GFR is 20 ml/min, or an 80% decline in renal function, the adjustment factor for ceftazidime which is 6-8 in ESRD would be 4.8-6.4. The extrapolated adjustment factor is then multiplied times the normal interval between doses to obtain a new interval for the same dose. Alternatively, the usual dose can be divided by the adjustment factor to be given at the usual interval.

Dose interval = normal interval x adjustment factor
    or

$$\text{Dose} = \frac{\text{normal dose}}{\text{adjustment factor}}$$

In practice, it is better to compromise and adjust both the individual dose and the interval to optimize peak and trough levels. This requires a working knowledge of the principles discussed at the beginning of this chapter. The data contained in the tables have been compiled from the work of both William Bennett and Craig Brater.

Table 27-1 Antimicrobial Agents

Drug	Major Route of Elimination	VD (L/Kg)	Protein Binding	$T_{1/2}(h)$ Normal	$T_{1/2}(h)$ ESRD	Supplement after Hemodialysis	Adjustment Factor
ANTIBIOTICS							
Aminoglycosides							
Amikacin	Renal	0.21	0	2-2.5	30	50%	4-6
Gentamicin	Renal	0.25	0	2	26	50%	4-6
Netilmicin	Renal	0.25	0	2.5	40	50%	4-6
Streptomycin	Renal	0.25	0	2.5	100	50%	6-8
Tobramycin	Renal	0.26	0	2.5	55	50%	4-6
Vancomycin	Renal	0.70	0	6-11	150-250	0	14
Carbapenes - Combination of imipenem and cilastin. Cilastin inhibits renal metabolism in the proximal tubule and prolongs the half-life of imipenem.							
Imipenem	Renal	0.3	20%	1	3.5-4	100%	2-4
Cilastin	Renal	0.25	20%	1	13-17	50%	--
Cephalosporins							
Cefaclor	Renal	0.36	25%	0.2-0.8	2-3	33%	1.0
Cefamandole	Renal	0.19	74%	0.5-1.0	7.5-11	50%	1.5
Cefazolin	Renal	0.14	85%	1.6-2.3	24-50	33-50%	4-6
Cefotaxime	Renal	0.48	30%	1-1.5	3-11	50%	2-3
Cefotetan	Renal	0.12	85%	3.0	11.0	0	6-8
Cefoxitin	Renal	0.27	74%	0.7	13-22	100%	3-4
Ceftazidime	Renal	0.25	17%	1.5-3	15-25	50%	8-10
Ceftriaxone	Renal	0.16	90%	6	12	0	2-4
Cefuroxime	Renal	0.20	40%	1.2	15-22	100%	2-4
Cephalexin	Renal	0.33	15%	0.9-1.2	10-20	75%	6
Cephalothin	Renal	0.32	65%	0.5	18-20	50%	1.5-2
Macrolides							
Clindamycin	Hepatic	0.66	60-90%	2.5-3.5	Unchanged	0	1
Erythromycin	Hepatic	0.78	85%	1.1-2.0	3-7	0	1
Lincomycin	Hepatic	0.54	70%	4.7-5.6	10	0	2-3

Table 27-1 Antimicrobial Agents (continued)

Drug	Major Route of Elimination	VD (L/Kg)	Protein Binding	T½(h) Normal	T½(h) ESRD	Supplement after Hemodialysis	Adjustment Factor
Monobactams							
Aztreonam	Renal	0.2	50-60%	1.7	8	40%	3-4
Moxalactam	Renal	0.28	50-60%	2-4	19-30	30-50%	7-10
Penicillins							
Amoxicillin	Renal	0.66	17%	0.8-2.3	10-15	30%	4-6
Ampicillin	Renal	0.30	18%	0.8-1.5	20	50%	4-10
Carbenicillin	Renal	0.13	50%	1.0	10-20	50%	5-10
Cloxacillin	Hepatic	0.10	95%	0.5	1.0	0	1
Dicloxacillin	Hepatic	0.09	96%	0.7	1-2	0	1
Methicillin	Renal	0.45	40%	0.75	4	0	2
Mezlocillin	Renal	0.14	30%	0.6-1.2	2.5-5.4	25%	1.5
Nafcillin	Hepatic	0.35	90%	0.5	1.2	0	1
Oxacillin	Hepatic	0.30	92%	0.5	1	0	1
Penicillin	Renal	0.23	60%	1.0	4-10	100%	2
Piperacillin	Renal	0.20	21%	1.0	3.3	50%	2
Ticarcillin	Renal	0.20	50%	1.2-1.5	10-25	50%	3-4
Quinolones							
Ciprofloxacin	Renal	5.0	20%	3.5-6.5	8.5	N	2
Norfloxacin	Hepatic	0.5-1	14%	3.5-6.5	7.7	N	2
Sulfonamides							
Sulfamethoxazole	Renal	0.25	65%	9-11	30-60	50%	2
Sulfisoxazole	Renal	6.16	90%	5.5-6.0	11	0	2
Trimethoprim	Renal	2.1	70%	8-11	24-30	50%	2

Tetracyclines - These drugs have an antianabolic effect which raises blood urea nitrogen independent of renal function. In addition they are nephrotoxic and most compounds have renal elimination.

Drug	Major Route of Elimination	VD (L/Kg)	Protein Binding	T½(h) Normal	T½(h) ESRD	Supplement after Hemodialysis	Adjustment Factor
Doxycycline	Renal	.75	90%	16	Prolonged	0	Avoid
Minocycline	Hepatic	0.4	70%	12-16	12-18	0	Avoid
Tetracycline	Renal	1.5	65%	6	30-80	0	Avoid

Table 27-1 Antimicrobial Agents (continued)

Drug	Major Route of Elimination	VD (L/Kg)	Protein Binding	$T_{1/2}(h)$ Normal	$T_{1/2}(h)$ ESRD	Supplement after Hemodialysis	Adjustment Factor
Others							
Chloramphenicol	Hepatic	0.5-0.8	25-50%	3-5	3-5	0	1
ANTIFUNGAL AGENTS							
Amphotericin B	Hepatic	4	95%	15	15	0	1
Flucytosine	Renal	0.7	3-4%	3.5-5.0	30-100	50%	3-4
Ketoconazole	Hepatic	1.25	99%	4.5-7	4.5-7	0	1
Miconazole	Hepatic	21	98%	20-24	20-24	0	1
ANTIMALARIAL AGENTS							
Chloroquine	Renal	150	55%	6-50	Increased	0	5-10
Quinine	Hepatic	1.8	90%	8.5	8.5	0	1
ANTIPARASITICS							
Metronidazole	Hepatic	0.8-1.0	10%	8	10	25%	1
ANTITUBERCULOUS AGENTS							
Ethambutol	Renal	2.3	20-30%	3	8	100%	2
Isoniazid	Hepatic	0.6	0	0.7-2.0	4-8		2
Aminosalicylic acid	Renal	0.24	60%	0.7	20	--	20-25
Rifampin	Hepatic	1.0	90%	3.5	3.5	0	1
ANTIVIRAL AGENTS							
Acyclovir	Renal	0.7	9-22%	2-3	19.5	50%	5-10
Amantadine	Renal	5.1	0	Young, 12 Elderly, 29	7-13 days	0	5-10
Ganciclovir	Renal	0.47	0	3.7	28	50%	4-8

Table 27-2 Cardiovascular Drugs, Antihypertensives, Diuretics, Bronchodilators, Antianginals, and Antiarrhythmics

Drug	Major Route of Elimination	VD (L/Kg)	Protein Binding	$T_{\frac{1}{2}}(h)$ Normal	$T_{\frac{1}{2}}(h)$ ESRD	Supplement after Hemodialysis	Adjustment Factor
ANTIARRHYTHMICS							
Amiodarone	Hepatic	70	96%	25-50 days	Unchanged	0	1
Bretylium	Hepatic	5	8-10%	6-11	16-32	0	5
Disopyramide	Renal	0.9	50-70%	4-10	10-18	0	2-5
Lidocaine	Hepatic	1.6	50%	1.8	1.3	0	1
Mexiletine	Hepatic	5.9	50%	10	16	0	1
Procainamide	Hepatic/renal	2.4	15%	2.6-3.5	10-14	0	1
Acetyl-procainamide	Renal	1.6	10%	6	35-45	50%	2-4
Quinidine	Hepatic	2-3.5	70-95%	5-12	5-12	0	1
Tocainide	Hepatic	2.2	50%	12-14	17-27	25%	2
ANTIHYPERTENSIVES							
Angiotensin-converting enzyme inhibitors							
Captopril	Renal	2	30%	2	20	40%	2
Enalapril	Hepatic	?	50%	30*	50	50%	3-5
Lisinopril	Renal	124	0%**	12	55	--	2-4
Beta-blockers							
Acebutolol	Hepatic	1.2	15%	3-4	7	0	2-3
Atenolol	Renal	1.2	5%	8	42	50%	4
Labetolol	Hepatic	5.6	50%	3-3.5	Unchanged	0	1
Metoprolol	Hepatic	4.9	12%	2.5-4.5	Unchanged	0	1
Nadolol	Renal	1.5	25%	14-24	45	50%	3
Pindolol	Hepatic	2.1	57%	3-4	3-4	0	1
Propranolol	Hepatic	4-4.5	99%	2.5-50	Unchanged	0	1
Timolol	Hepatic	1.7	10%	3	4	0	1

* Effective half-life of 11 hours.
** Saturable binding to ACE, but not to other circulating serum proteins.

Table 27-2 Cardiovascular Drugs, Antihypertensives, Diuretics, Bronchodilators, Antianginals, and Antiarrhythmics (continued)

Drug	Major Route of Elimination	VD (L/Kg)	Protein Binding	$T_{1/2}(h)$ Normal	$T_{1/2}(h)$ ESRD	Supplement after Hemodialysis	Adjustment Factor
Calcium Channel Antagonists							
Diltiazem	Hepatic	5	80%	3.5-5	Unchanged	0	1
Nifedipine	Hepatic	0.8	95%	3.5-4	Unchanged	0	1
Nitrendipine	Hepatic	2-6	98%	12-24	Unchanged	0	1
Verapamil	Hepatic	5-6	90%	3-5	Unchanged	0	1
Central Agents: Alpha₂-Agonists							
Methyldopa	Hepatic	5	10%	1.3-1.8	3.6	0	2
Clonidine	Renal	4.0	25%	7-18	30-40	2-3	
Guanabenz	Hepatic	5	90%	4.3	6.4	50%	1
Guanfacine	Hepatic	5	65%	12-23	Unchanged	0	1
Diuretics							
Amiloride	Renal	350	0-10%	22	100	--	Avoid
Bumetanide	Renal	0.5	96%	1.2	1.5	--	↑
Chlorthalidone	Renal	3-13	98%	50-80	100	--	2
Ethacrynic acid	Hepatic	0.1	95%	2-4	Increased	0	↑
Furosemide	Renal	0.15	95%	0.3-1.6	1.3-1.4	0	↑
Mannitol	Renal	0.5	0	1.2	36	--	Avoid
Metalozone	Renal	1.6	95%	6.0	Increased	0	↑
Spironolactone	Hepatic	--	98%	10-35	10-35	--	Avoid
Thiazides	Renal	1.5	95%	1.5	5	--	Avoid
Triamterene	Renal	13	50%	1.5-2.5	10	--	Avoid

↑ = Decreased drug effect in renal failure. The dose must be increased to obtain the same effect.

Table 27-2 Cardiovascular Drugs, Antihypertensives, Diuretics, Bronchodilators, Antianginals, and Antiarrhythmics (continued)

Drug	Major Route of Elimination	VD (L/Kg)	Protein Binding	$T_{1/2}(h)$ Normal	$T_{1/2}(h)$ ESRD	Supplement after Hemodialysis	Adjustment Factor
Vasodilators							
Hydralazine	Hepatic	6-8	90%	1.0	Unchanged	0	1
Minoxidil	Hepatic	12	0	3-4	Unchanged	30%	1
Prazosin	Hepatic	0.57	90%	3.0	Unchanged	0	1
Terazosin	Hepatic	--	90%	10	Unchanged	0	1
Inotropes							
Amrinone	Hepatic	1.4	40%	2.0-4.4	Unchanged	0	1
Digitoxin	Hepatic	0.73	90%	6-8	7	0	1
Digoxin	Renal	5-8	25%	42	80-100	0	1

Table 27-3 Drugs Used in Psychiatry and Neurology

Drug	Major Route of Elimination	VD (L/Kg)	Protein Binding	$T_{\frac{1}{2}}(h)$ Normal	$T_{\frac{1}{2}}(h)$ ESRD	Supplement after Hemodialysis	Adjustment Factor
Antidepressant Agents							
Amitriptyline	Hepatic	14	95%	16	Unchanged	0	1
Desipramine	Hepatic	20-60	90%	15-60	Unchanged	0	1
Doxepin	Hepatic	9-33		8-25	Unchanged	0	1
Imipramine	Hepatic	20-40	95%	10-20	Unchanged	0	1
Nortriptyline	Hepatic	20-30	95%	20-30	Unchanged	0	1
Protriptyline	Hepatic	20-55	95%	55-200	Unchanged	0	1
Anticonvulsants							
Carbamazepine	Hepatic	1	75%	Variable	Unchanged	0	1
Phenytoin	Hepatic	0.6	90%	24	Unchanged	0	1
Valproic Acid	Hepatic	0.2	90%	6-15	Unchanged	0	1
Antipsychotics							
Chlorpromazine	Hepatic	20	95%	30	Unchanged	0	1
Haloperidol	Hepatic	14-21	92%	20	Unchanged	0	1
Barbiturates							
Phenobarbital	Hepatic	0.9	50%	24-140	Unchanged	0	1
Secobarbital	Hepatic			20-35	Unchanged	0	1
Benzodiazepines							
Alprazolam	Hepatic	1.3	70%	10-20	Unchanged	0	1
Chlordiazepoxide	Hepatic	0.5	95%	6-25	Unchanged	0	1
Diazepam	Hepatic	1-2	98%	20-70	Unchanged	0	1
Flurazepam	Hepatic	22	97%	50-100	Unchanged	0	1
Lorazepam	Hepatic	0.7-1.0	85%	10-20	Unchanged	0	1
Oxazepam	Hepatic	1.0	97%	10	25	0	1
Temazepam	Hepatic	1.1	97%	2-4.5	Unchanged	0	1

Table 27-3 **Drugs Used in Psychiatry and Neurology**

Drug	Major Route of Elimination	VD (L/Kg)	Protein Binding	$T_{1/2}(h)$ Normal	$T_{1/2}(h)$ ESRD	Supplement after Hemodialysis	Adjustment Factor
Others							
Chloral hydrate	Hepatic	0.6	75%	4-10	Unchanged	0	1
Lithium	Renal	0.7	0	8-41	Prolonged	100%	2-3
Levodopa	Nonrenal	0.6	5-8%	0.8-1.6	Unchanged	0	1
Bromocriptine	Hepatic	--	90%	3	Unchanged	0	1

Table 27-4 Analgesics, Anti-inflammatory Drugs, Antineoplastics, Hypouricemics, Immunosuppressives

Drug	Major Route of Elimination	VD (L/Kg)	Protein Binding	$T_{1/2}(h)$ Normal	$T_{1/2}(h)$ ESRD	Supplement after Hemodialysis	Adjustment Factor
Analgesics							
Acetaminophen	Hepatic	1.0	0	2-4	Unchanged	0	1
Codeine	Hepatic	1-3.4	7	2-4	--	0	1
Meperidine	Hepatic	4.2-5.2	70%	3-7	Unchanged	0	2
Methadone	Hepatic	3.6	75%	20-30	Unchanged	0	1
Morphine	Hepatic	2-3.5	35%	1.7-4.5	Unchanged	0	1
Propoxyphene	Hepatic	16	80%	12-20	12-20	0	3
Salicylates	Hepatic	0.15	85%	2-3 hr	Prolonged at high dosage	0	1
Anti-inflammatory Agents							
Diclofenac	Hepatic	0.55	99	2	Unchanged	0	1
Fenoprofen	Hepatic	0.1	99	2-3	Unchanged	0	1
Ibuprofen	Hepatic	0.15	99	2-2.5	Unchanged	0	1
Indomethacin	Hepatic	0.12	99	6	Unchanged	0	1
Mefenamic Acid	Hepatic	--	99	3	Unchanged	0	1
Naproxen	Hepatic	0.1	99	12-15	Unchanged	0	1
Piroxicam	Hepatic	0.13	99	45	Unchanged	0	1
Sulindac	Hepatic		95	16	Unchanged	0	1
Tolectin	Hepatic	0.1-0.14	99	1-1.5	Unchanged	0	1

Table 27-4 Analgesics, Anti-inflammatory Drugs, Antineoplastics, Hypouricemics, Immunosuppressives (continued)

Drug	Major Route of Elimination	VD (L/Kg)	Protein Binding	$T_{1/2}(h)$ Normal	$T_{1/2}(h)$ ESRD	Supplement after Hemodialysis	Adjustment Factor
Antineoplastic and Immunosuppressive Drugs							
Azathioprine	Hepatic	.55	20%	1	Unchanged	Yes	1.5
Bleomycin	Renal	0.3	9	1.3-9	20	0	2
Cisplatin	Renal	0.5	90%	2-72	1-240	Yes	2
Cyclophosphamide	Hepatic	0.62	60%	4-7.5	10	50%	1
Cyclosporine	Hepatic	3.5	96%	12-24	Unchanged	0	1
Doxorubicin	Hepatic	52	85%	16-24	Unchanged	0	1
Fluorouracil	Hepatic	0.25	10%	0.2	Unchanged	Yes	1
Melphalan	Nonrenal	0.6		2	4-6	?	1.5
Methotrexate	Renal	0.76	45%	8-12	Increased	Yes	1.5
Vinblastine	Hepatic	24	75%	1-1.5	Unchanged	0	1
Steroids							
Methyl-prednisolone	Hepatic	1.2	50%	3-6	Unchanged	0	1
Prednisolone	Hepatic	0.48	90%	2.5-3.5	Increased	Yes	1
Prednisone	Hepatic	0.97	50-80%	2.5-3.5	Increased	Yes	1
Hypouricemic Drugs							
Allopurinol	Renal	0.6	5%	2-8	Prolonged	Yes	2-3
Colchicine	Hepatic	2.2	31%	19	40	?	2
Probenecid	Hepatic	.15	85%	5-8	Unchanged	0	Avoid

SUGGESTED READING

Brater DC. Drug use in clinical medicine. 3rd ed. Toronto: BC Decker Inc, 1987.

Gilman AG, Goodman LS, Gilman A. The pharmacological basis of therapeutics. 7th ed. New York: Mamillard Publishing Co, 1980.

Greenblatt DJ, Koch-Weser JL. Clinical pharmacokinetics, parts 1 and 2. N Engl J Med 1975;293:702-705, 964-970.

Johnson CA, Zimmerman SW, Rogge M. The pharmacokinetics of antibiotics used to treat peritoneal dialysis-associated peritonitis. Am J Kid Dis 1984;4:3-17.

Paton TW, Cornish WR, Manuel MA, Hardy BG. Drug therapy in patients undergoing peritoneal dialysis, clinical pharmacokinetic considerations. Clin Pharm 1985;10:404-426.

Perucca E, Grimaldi R, Cieme A. Interpretation of drug levels in acute and chronic disease states. Clin Pharm 1985;10:498-513.

Reidenberg MM, Drayer DE. Alteration of drug-protein binding in renal disease. Clin Pharm 1984;9(Suppl 1):18-26.

Rose B. Pathophysiology of renal disease. 2nd ed. New York: McGraw-Hill Book Co, 1987.

Chapter 28

Clinical Use of Diuretics

Christopher S. Wilcox

Diuretics are among the drugs of first choice in the treatment of hypertension or edema. Knowledge of their sites and mechanisms of action helps to predict their specific uses, adverse effects, and drug interactions. Since loop diuretics and thiazides share many adverse effects, these will be considered together.

CLASSIFICATION

CARBONIC ANHYDRASE INHIBITORS

Site and Mechanism of Action

These drugs inhibit the dehydration of carbonic acid to H^+ and HCO_3, primarily in the proximal tubule. Consequently, they diminish the production of H^+ ions required for tubular H^+ secretion and HCO_3 reabsorption. During prolonged therapy, mild to moderate metabolic acidosis develops which curtails further diuretic action. Hypokalemia is infrequent because kaliuresis is transient and metabolic acidosis redistributes K from cells to extracellular fluid. These drugs also reduce aqueous humor formation.

Clinical Indications

Glaucoma. These drugs are used widely to treat glaucoma. Acetazolamide (Diamox) can be given as a 500-mg sustained release preparation each 12 hr. Alternatively, methazolamide (Neptazane, 100-300 mg daily) can be prescribed.

Other. These drugs are used occasionally to treat metabolic alkalosis, epilepsy, and hypokalemic periodic paralysis, and they are prescribed for prophylaxis of mountain sickness.

Adverse effects

Patients develop a metabolic acidosis which can cause paresthesias, malaise, and decreased libido. Nausea and gastrointestinal distress are frequent. These drugs are contraindicated in liver disease because they increase blood ammonia and in pregnancy because they are teratogenic in animals.

OSMOTIC DIURETICS

Site and Mechanism of Action

Osmotic diuretics [e.g., mannitol (Osmitrol^R)] are filtered at the glomerulus but are not reabsorbed. Sodium (Na) and fluid reabsorption concentrates osmotic diuretics in the tubule fluid sufficiently to impair further Na and fluid reabsorption from the proximal tubule and loop of Henle. The resulting increase in distal delivery of fluid stimulates K secretion. Blood flow to the renal medulla is increased and washes out the osmotic gradient required for urinary concentration. The result is a considerable diuresis and kaliuresis of isotonic fluid. The infusion of an osmotically active solute abstracts fluid from cells. Consequently, mannitol can expand the extracellular fluid by a larger degree than the volume of fluid administered.

Clinical Indications

Prophylaxis of acute tubular necrosis (ATN). There is a high incidence of ATN following cardiothoracic or aortic operations, operations on jaundiced, traumatized, or shocked patients, mismatched blood transfusions, or radiocontrast dye administration. The risks are increased in patients with poor renal function, the aged, or those with diabetes mellitus. Hydration to maintain a urine flow of 1-2 ml/min reduces the risk of ATN, which can be reduced further by administration of mannitol (12.5-25 g). Continuous assessment of urine output, volume status, and electrolytes is mandatory since a very rapid extracellular volume (ECV) expansion leading to pulmonary edema can occur if renal failure supervenes.

Conversion to nonoliguric acute renal failure. A diuresis can be achieved in about half of the patients with oliguric acute renal failure. While this does not influence the duration of renal failure, nor the mortality, it reduces the need for dialysis caused by fluid overload, hyperkalemia, or acidosis. Mannitol (200 mg/kg) is given and if a diuresis is not obtained, a loop diuretic (e.g., furosemide, 80-400 mg) is added. If successful, the diuresis can usually be maintained with a loop diuretic alone.

Cerebral edema. Mannitol or urea reduce cell volume and are helpful in the acute management of cerebral edema.

Adverse Effects

ECV expansion. This occurs predictably when renal elimination is impaired, and it can precipitate pulmonary edema.

Hyponatremia, hyperkalemia, and metabolic acidosis. These consequences of cellular dehydration occur when renal elimination is impaired.

LOOP DIURETICS

Site and Mechanism of Action

These drugs, (furosemide, bumetanide, and ethacrynic acid) act primarily in the loop of Henle where they inhibit the coupled reabsorption of Na, K and Cl. The resultant loss of Cl in excess of HCO_3 generates a "contraction" metabolic alkalosis. Reabsorption of Ca is secondary to Na reabsorption; therefore, loop diuretics also increase Ca excretion. Since reabsorption of Na in the loop of Henle is critical both for the dilution of tubular fluid and for the development of the medullary concentration gradient, these drugs impair urinary dilution and concentration. Their natriuretic action depends in part on renal prostaglandin production.

Acute intravenous administration causes venodilatation secondary to prostaglandin generation and arterial vasoconstriction secondary to renin release and angiotensin II formation. Renal blood flow and glomerular filtration rate (GFR) increase modestly with the diuresis. During prolonged therapy, GFR is usually well maintained unless severe volume depletion develops which leads to prerenal azotemia.

Pharmacokinetics and Drug Interactions

Loop diuretics are readily absorbed and strongly bound to plasma proteins. There is some hepatic metabolism (especially of bumetanide), but about one-third to one-half of an oral dose is eliminated in active form by the kidney where it is secreted by the proximal tubule. These drugs are active only from the tubule lumen. Therefore, the dose of a loop diuretic required in renal failure increases in proportion to the fall in GFR (i.e., doses should be doubled where the creatinine clearance is half normal). Nonsteroidal anti-inflammatory agents (aspirin, indomethacin) which prevent prostaglandin formation impair the actions of diuretics.

Clinical Indications

Edema. These powerful diuretics are frequently used in patients with severe edema or those refractory to thiazides. These are the only diuretics which retain their efficacy in moderate and severe renal failure.

Conversion of oliguric to nonoliguric acute renal failure. High doses of loop diuretics are used often with osmotic diuretics.

Short-term treatment of hypercalcemia. Loop diuretics are used after vigorous volume repletion and during quantitative replacement of urinary Na, K, and fluid losses.

Other. Other uses are with isotonic or hypertonic NaCl to treat hyponatremia, and to treat distal hyperkalemic renal tubular acidosis.

Adverse Effects

ECV depletion. Prerenal azotemia, hyponatremia, and orthostatic hypotension are signs of excessive fluid depletion.

Acid-base and electrolyte disturbances. A hypokalemic metabolic alkalosis is common. Some patients develop hypomagnesemia.

Metabolic disturbances. Hyperuricemia is common. Some patients develop carbohydrate intolerance which progresses occasionally to diabetes mellitus. Most have a rise in serum cholesterol.

Drug allergy. This is related to the sulfonamide component and is less common with ethacrynic acid which does not have this chemical configuration. Fever, skin rash, eosinophilia, and thrombocytopenia are signs of drug allergy. Rarely, patients develop an interstitial nephritis with decreased renal function, increased renal size, eosinophilia, and an active urine sediment that often contains eosinophils.

Ototoxicity. Hearing loss, which is occasionally irreversible, can occur when high doses are given to patients with impaired elimination due to renal failure.

Individual Drugs

Furosemide (Lasix, initially 20 to 40 mg once or twice daily)

Bumetanide (Bumex, initially 1 to 2 mg once or twice daily)

Ethacrynic acid (Edecrin, 25 to 50 mg once or twice daily)

THIAZIDES

Site and Mechanism of Action

Thiazides act predominantly in the early distal convoluted tubule where they inhibit the coupled reabsorption of NaCl. Since the early distal convoluted tubule dilutes the tubular fluid further, thiazides can lead to hyponatremia. In contrast to loop diuretics, thiazides increase distal Ca reabsorption and decrease Ca excretion.

Pharmacokinetics

They are actively secreted by the proximal tubule. Thiazides become less effective with advancing renal failure (plasma creatinine, 2 to 4 mg/dl or greater).

Clinical Indications

Hypertension. They are among the drugs of first choice for treatment of patients with hypertension in the presence of normal renal function.

Edema. They are widely used for management of mild edema.

Nephrolithiasis. They can prevent recurrent nephrolithiasis, especially in patients with idiopathic hypercalciuria.

Diabetes insipidus. In the presence of Na restriction, they decrease urine volume in both central and nephrogenic diabetes insipidus.

These uses are described in detail below under Clinical Use of Diuretics.

Individual Drugs

Hydrochlorothiazide (HydroDIURIL, initial dosage, 12½ to 25 mg daily). Has a duration of action of 6 to 10 hr.

Chlorthalidone (Hygroton, initial dose, 12½ to 25 mg daily). Has a more prolonged duration of action of 24-36 hr.

Metolazone (Zaroxolyn, initial dose, 2.5 to 5 mg daily). Has some additional action on the proximal nephron and, therefore, may be somewhat more effective in patients with renal impairment.

DISTAL POTASSIUM-SPARING DIURETICS AND ALDOSTERONE ANTAGONISTS

Sites and Mechanism of Action

These drugs, which include triamterene, amiloride, and spironolactone, act in the cortical collecting duct where they inhibit reabsorption of Na and secretion of K and protons. Although they are weak diuretics, they have major actions in reducing K and proton secretion. Therefore, they are used most frequently either to promote a gentle diuresis or to counter hypokalemic metabolic alkalosis. Spironolactone is a competitive antagonist of aldosterone; its clinical effects are similar to triamterene and amiloride.

Pharmacokinetics

Triamterene is partly metabolized by the liver; it accumulates in cirrhosis because of decreased hydroxylation and biliary secretion. Amiloride is excreted by the kidney in active form. Both drugs accumulate in renal failure. Spironolactone takes 24-48 hr for maximal action.

Clinical Indications

Prevention of hypokalemia and metabolic alkalosis. They are used in combination with a thiazide or loop diuretic to counter these adverse metabolic effects.

Hyperaldosteronism. These drugs are useful in patients with hyperaldosteronism (e.g., primary hyperaldosteronism in Conn's syndrome and idiopathic adrenal hyperplasia) or secondary hyperaldosteronism (poorly compensated edema, renal artery stenosis, or vigorous salt-depletion therapy). Large doses of spironolactone (up to 400-600 mg daily) are needed to reduce blood pressure (BP) in patients with very high levels of aldosterone.

Cirrhosis of the liver with ascites. The slow and modest diuretic action of spironolactone or amiloride, combined with retention of K and protons, is valuable.

Adverse Effects

Hyperkalemia and metabolic acidosis. They decrease renal K excretion and increase efflux of K from cells due to the production of a metabolic acidosis. Therefore, S_K and electrolytes must be monitored. Patients at high risk of developing hyperkalemia are those with impaired renal function (especially the aged), those with diabetes mellitus with acidosis (especially hyporeninemic hypoaldosteronism), and those with a high catabolic rate (trauma or postoperative). Hyperkalemia can be precipitated by ongoing administration of KCl, an angiotensin-converting enzyme (ACE) inhibitor (e.g., captopril, enalopril, lisinopril), or large quantities of K-containing drugs (e.g., some antibiotics); these usually need to be stopped in patients receiving these diuretic agents.

Renal failure. Triamterene and nonsteroidal anti-inflammatory agents (e.g., aspirin, indomethacin) can induce renal failure.

Nephrolithiasis. Triamterene can cause nephrolithiasis.

Other. All may cause gastrointestinal upset, while spironolactone can cause gynecomastia and postmenopausal bleeding.

Individual Drugs and Doses

Triamterene (Dyrenium, 50-100 mg once or twice daily).

Amiloride (Midamor, 5-10 mg daily).

Spironolactone (Aldactone, 50-100 mg daily). Doses up to 600 mg daily are sometimes required in patients with severe hyperaldosteronism.

Combination of these drugs with a thiazide is convenient, e.g., Maxzide and Dyazide (hydrochlorothiazide and triamterene); Moduretic (hydrochlorothiazide and amiloride) and Aldactazide (hydrochlorothiazide and spironolactone).

ADVERSE EFFECTS OF LOOP AND THIAZIDE DIURETICS

ELECTROLYTE ABNORMALITIES

Azotemia

A rise in blood urea nitrogen usually implies that the diuresis has been too abrupt or extensive. Diuretic-induced azotemia is best managed by permitting some ECV re-expansion (by decreasing diuretic dosage and liberalizing salt and fluid intake). Development of azotemia with proteinuria and an active urinary sediment may indicate diuretic-induced interstitial nephritis.

Hyponatremia

Thiazides promote Na loss and diminish urinary dilution. Severe hyponatremia (S_{Na} 120 mEq/l or below) is a serious complication which occurs particularly in elderly women with well-preserved renal function who have received thiazide diuretics for a short period. Such patients can develop hyponatremia on rechallenge with thiazides. Management is discussed in Chapter 6.

Hypokalemia

Serum K falls by an average of 0.6 mEq/l in hypertensive patients receiving thiazides. KCl supplementation reduces but rarely prevents this fall. Loop diuretics and thiazides increase tubular fluid flow through the terminal nephron which stimulates K secretion. They also increase renin release and aldosterone secretion; hyperaldosteronism promotes distal K secretion further.

Severe hypokalemia (S_K 3.0 mEq/l or below) is associated with dangerous ventricular ectopy. Milder hypokalemia (S_K 3.0-3.5 mEq/l) may cause dangerous arrhythmias in patients with myocardial ischemia or in those receiving cardiac glycosides. Hypokalemia may contribute to diuretic-induced carbohydrate intolerance and hyperlipidemia. Therefore, most physicians aim to maintain S_K at 3.5 mEq/l or above.

Diuretic-induced hypokalemia can be managed by administration of KCl tablets. Patients usually require 2 to 6 tablets daily. KCl tablets can cause gastrointestinal erosion and are best administered as slow release formulations given with meals.

ACE inhibitors which blunt diuretic-induced increases in angiotensin II (AII) concentration can potentiate the antihypertensive and salt-depleting actions of diuretics. Since prevention of AII generation also blocks hyperaldosteronism, ACE inhibitors will also diminish hypokalemia and alkalosis. Therefore, careful use of ACE inhibitors and diuretics can provide enhanced efficacy with decreased toxicity. This combined therapy can cause hypotension and prerenal azotemia and is reserved for patients refractory to diuretics alone. It requires careful monitoring.

Distal K-sparing diuretics (amiloride, triamterene, or spironolactone) also can promote the salt-depleting actions of loop and thiazide diuretics while countering their adverse effects on K and proton depletion.

Hypomagnesemia

Loop diuretics and thiazides increase Mg excretion. Occasionally patients who develop overt hypomagnesemia manifest depression, muscular weakness, and cardiac arrhythmias or failure. Distal K sparing agents, and probably spironolactone, diminish Mg excretion.

Metabolic Alkalosis

The plasma [HCO_3] usually increases 2-5 mEq/l with thiazides or loop diuretics. Occasionally, more severe metabolic alkalosis develops, especially in edematous subjects receiving large doses of diuretics. Alkalosis predisposes to arrhythmias and diminishes ventilatory drive in patients with chronic obstructive pulmonary disease. It is best managed by administration of KCl.

METABOLIC DISTURBANCES

Hyperglycemia and Hyperlipidemia

Loop diuretics, and particularly thiazides, can impair carbohydrate tolerance. This has been ascribed to hypokalemia, which impairs insulin release. Diuretics should be avoided when possible in patients with hyperglycemia, obesity, or overt diabetes mellitus.

Loop diuretics or thiazides often raise plasma cholesterol concentrations, but these revert toward normal during prolonged therapy.

Hyperuricemia

Loop diuretics and thiazides increase plasma urate levels by 1-3 mg/dl. Diuretics should be avoided in patients prone to gout or in those with serum urate levels above 10-12 mg/dl.

CLINICAL USE OF DIURETICS

EDEMATOUS CONDITIONS

Congestive Heart Failure (CHF)

Mild chronic CHF can be managed by dietary salt restriction (goal: Na intake of 80 to 120 mEq/day) and a thiazide. Since the risks of hypokalemia and hypomagnesemia are increased, particularly in those receiving digitalis glycosides, measures to prevent these changes should be instituted. More severe CHF, particularly when complicated by decreased renal function, requires therapy with loop diuretics, which are often combined with distal K-sparing agents. ACE inhibitors can increase cardiac output and may decrease mortality in severe cardiac failure. Therefore, these drugs are often combined with diuretics for management of advanced refractory CHF. However, this combination can cause prolonged hypotension and prerenal azotemia. Thus, therapy should be initiated with small doses of a short-acting ACE inhibitor (e.g., captopril, 6.25 mg twice daily) under close clinical and biochemical surveillance. Later, the dose can be increased. ACE inhibitors usually improve renal function. Renal failure occurs in the setting of an abrupt or severe fall in BP or excessive volume depletion.

Nephrotic Syndrome

Nephrotic edema is best managed by dietary salt and fluid restriction. When required, most patients respond to a thiazide (e.g., hydrochlorothiazide, 12.5-25 mg daily initially). In the presence of renal failure, loop diuretics are required. Overvigorous diuresis can reduce renal function further.

NONEDEMATOUS CONDITIONS

Hypertension

The use of diuretics in hypertension is described in Chapter 19, "Treatment of Hypertension."

Renal Tubular Acidosis (RTA)

Furosemide can increase renal K and proton excretion in patients with hyperkalemic distal RTA. Furosemide therapy for hyporeninemic hypoaldosteronism is reserved for patients who are unresponsive or unsuitable because of hypertension for the preferred management with mineralocorticosteroids and NaCl.

Hypercalcemia

Most hypercalcemic patients are severely ECV depleted and initial therapy is vigorous rehydration. Thereafter, an intravenous loop diuretic (e.g., furosemide, 40 to 80 mg) can be given each 1 to 2 hr with replacement of urinary losses with isotonic saline.

Nephrolithiasis

Thiazides decrease Ca excretion in normal subjects and those with idiopathic hypercalciuria. Hydrochlorothiazide (12.5-25 mg twice daily) can be prescribed with amiloride (5 mg) to prevent hypokalemia or alkalosis.

Diabetes Insipidus (DI)

Thiazide diuretics can reduce urine flow by up to 50% in patients with central or nephrogenic DI. This is ascribed to ECV depletion, which reduces GFR and increases proximal fluid reabsorption, thereby limiting the supply of filtrate to the diluting segment. Therefore, thiazide therapy should be accompanied by dietary salt restriction.

DIURETIC RESISTANCE

This implies an inadequate fluid depletion produced by a full dose of diuretic.

CAUSES

Incorrect Diagnosis

Diuretics do not clear lymphatic or venous edema.

Inadequate Diuretic Reaching the Tubule Lumen

Poor compliance. Check with measurements of diuretic in urine.

Inadequate dose. Increased doses are required during regular therapy to counteract the compensatory mechanisms which prevent ECV losses.

Renal failure. Doses of loop diuretics must be increased in proportion to the reduction in creatinine clearance. Thiazides are ineffective at a plasma creatinine above 2-4 mg/dl.

Inadequate Tubular Response to the Diuretic

Nonsteroidal anti-inflammatory drugs (NSAIDs). Such drugs (e.g., aspirin, indomethacin) impair the response to all diuretics, particularly in volume-depleted patients or in those with edema.

Inappropriate dietary salt intake. Even powerful loop diuretics require dietary salt restriction. Therefore, salt intake should be assessed from measurements of 24-hr renal Na excretion. Dietary Na must be restricted severely (50-80 mEq daily) in patients with resistant edema.

Advanced edema. Patients with uncompensated CHF, cirrhosis, or nephrosis are resistant to diuretics and require increasing doses.

Physiological adaptation to diuretics. Prolonged therapy with one diuretic leads to humoral and renal adaptations that limit the response. However, patients remain very responsive to diuretics of a different class.

MANAGEMENT

When an obvious cause for diuretic resistance is not discovered, it can be managed by addition of a second drug. Administration of a thiazide to therapy with a loop diuretic is often highly effective but can precipitate severe fluid and electrolyte depletion, notably hypokalemia. Administration of a distal K-sparing diuretic or spironolactone to therapy with a thiazide or loop diuretic produces less hypokalemia and alkalosis. When diuretic resistance is due to overactivity of the renin-angiotensin-aldosterone system, addition of an ACE inhibitor is logical. However, there is increased risk of hypotension and prerenal azotemia. Combined drug administration requires very close surveillance.

SUGGESTED READING

Dirks JH, Sutton RAL. Diuretics: physiology, pharmacology, and clinical use. Philadelphia: WB Saunders Co, 1986.

Eknoyan G, Martinez-Maldonado M, eds. The physiologic basis of diuretic therapy in clinical medicine. Orlando: Grune and Stratton Inc, 1986.

Wilcox, CS. Diuretics and potassium. In: Seldin DW, Giebish G, eds. The regulation of potassium balance. New York: Raven Press, 1989:325-346.

Chapter 29

Anatomy of the Kidney

Kirsten M. Madsen

GROSS ANATOMY

The kidneys are located retroperitoneally from the twelfth
thoracic to the third lumbar vertebra. The right kidney is positioned
a little lower than the left. Each kidney measures approximately 11-12
cm in length, 5-7.5 cm in width, and 2.5-3 cm in thickness. The kidney
weight in adult men is 125 to 170 g and in adult women 115 to 155 g.
On the medial margin is a cleft, the hilus, through which the renal
pelvis, the renal artery and vein, lymphatics, and a nerve plexus pass
into the sinus of the kidney (Fig. 29-1). The renal pelvis, an

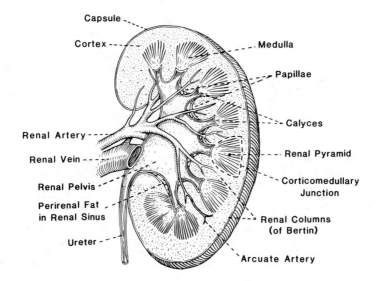

Figure 29-1   Schematic drawing illustrating the cut surface of a
bisected kidney.

expansion of the upper end of the ureter, continues into funnel-shaped tubes called the calyces which connect with the renal papillae. The kidney is covered by a tough fibrous capsule which is normally smooth and easily removable.

The kidney can be divided into cortex and medulla. In the human, the medulla forms 8-18 renal pyramids, the bases of which are located at the corticomedullary junction (Fig. 29-1). The apices of the pyramids extend toward the renal pelvis each forming a papilla. From the base of the pyramids medullary rays consisting of collecting ducts and the straight portions of proximal and distal tubules extend into the cortex. Based on the segmentation of the nephron (Fig. 29-2), the medulla can be divided into an outer medulla, which in turn can be subdivided into an outer and inner stripe, and an inner medulla, which includes the renal papillae.

The functional unit of the kidney is the nephron, which consists of a renal corpuscle or glomerulus and its associated tubule (Fig.29-2). The tubular portion of the nephron is composed of three major subdivisions: the proximal convoluted tubule (PCT), the loop of Henle, and the distal convoluted tubule (DCT). The latter continues into the collecting duct system, which is derived from the ureteric bud and, strictly speaking, is not part of the nephron. The loop of Henle consists of the proximal straight tubule (PST) (pars recta of the proximal tubule), the thin limb segments, and the thick ascending limb (TAL) (pars recta of the distal tubule).

Each human kidney contains approximately 1.2 million nephrons. Those originating from outer and midcortical glomeruli have short loops of Henle that bend in the inner stripe of the outer medulla. Juxtamedullary nephrons originating from glomeruli located near the corticomedullary junction have long loops of Henle that reach into the inner medulla. In the human kidney 10-15% of the glomeruli belong to long-looped nephrons.

MICROSCOPIC ANATOMY

GLOMERULUS

The glomeruli are located in the cortex. The human glomerulus measures approximately 200 μm in diameter and it includes a capillary tuft and the surrounding parietal epithelium of Bowman's capsule. The glomerulus is responsible for the formation of an ultrafiltrate of plasma. It consists of a capillary network lined by a thin fenestrated endothelium, a central mesangial region, and the visceral epithelium with its associated basement membrane (Fig. 29-3A). The filtration barrier between the blood and the urinary space is composed of the fenestrated endothelium, the peripheral glomerular basement membrane, (GBM), and the slit pores between the foot processes of the visceral epithelial cells (Fig. 29-3B).

Figure 29-2 Diagram illustrating the relationships between the various segments of the nephron and the zones of the kidney. PCT, proximal convoluted tubule; PST, proximal straight tubule; TL, thin limb of Henle's loop; MTAL, medullary thick ascending limb; CTAL, cortical thick ascending limb; DCT, distal convoluted tubule; CNT, connecting segment; CCD, cortical collecting duct; OMCD, outer medullary collecting duct; IMCD, inner medullary collecting duct.

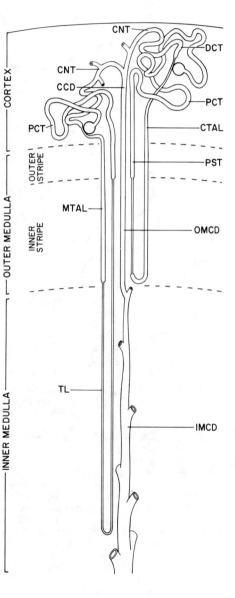

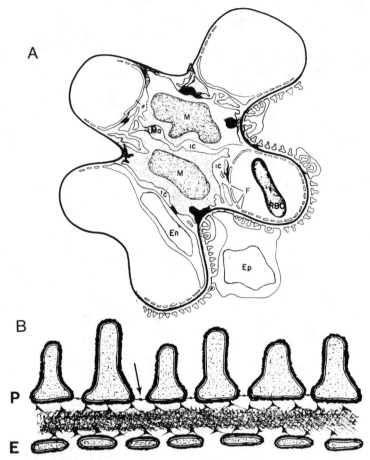

Figures 29-3A and 29-3B   A)Schematic drawing illustrating the relationship between endothelial cells (En), epithelial cells (Ep), and mesangial cells (M) of the glomerulus. F, endothelial fenestrae; Ma, mesangial matrix; IC, intercellular channels. From Latta H. Ultrastructure of the glomerulus and juxtaglomerular apparatus. In: Geiger SR, ed.   Handbook of physiology.   Baltimore: Williams & Wilkins, 1973:1-30.   B)Schematic drawing illustrating the GBM with adjoining endothelial fenestrae (E) and epithelial foot processes (P) with slit pores (arrow). From Kanwar YS, Farquhar MG.   J Cell Biol 1979;81:137.   Reprinted by copyright permission of the Rockefeller University Press.

The thin **endothelium** is perforated by pores or fenestrae measuring approximately 70 to 100 nm in diameter. It constitutes the initial barrier to the passage of blood constituents but is not believed to represent a significant barrier to the passage of macromolecules.

The **GBM** is located between the endothelium and the visceral epithelium and measures approximately 300 nm in thickness. It is composed of three layers: a central dense layer, the lamina densa, and two electronlucent layers, the lamina rara externa and the lamina rara interna. The GBM is believed to constitute the size-selective as well as the charge-selective barrier to the passage of macromolecules. It is composed of various glycoproteins, including type IV and type V collagen, laminin, fibronectin, and negatively charged glycosaminoglycans rich in heparan sulfate. These anionic sites appear to be important in establishing the charge-selective filtration barrier.

The **visceral epithelial cells** (or podocytes) have long cytoplasmic processes that divide into foot processes or pedicles that are in close contact with the GBM. The space between adjacent foot processes is called the filtration slit or slit pore and it is closed by a thin membrane, the slit diaphragm. The foot processes are covered with negatively charged sites which are rich in sialic acid and appear to be important for maintaining the normal structure and function of the filtration barrier. Removal of these anionic sites causes the foot processes to disappear and to be replaced by a continuous band of cytoplasm along the GBM. Similar changes called "foot process fusion" or "effacement" are observed in various proteinuric conditions.

The **mesangium** is separated from the capillary lumen by the endothelium and consists of mesangial cells and surrounding mesangial matrix. These cells provide structural support for the capillary loops. They contain numerous filaments and have contractile as well as phagocytic properties. Cell contraction is believed to limit filtration, perhaps by reducing the area of the glomerular filter. It is stimulated by angiotensin II, arginine vasopressin, and thromboxane, but it is inhibited by prostaglandin E_2. Mesangial cells are phagocytic and in certain forms of glomerulonephritis appear to be involved in the sequestration of immune complexes from the glomerular tuft.

The **parietal epithelium** of Bowman's capsule is continuous with the visceral epithelium at the vascular pole. At the urinary pole there is an abrupt transition from the parietal epithelium to the epithelium of the proximal tubule.

JUXTAGLOMERULAR APPARATUS

The juxtaglomerular apparatus which is located at the vascular pole of the glomerulus has vascular components and a tubular component. The vascular components include the terminal portion of the afferent arteriole, the initial portion of the efferent arteriole, and the extraglomerular mesangium between the arterioles. The tubular component is a specialized part of the TAL called the macula densa. Some of the cells in the vascular portion of the juxtaglomerular apparatus contain numerous granules. These granular cells secrete renin which, through the formation of angiotensin, is involved in the regulation of tubuloglomerular feedback and in the control of aldosterone-stimulated sodium and potassium transport. Therefore, the juxtaglomerular apparatus is an important focal point for control of renal hemodynamics and salt excretion.

PROXIMAL TUBULE

The proximal tubule includes an initial pars convoluta, or PCT, and a pars recta, or PST, which is located in the medullary ray (Fig. 29-2). The PCT has numerous lateral cell processes that extend from the apical to the basal surface of the cell and interdigitate with similar cell processes from adjacent cells (Fig. 29-4). Mitochondria are located in these processes in close proximity to the cell membrane. The presence of these lateral cell processes and interdigitations gives rise to a complex extracellular compartment between the cells. The intercellular space is separated from the tubule lumen by the tight junction or zonula occludens. A prominent endocytic apparatus and many lysosomes are present in the cells and these play an important role in the reabsorption and catabolism of proteins from the tubule fluid. Based on morphologic differences, the proximal tubule can be subdivided into three distinct segments. The S_1 segment corresponds to the initial PCT; the S_2 segment corresponds to the terminal PCT and the initial PST; and the S_3 segment constitutes the remainder of the PST.

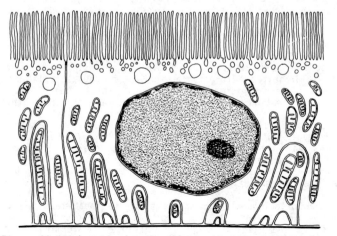

Figure 29-4 Schematic drawing illustrating proximal tubule cell.

The main function of the proximal tubule is the reabsorption of sodium, chloride, bicarbonate, potassium, water, and organic solutes such as glucose and amino acids, and the secretion of organic acid and base, including common drugs such as salicylates, barbiturates, penicillin, and most diuretics. Much of sodium reabsorption is an active process mediated by the Na-K-ATPase or sodium pump which is located in the basolateral plasma membrane. The transport of the various anions and organic solutes across the luminal membrane is coupled to the reabsorption of sodium down its concentration gradient. Fluid reabsorption is accomplished primarily by isosmotic water flow through the cell and the intercellular spaces.

THIN LIMB OF HENLE'S LOOP

The thin limb of Henle's loop extends from the proximal tubule to the TAL (Fig. 29-2). Short-looped nephrons have only a short descending thin limb segment that is located in the inner stripe of the outer medulla. Long-looped nephrons have both a long descending and a long ascending thin limb. Four morphologically distinct segments can be identified in the thin limb. They are all lined by a flat epithelium containing few cell organelles.

The thin limb of Henle's loop plays an important role in the countercurrent multiplication mechanism. The descending limb is permeable to water but impermeable to sodium, whereas the ascending limb is almost impermeable to water but highly permeable to sodium and modestly permeable to urea. Accordingly, water diffuses out of the descending limb and, subsequently, sodium exits the ascending limb down its concentration gradient. Thus, the countercurrent mechanism plays a role in the maintenance of a hypertonic medullary interstitium and in the formation of a dilute tubule fluid.

DISTAL TUBULE

The distal tubule consists of the TAL which can be subdivided into a medullary and a cortical segment, the macula densa, and the distal convoluted tubule (DCT) (Fig. 29-2). The transition from the TAL to the DCT occurs shortly after the macula densa. The cells of both the TAL and the DCT possess extensive invaginations of the basolateral plasma membrane and interdigitations of cell processes between adjacent cells. Numerous elongated mitochondria are located in the lateral cell processes in close proximity to the plasma membrane. In contrast to the proximal tubule, the luminal membrane of the distal tubule does not possess a brush border (Fig. 29-5).

The ultrastructural composition of the distal tubule is characteristic of an epithelium involved in active transport. Both the TAL and the DCT are responsible for active reabsorption of sodium chloride, which plays an important role in the countercurrent multiplication process and the urinary concentrating and diluting mechanism. Since the TAL is relatively impermeable to water, the active reabsorption of sodium chloride creates a hypertonic inter-stitium and ensures the delivery of a hypotonic tubule fluid to the DCT. The TAL is the site of action of the loop diuretics (e.g., furosemide), whereas thiazide diuretics exert their effect mainly on the DCT.

The **connecting segment** is located between the distal tubule and the collecting duct (Fig. 29-2). It is a transition region where a mixture of cells from adjacent regions can be encountered including DCT cells, connecting tubule cells, and collecting duct cells (intercalated and principal cells).

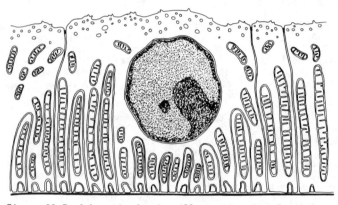

Figure 29-5 Schematic drawing illustrating distal tubule cell.

COLLECTING DUCT

The collecting duct system can be divided into the cortical (CCD), outer medullary (OMCD), and inner medullary collecting duct (IMCD) (Fig. 29-2). The CCD consists of the initial collecting tubule and the segment located in the medullary ray. The epithelium of both the CCD and the OMCD is composed of two different cell types, principal cells and intercalated cells, the latter constituting approximately one third of the cells. Principal cells have a light cytoplasm with few cell organelles and a relatively smooth luminal surface (Fig. 29-6), whereas intercalated cells have a dark staining cytoplasm with many mitochondria and numerous small vesicles in the apical region (Fig. 29-7). The luminal surface of intercalated cells is covered with microprojections that are either microvilli or microplicae. Two different configurations of intercalated cells have been observed, type A cells which are believed to be involved in hydrogen ion secretion and type B cells that may secrete bicarbonate. A main function of principal cells in the CCD is potassium secretion.

Intercalated cells gradually disappear in the early portion of the IMCD and are absent in the papillary portion. Most IMCD cells have a very light cytoplasm and few organelles. They increase in height as the collecting duct descends toward the papillary tip. The principal cells and the IMCD cells are responsive to antidiuretic hormone (ADH). In the presence of ADH water is reabsorbed from the collecting duct which leads to the formation of a hypertonic urine. In the absence of ADH the collecting duct is relatively impermeable to water and a hypotonic urine is formed.

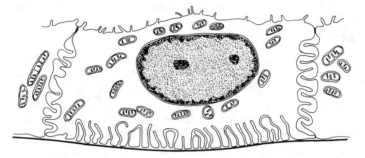

Figure 29-6 Schematic drawing illustrating principal cell.

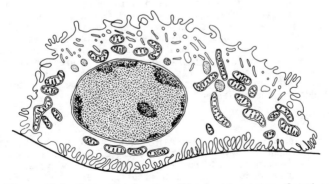

Figure 29-7 Schematic drawing illustrating intercalated cell.

INTERSTITIUM

The interstitium is composed of interstitial cells and a loose flocculent extracellular material rich in glucosaminoglycans. Interstitial tissue is sparse in the cortex where two types of interstitial cells have been described, one that resembles a fibroblast and another less common mononuclear cell. In the medulla there is a gradual increase in the amount of interstitial tissue from the outer medulla to the papillary tip. Three different types of interstitial cells have been described in the medulla: type I, the typical renomedullary interstitial cell; type II, a mononuclear cell; and type III, a pericyte. The renomedullary (type I) cells are very prominent in the inner medulla, where they are arranged in rows between adjacent tubules and vessels resembling rungs on a ladder. These cells have numerous lipid inclusions or droplets whose function is not known with certainty. The renomedullary cells are important sites of prostaglandin E_2 production.

VASCULATURE

The blood flow to the kidneys is large, amounting to approximately 1200 ml/min (20-25% of cardiac output). The renal artery divides into anterior and posterior segmental branches at the hilus of the kidney (Fig. 29-1). From the segmental arteries lobar arteries run toward the papillae where they divide into interlobar arteries which ascend along the sides of the renal pyramids. At the corticomedullary junction they continue into the arcuate arteries which run parallel to the surface of the kidney. From the arcuate arteries, interlobular arteries ascend into the cortex where they give off afferent arterioles to the glomeruli. Blood leaves the glomeruli through the efferent arterioles which continue on to form the peritubular capillary networks in the cortex. The efferent arterioles from juxtamedullary glomeruli descend into the outer medulla where they form vascular bundles containing the vasa recta through which the outer and inner medulla is supplied. Blood from the capillaries drains into the interlobular, arcuate, and interlobar veins, which accompany the arteries of the same name, and finally leaves the kidney through the renal vein. Networks of lymphatics are present in the renal cortex and the renal capsule, but lymphatics have not been described in the medulla. In the cortex they follow the arteries and are embedded in the periarterial interstitial tissue.

INNERVATION

The kidneys are innervated mainly via the celiac plexus and the greater splanchnic nerve. Both adrenergic and cholinergic nerve fibers have been described and they follow the blood vessels in the cortex and outer stripe of the outer medulla. Nerve endings have also been described in contact with both proximal and distal tubules in the cortex and with various components of the juxtaglomerular apparatus.

SUGGESTED READING

Clapp WL, Tisher CC. Gross anatomy of the kidney. In: Tisher CC, Brenner BM, eds. Renal pathology with clinical and functional correlations. Philadelphia: JB Lippincott Co, 1989:92-110.

Kriz W, Kaissling B. Structural organization of the mammalian kidney. In: Seldin D, Giebisch G, eds. The kidney: physiology and pathophysiology. New York: Raven Press, 1985:265-306.

Madsen KM, Brenner BM. Structure and function of the renal tubule and interstitium. In: Tisher CC, Brenner BM, eds. Renal pathology with clinical and functional correlations. Philadelphia: JB Lippincott Co, 1989:606-641.

Tisher CC, Brenner BM. Structure and function of the glomerulus. In: Tisher CC, Brenner BM, eds. Renal pathology with clinical and functional correlations. Philadelphia: JB Lippincott Co, 1989:92-110.

Tisher CC, Madsen KM. Anatomy of the kidney. In: Brenner BM, Rector FC, Jr, eds. The kidney. Philadelphia: WB Saunders Co, 1986:3-60.

Index

Page numbers in *italics* denote figures; those followed by "t" denote tables.